Surgical Advances in Plastic Surgery

Guest Editor

MAREK K. DOBKE, MD, PhD

CLINICS IN PLASTIC SURGERY

www.plasticsurgery.theclinics.com

October 2012 • Volume 39 • Number 4

SAUNDERS an imprint of ELSEVIER, Inc.

W.B. SAUNDERS COMPANY
A Division of Elsevier Inc.

1600 John F. Kennedy Boulevard • Suite 1800 • Philadelphia, Pennsylvania 19103-2899

http://www.theclinics.com

CLINICS IN PLASTIC SURGERY Volume 39, Number 4
October 2012 ISSN 0094-1298, ISBN-13: 978-1-4557-4927-0

Editor: Joanne Husovski

Clinics in Plastic Surgery (ISSN 0094-1298) is published quarterly by Elsevier Inc., 360 Park Avenue South, New York, NY 10010-1710. Months of issue are January, April, July, and October. Business and Editorial Offices: 1600 John F. Kennedy Blvd., Suite 1800, Philadelphia, PA 19103-2899. Periodicals postage paid at New York, NY and additional mailing offices. Subscription prices are $448.00 per year for US individuals, $666.00 per year for US institutions, $221.00 per year for US students and residents, $509.00 per year for Canadian individuals, $779.00 per year for Canadian institutions, $578.00 per year for international individuals, $779.00 per year for international institutions, and $279.00 per year for Canadian and foreign students/residents. To receive student/resident rate, orders must be accompanied by name of affiliated institution, date of term, and the *signature* of program/residency coordinator on institution letterhead. Orders will be billed at individual rate until proof of status is received. Foreign air speed delivery is included in all *Clinics* subscription prices. All prices are subject to change without notice. **POSTMASTER:** Send address changes to *Clinics in Plastic Surgery*, Elsevier Health Sciences Division, Subscription Customer Service, 3251 Riverport Lane, Maryland Heights, MO 63043. **Customer Service: 1-800-654-2452 (US and Canada). From outside of the United States and Canada, call 314-447-8871. Fax: 314-447-8029. E-mail: JournalsCustomerService-usa@elsevier.com (for print support); JournalsOnlineSupport-usa@ elsevier.com (for online support).**

Reprints. For copies of 100 or more of articles in this publication, please contact the Commercial Reprints Department, Elsevier Inc., 360 Park Avenue South, New York, New York 10010-1710. Tel.: (+1) 212-633-3812; Fax: (+1) 212-462-1935; E-mail: reprints@elsevier.com.

Clinics in Plastic Surgery is covered in *Current Contents, EMBASE/Excerpta Medica, Science Citation Index, MEDLINE/ PubMed (Index Medicus), ASCA,* and *ISI/BIOMED.*

Printed and bound by CPI Group (UK) Ltd, Croydon, CR0 4YY
Transferred to digital print 2012

Contributors

GUEST EDITOR

MAREK K. DOBKE, MD, PhD
Professor of Surgery, Division of Plastic and Reconstructive Surgery, University of California at San Diego; Department of Surgery, Division of Plastic and Reconstructive Surgery, University of California at San Diego, San Diego, California

AUTHORS

LIONEL ARRIVE, MD
Professor, Department of Radiology, Hopital Saint-Antoine, Paris, France

BERNARDO N. BATISTA, MD
Department of Plastic Surgery, Lymphedema Centre, Paris, France

CORINNE BECKER, MD
Department of Plastic Surgery, Lymphedema Center, Paris, France

JAMES CHANG, MD
Chief, Division of Plastic and Reconstructive Surgery, Professor, Department of Surgery, Stanford University Hospital and Clinics, Palo Alto, California

CONSTANCE M. CHEN, MD
Department of Plastic Surgery, New York Eye and Ear Infirmary, New York, New York

STEVEN R. COHEN, MD, FACS
Clinical Professor, Division of Plastic and Reconstructive Surgery, Department of Surgery, University of California; Director, Craniofacial Surgery, Rady Children's Hospital; Private Practice, FACES+ Plastic Surgery, Skin and Laser, San Deigo, California

MAREK K. DOBKE, MD, PhD
Professor of Surgery, Division of Plastic and Reconstructive Surgery, University of California at San Diego; Department of Surgery, Division of Plastic and Reconstructive Surgery, University of California at San Diego, San Diego, California

ULF DORNSEIFER, MD
Attending Surgeon, Department of Plastic, Reconstructive, Hand and Burn Surgery, Klinikum Bogenhausen, Städtisches Klinikum München GmbH, Munich, Germany

GREGORY R.D. EVANS, MD, FACS
Professor of Surgery and Biomedical Engineering, Chief, Aesthetic and Plastic Surgery Institute, University of California, Irvine, Irvine, California

PAOLO FANZIO, MD
Lymphedema Center, Paris, France

GEORGIOS GAKIS, MD
Attending Surgeon, Department of Urology, Eberhard-Karls University, Tuebingen, Germany

MICHEL GERMAIN, MD
Professor, Lymphedema Center, Paris, France

MOUSTAPHA HAMDI, MD, PhD
Professor and Chairman, Department of Plastic
and Reconstructive Surgery, Brussels
University Hospital, Free University of Brussels,
Brussels, Belgium

ALADDIN H. HASSANEIN, MD, MMSc
Resident, Division of Plastic Surgery,
University of California San Diego,
San Diego, California

THOMAS HITCHCOCK, PhD
Senior Manager, Medical Affairs, Ulthera, Inc.,
Mesa, Arizona

JEFF J. KIM, BS
University of California, School of Medicine,
Irvine, California

JOSHUA L. LEVINE, MD
Department of Plastic Surgery, New York Eye
and Ear Infirmary, New York, New York

SARAH LORENZ, MD
Resident, Department of Plastic,
Reconstructive, Hand and Burn Surgery,
Klinikum Bogenhausen, Städtisches Klinikum
München GmbH, Munich, Germany

BRIAN A. MAILEY, MD
Resident, Division of Plastic and
Reconstructive Surgery, Department of
Surgery, University of California, San Diego,
California

STEPHEN H. MILLER, MD, MPH
Voluntary Clinical Professor of Surgery and
Family Medicine, University of California at San
Diego, San Diego, California

LISA MISELL, PhD
Vice President, Clinical and Medical Affairs,
Ulthera, Inc., Mesa, Arizona

MARINA NINKOVIC, MD, PhD
Assistant Professor, Chief, Unit of Physical
Medicine and Rehabilitation, Center of
Operative Medicine, Innsbruck Medical
University, Innsbruck, Austria

MILOMIR NINKOVIC, MD, PhD
Head, Department of Plastic, Reconstructive,
Hand and Burn Surgery, Klinikum
Bogenhausen, Städtisches Klinikum München
GmbH, Munich, Germany

SALVATORE J. PACELLA, MD, MBA
Division Head, Plastic and Reconstructive
Surgery, Scripps Clinic and Green Hospital,
La Jolla, California

GAEL PIQUILLOUD, MD
Lymphedema Center, Paris, France

**MOHAMED ZULFIKAR RASHEED, MBBS,
MRCSEd, MMed(Surgery)**
Clinical Fellow, Department of Plastic and
Reconstructive Surgery, Brussels University
Hospital, Free University of Brussels,
Brussels, Belgium; Associate Consultant,
Department of Plastic, Reconstructive and
Aesthetic Surgery, Singapore General
Hospital, Singapore

HANS-OLIVER RENNEKAMPFF, MD
Professor of Plastic and Reconstructive
Surgery, Department of Plastic, Hand and
Reconstructive Surgery, Hannover Medical
School, Hanover, Germany

MARC RIQUET, MD
Department of Thoracic Surgery, European
Hospital Georges Pompidou, Paris, France

ANNE SAARISTO, MD
Plastic Surgery Department, Turku University
Hospital, Turku, Finland

SALIM C. SABA, MD
Chief Resident, Department of Plastic and
Reconstructive Surgery, Division of Plastic
and Reconstructive Surgery,
University of California at San Diego, San
Diego, California

GORDON H. SASAKI, MD, FACS
Clinical Professor Plastic Surgery, Private
Practice, Loma Linda Medical University
Center, Pasadena, California

TALIAH SCHMITT, MD
Division of Plastic and Reconstructive Surgery,
Department of Surgery, Stanford University
Hospital and Clinics, Palo Alto, California

MARIA SIEMIONOW, MD, PhD, DSc
Professor of Surgery, Cleveland Clinic
Lerner College of Medicine of Case Western
Reserve University, Cleveland Clinic; Director
of Plastic Surgery Research, Department of
Plastic Surgery, Cleveland Clinic,
Cleveland, Ohio

ARNULF STENZL, MD, PhD
Head, Department of Urology, Eberhard-Karls
University, Tuebingen, Germany

REBECCA M. STUDINGER, MD
Department of Plastic Surgery, New York Eye
and Ear Infirmary, New York, New York

JOHN TALLEY, MD
Division of Plastic and Reconstructive Surgery,
Department of Surgery, Stanford University
Hospital and Clinics, Palo Alto, California

MAYER TENENHAUS, MD, FACS
Professor of Plastic and Reconstructive
Surgery, Division of Plastic and Reconstructive
Surgery, University of California San Diego
Medical Center, San Diego, California

JULIE V. VASILE, MD
Department of Plastic Surgery, New York Eye
and Ear Infirmary, New York, New York

SEBASTIAN VOIGT, MD
Resident, Department of Plastic,
Reconstructive, Hand and Burn Surgery,
Klinikum Bogenhausen, Städtisches
Klinikum München GmbH, Munich,
Germany

TALJAH SCHMITT, MD
Division of Plastic and Reconstructive Surgery,
Department of Surgery, Stanford University
Hospital and Clinics, Palo Alto, California

MARIA SIEMIONOW, MD, PhD, DSc
Professor of Surgery, Lerner
Lerner College of Medicine of Case Western
Reserve University, Cleveland Clinic; Director
of Plastic Surgery Research, Department of
Plastic Surgery, Cleveland Clinic,
Cleveland, Ohio

ATHULE STREIZL, MD, PhD
Department of Urology, Boston, Massachusetts
Boston University School of Medicine

JOHN TALLEY, MD
Division of Plastic and Reconstructive Surgery,
Department of Surgery, Stanford University
Hospital and Clinics, Palo Alto, California

MAYER TENENHAUS, MD, FACS
Professor of Plastic and Reconstructive
Surgery, Division of Plastic and Reconstructive
Surgery, University of California, San Diego
Medical Center, San Diego, California

JULIE V. VASILE, MD
Department of Plastic Surgery, New York Eye
and Ear Infirmary, New York, New York

SEBASTIAN VLHOT, MD
Division of Plastic and Reconstructive
Surgery, Head and Neck Surgery,
Department of Reconstructive Plastic
Surgery, München-Gross, Munich,
Germany

Contents

The expansion of the application of biomaterials in plastic surgery has led to the increased availability of commercial products in recent years. This overview discusses soft tissue fillers, bioengineered skins, acellular dermal matrices, biomaterials for craniofacial surgery, and peripheral nerve repair. We summarize indications, properties, uses, types, advantages and disadvantages of some of the currently available products from each category. Finally, the current state of development in drug delivery system is also briefly summarized.

Lymphedema is a pathologic condition that results from a disturbance of the lymphatic system, with localized fluid retention and tissue swelling. Primary lymphedema is a congenital disorder, caused by a malformation of lymph vessels or nodes. Major progress has been achieved in the radiologic diagnosis of patients affected by lymphedema. The ideal treatment of the affected limb should restore function and cosmetic appearance. Surgical treatment is an alternative method of controlling chronic lymphedema. Free lymph nodes autologous transplantation is a new approach for lymphatic reconstruction in hypoplastic forms of primary lymphedema. The transferred nodes pump extracellular liquid out of the affected limb and contain germinative cells that improve immune function.

Lymphedema is a chronic and progressive condition that occurs after cancer treatment. Autologous lymph node transplant, or microsurgical vascularized lymph node transfer (ALNT), is a surgical treatment option that brings vascularized vascular endothelial growth factor-C–producing tissue into the operated field to promote lymphangiogenesis and bridge the distal obstructed lymphatic system with the proximal lymphatic system. Operative techniques for upper- and lower-extremity ALNT are described with 3 donor lymph node flaps (inguinal, thoracic, cervical). Surgical technique is described for the combination of ALNT with abdominal flaps and nonabdominal flaps. Imaging showing restoration of lymphatic drainage after ALNT is shown.

Energy-based noninvasive surgical tools can be used for ablative bio-stimulation (eg, collagen production) or tissue restructuring functions (eg, tightening or lifting) and are the subject of this review. The authors present the various methods and tools for noninvasive cosmetic surgery (ultrasound, radiofrequency, cryolipolysis, and lasers) and present the clinical outcomes of each. They summarize techniques and methods and their indications, physical parameters and tissue target, and consistency.

This article reports on the early experience with the 1440-nm wavelength, using a specially designed side-firing fiber, in a four-step approach, primarily to the lower third of the midface and neck. The author presents the clinical protocol, procedure steps, outcomes, and adverse events of use of the laser. Outcomes are described at 3 months, 6 months, and 18 months.

Robot assisted surgery is a technology that is being used frequently among multiple surgical specialties; robot assisted microsurgery (RAMS) and transoral robotic surgery (TORS) are applications relevant to plastic surgery that are being studied and clinically utilized. Advantages of RAMS include elimination of tremor and the ability to provide enhanced exposure. TORS facilitates oropharyngeal tumor excision and reconstruction without mandibular splitting. This article investigates current and potential uses of the surgical robot in plastic surgery as well as obstacles to its application.

This article summarizes the current knowledge on the new developing field of reconstructive transplantation. A brief outline of vascularized composite allografts (VCA) such as human hand, face, larynx, and abdominal wall transplants is provided. The clinical applications and indications for these new reconstructive transplantation procedures are outlined. The advantages, disadvantages, and complications and concerns surrounding clinical VCA are discussed. Finally, the impact of reconstructive transplantation on the future of plastic and reconstructive surgery is presented.

This article introduces and discusses several biophysical and cellular modalities that are being tested or used in clinical practice to optimize wound bed preparation, effect soft tissue coverage, and improve the quality of the inevitable and resultant scar. Among these promising technologies is the use of electrical stimulation to mimic a physiologic current of injury in an effort to accelerate re-epithelialization and the wound healing process. Over the past several years an on-site individualized regenerative medicine kit has become commercially available (ReCell, Avita Medical), utilizing well-established laboratory techniques of cell separation without the need for cell cultivation in an effort to expand and promote wound coverage and end result.

Complex traumatic injuries and degenerative conditions of the hand continue to lead to significant impairment and disability. From technical innovations to regenerative concepts, this article presents the latest advances in the dynamic field of hand surgery in which worldwide efforts are made around the globe to repair, regenerate, or restore each composite tissue forming the hand. The systematic method by which finger replantation is performed, from bony fixation to skin closure, provides a platform for discussion of the newest innovations available to reconstructive hand surgeons.

The identification of regenerative cells in adult human fat has invigorated the field of facial fat grafting. This article reviews traditional and cell-enriched fat grafting methods and the use of fat to create or refine aesthetic results. The rationale and potential applications of adipocyte-derived stem and regenerative cells in facial surgery are also described. The reader is presented with surgical techniques for harvesting and delivering fat grafts to optimize engraftment. Mesotherapy and related applications currently under investigation are also discussed.

An overview of advances and controversies in the management of breast cancer and their impact on plastic breast surgery is presented, including prophylactic mastectomy for women at high risk of breast cancer, size and location of the primary tumor and feasibility of breast-conserving surgery and oncoplastic approach, the management of the axilla, postmastectomy radiation and chemotherapy, emerging breast reconstructive techniques and cancer risk, and oncological follow-up and imaging of the reconstructed breast. This material should help plastic surgeons to understand multiple specialty considerations regarding breast cancer and provide comprehensive surgical care and interventions in aesthetic and reconstructive settings.

This article presents an overview of pedicled perforator flaps available in breast surgery. The indications, classification, surgical anatomy, and techniques for safe flap elevation are described. Clinical outcomes and complications are discussed, and illustrative case examples are presented.

The main goal of reconstructive microsurgery must be an optimal functional and esthetic reconstruction meeting the individual trauma site requirements with minimal donor site morbidity. The authors discuss new microsurgical options for extremity salvage: indications for reconstruction versus amputation, timing of free tissue transfer, reconstruction of soft tissue and bone, and functional muscle transfer. They discuss indications and contraindications for these procedures, along with emphasizing the important points of each.

Patients with bladder acontractility caused by lower motor neuron lesion are generally dependent on lifelong clean intermittent catheterization with all of its inherent risks. The functional neurovascular transfer of the latissimus dorsi muscle to the pelvis allows the restoration of voluntary voiding. This article describes the operative technique, indications, preoperative considerations, and postoperative care. The literature is reviewed and the latissimus detrusor myoplasty is compared with other functional muscle transfers to restore voluntary micturition.

The purpose of this article is to examine how plastic surgeons learn to use novel technology in their practices. In addition, a critical evaluation of current teaching methods as they relate to surgeon competence in these new technologies is discussed.

CLINICS IN PLASTIC SURGERY

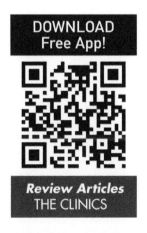

CLINICS IN PLASTIC SURGERY

Preface
Are We Witnessing the Emergence of a Superspecialty?

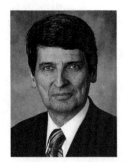

Marek K. Dobke, MD, PhD
Guest Editor

Few areas in surgery have witnessed such a steep growth trajectory as advancements in plastic surgery. Conceptual and technical advances in our specialty through evolutionary and revolutionary mechanisms, now firmly entrenched in medical evidence, are some of the most illustrious and diversified in the history of medicine. It is no wonder that so many medical students very early in their clinical upbringing develop a passion for plastic surgery and choose to devote their careers to this uniquely diverse specialty.

While many specialties are being divided into smaller entities, plastic surgery expands as both a surgical and a medical clinical specialty developing devices, cosmeceuticals, and noninvasive techniques. Years ago, during my general surgery residency, one of my mentors, a very senior general surgeon, defined plastic surgery as "general surgery done well." For a long time I could not decide whether or not he intended this as a joke. Finally, I concluded that there was a serious message in his humor with respect to our specialty of plastic surgery. I take the metaphor of superfruits—superfruits are defined by their unusually high nutritional value, high antioxidant capacity, and high consumer appeal; by extrapolating this to a specialty with explosive growth of basic and clinical science

behind it, tremendous capacity to turn people's life around, and high consumers respect, we can assert that plastic surgery becomes a superspecialty!

The content of this volume exemplifies "the power" of modern plastic surgery. The rich and diverse experience of the group of plastic surgery leaders who have collaborated to make it possible to share their technical mastery and vision of key recent advances allowed us to prepare a volume of *Clinics in Plastic Surgery* devoted to "Technical Advances in Plastic Surgery." In addition, considering the growth and increasing complexity of technology, invasive and noninvasive techniques, publications, journals and handbooks, electronic materials, and workshops, we emphasize that the teaching and mastering of plastic surgery cannot be effective anymore without an appropriate infrastructure that is dedicated to modern education. This challenge was taken very seriously at my alma mater. At UC San Diego Center for the Future of Surgery, dedicated solely to education and telemedicine, surgeons and scientists are advancing surgical techniques by investigating, developing, testing, and teaching procedures that will revolutionize the field of surgery and foster multispecialty interactions as new developments are taken from the Teaching Lab to the patient (**Fig. 1**).

Clin Plastic Surg 39 (2012) xiii–xiv
http://dx.doi.org/10.1016/j.cps.2012.07.019

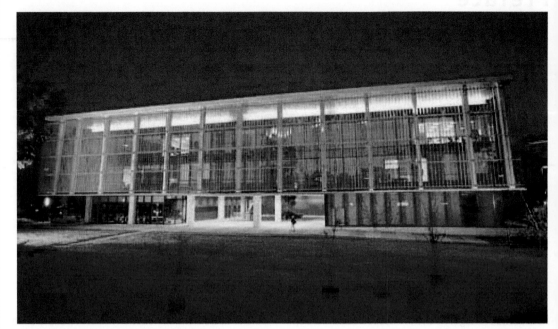

Fig. 1. The Center for the Future of Surgery is situated in newly opened Medical Education and Telemedicine Building in UC San Diego La Jolla Campus.

Contributions in this volume represent a mix of cutting-edge clinical practice. Some are in clinical trials or provided as an experimental treatment and need further evaluations and refinements, and some are in the early stage of development, but a common denominator for all of them is that there is already acknowledged evidence of their substantial impact on patient care.

The editor is grateful to all contributors for their creative work and support and to Amy Patterson (UCSD) and Joanne Husovski (Elsevier) for their encouragement and assistance in bringing this volume to you.

Marek K. Dobke, MD, PhD
Department of Surgery
Division of Plastic Surgery
University of California San Diego
San Diego, CA 92103, USA

E-mail address:
mdobke@ucsd.edu

Applications of Biomaterials in Plastic Surgery

Jeff J. Kim, BS, Gregory R.D. Evans, MD*

KEYWORDS

• Biomaterials • Acellular dermal matrix • Wound healing • Drug delivery

KEY POINTS

- Biomaterials preserve, to some degree, the native biologic properties and extracellular matrix structure of that tissue they become incorporated into or remodeled by the recipient host, limiting the immunologic and inflammatory response of introducing non-native materials into the body.
- Biomaterials serve initially as a functional mechanical bridge or reinforcement and act as a biologic scaffford that may be remodeled with the host tissue.
- Tailored bioengineered skins for wound-specific coverage improve healing time and quality.
- Use of acellular dermal matrix has revolutionized approaches to many difficult clinical scenarios involving breast and abdominal procedures.
- Injectable scaffold systems can potentially deliver water soluble drugs and growth factors in combination with cells to a tissue defect in a manner that provides an adequate environment for long term cell survival proliferation and differentiation.

INTRODUCTION

Biomaterials differ from purely synthetic materials in that they are derived from animal or human tissue and preserve, to some degree, the native biologic properties and extracellular matrix structure of that tissue. This preservation allows for the advantage of becoming incorporated into or remodeled by the recipient host, limiting the immunologic and inflammatory response of introducing non-native materials into the body. In general, these materials not only serve initially as a functional mechanical bridge or reinforcement, but after implantation, also act as a biologic scaffold that may be remodeled with the host tissue.

WOUND HEALING

Over the past 2 decades, wound healing and tissue repair have witnessed tremendous advances resulting from greater clinical understanding of wounds and their pathophysiology. Several modalities, including engineered human skin substitutes,

growth factors, and dressings, have been devised in recent years to address the problems of chronic wounds, which are a significant medical burden to the US health system, costing more than $25 billion per year.[1] These wounds often fail to normally progress through stages of healing because they are complicated by a proinflammatory milieu caused by increased proteinases, hypoxia, and bacterial burden. As a result, efforts have been directed toward correcting the chronic wound environment through these different modalities.[2]

Engineered Skin

Bioengineered skin constructs provide a possible off-the-shelf solution to the problem of donor graft shortage to offer protection from fluid loss and contamination while also delivering dermal matrix components, cytokines, and growth factors to the wound bed, enhancing the natural host wound healing responses.[3] These constructs have resulted in a substantial and demonstrable improvements in

Aesthetic and Plastic Surgery Institute, University of California, School of medicine, Irvine, 200 South Manchester, Suite 650, Orange, CA 92868, USA
* Corresponding author. Aesthetic and Plastic Surgery Institute, The University of California, Irvine, 200 South Manchester, Suite 650, Orange, CA 92868.
E-mail address: gevans@uci.edu

Clin Plastic Surg 39 (2012) 359–376
http://dx.doi.org/10.1016/j.cps.2012.07.007
0094-1298/12/$ – see front matter Published by Elsevier Inc.

wound care and some of these constructs are now approved by the Food and Drug Administration (FDA).[4]

Useful classifications of these constructs are based on[5-7]

1. Anatomic structure: epidermal, dermal, or composite
2. Duration of the cover: temporary, semipermanent, or permanent
3. Cellular composition: cellular or acellular
4. Material type: biologic or synthetic

Table 1 provides summary information of the different types of products currently being used.

Dressings

There are 2 general categories of wound dressings: passive wound dressings mainly control wound moisture levels, whereas active dressings locally alter the wound's biochemical environment.

Passive wound dressings mainly control wound moisture levels. The synthetic polymers in these dressings afford customization in terms of absorbency, physical form, and gas permeability. Some examples include alginates, which draw out contaminates, and excess exudate in heavily draining wounds. Hydrocolloids have a highly occlusive property made of a mixture of gelatin, pectin, and Polycarboxymethyl cellulose. Hydrogels are glycerin-based cross-linked polymer gels that enhance secondary absorption and compression in the relief of burns and excoriated wounds.[8-10]

The development of *active dressings*, which manipulate the local biochemical environment, has stemmed from the altered biology of chronic wound.[11-14] Potential targets include increased bacterial load and excessive protease levels, which have led to the development of antimicrobial, protease inhibitor,[15] and collagen dressings.[8] Some examples of commercially available active dressing products include Acticoat (Smith & Nephew, London, United Kingdom), Algicell (Derma Sciences, Princeton, New Jersey), Promogran wound matrix (Systagenix, North Yorkshire, United Kingdom), Oasis Wound Matrix (Cook Biotech, Fort Worth, Texas), Medifill (Human BioSciences, Gaithersburg, Maryland), and CellerateRX (Wound Care Innovations, Fort Lauderdale, Florida).[2] **Tables 2** and **3** provide a summary of these products.

SOFT TISSUE HEALING

The role of injectable soft tissue augmentation in both reconstructive and aesthetic plastic surgery continues to expand, with continued search for safer, more effective, long-lasting, biocompatible dermal filler materials.[16] Ideally, an injectable implant should have a lack of any significant inflammatory response, be easily introduced into the recipient site by injection, and produce an acceptably long period of volume retention.[17]

Many products that include synthetic polymers and autologous tissue have emerged in recent years that attempt to meet these criteria. **Table 4** provides an overview of some of the currently available products in various classes of fillers, including the composition, indications, clinical characteristics, and advantages/disadvantages.

BREAST/ABDOMINAL WALL

Although synthetic materials providing coverage, such as Marlex mesh, polytetrafluoroethylene, titanium implants, or methylmethacrylate, have been useful for implantation and structural support in a variety of surgical settings, including breast and abdominal wall surgeries, they all have several limitations.[34] They do not stimulate wound healing to amplify the wound healing process. Furthermore, the inability of permanent prostheses to become completely incorporated predisposes them to the risk for infection, extrusion, and invasion into surrounding tissue.[35,36]

The application of biosynthetic material in such situations has provided a unique advantage of integrating the supporting material into the native tissue, offering a more biocompatible solution. Specifically, the development of acellular dermal matrix (ADM) has revolutionized approaches to many difficult clinical scenarios.[35]

Abdominal Wall Procedures

There has always been interest in an implant material that would add strength to the abdominal closure while resisting infection. Permanent mesh is unusable in these situations, and temporary synthetic meshes often do not provide adequate or lasting tensile strength to prevent hernia formation.

The advantage of bioprosthetics, such as ADM, is that these heal by a more regenerative process rather than by scar-tissue formation.[36] Once remodeled with autologous tissue, there is theoretically no ongoing foreign body response, reducing the risk of chronic infection and subsequent erosion through the skin or viscera. Cutaneous exposure of ADM is usually managed with local wound care rather than by removal.[37] Many surgeons feel more comfortable placing biosynthetic mesh into a contaminated field because they seem to tolerate contamination better. Adhesions to abdominal viscera have also been reported to be markedly less for bioprosthetics than for synthetic materials like polypropylene

Table 1
General summary of some bioengineered skin products and representative properties

Products/ Company	Structure/Characteristics	Uses	Advantages/ Disadvantages
Epidermal Constructs			
Bioseed-S (BioTissue Technologies, Freiburg, Germany)	Autologous keratinocytes suspended in a fibrin glue	Venous leg ulcers	Simple handling; the gel-like construct is applied to the wound with a syringe
CellSpray (Avita Medical, Woburn, Massachusetts)	Subconfluent keratinocytes are harvested in their most active proliferating state; they are then applied to the wound bed by spraying	Partial-thickness and graft donor-site wounds	Convenient way (spray) of delivering keratinocytes to the wound bed at earlier stages after wounding
Epicel (Genzyme Corp, Cambridge, Massachusetts)	Cultured autograft comprised of living keratinocytes cultured for 3 wk; no dermal component; delivered on a petrolatum gauze backing	Deep dermal and full-thickness burns; grafting after congenital nevus removal	No apparent rejection; 1-d shelf life; requires dermal support and a 3-wk cultivation period
MySkin (Altrika, Sheffield, United Kingdom)	Cultured autograft comprised of living keratinocytes, grown on a silicone support layer with surface coating; cultured from biopsy specimen of patient's own skin	Partial-thickness burns; skin graft sites; diabetic, neuropathic, and pressure ulcers	No apparent rejection; delay in preparation because of graft cultivation; currently available in the United Kingdom only
VivoDerm (ER Squibb and Co, Princeton, New Jersey)	Hyaluronic acid-containing material is perforated and seeded on both sides with autologous keratinocytes from a biopsy specimen of the patient's own skin; pores enhance drainage	Partial-thickness burns; venous and pressure ulcers; vitiligo treatment	No apparent rejection; 2-d shelf life; delay in preparation because of graft cultivation
Dermal Constructs			
AlloDerm (LifeCell Corp, Branchburg, New Jersey)	Cadaveric freeze-dried acellular dermal matrix	Full-thickness acute and chronic wounds, burns; as cosmetic and reconstructive implants	No apparent rejection; 2-y shelf life; immediate availability; minimal wound contracture/ scarring
Biobrane (Smith & Nephew, Hull, United Kingdom)	Porcine collagen chemically bound to nylon/silicone membrane	Partial-thickness burns/ donor sites; treatment of toxic epidermal necrolysis	3-y shelf life; good fluid exchange/barrier function; decreased wound contracture; immediate availability; temporary dressing, needs removal after application

(continued on next page)

Table 1
(continued)

Products/Company	Structure/Characteristics	Uses	Advantages/Disadvantages
Dermagraft (Advanced BioHealing, Inc, LaJolla, California)	Living allogeneic fibroblasts from neonatal skin on a biodegradable polyglactin mesh; fibroblasts remain viable after implantation, continue to secrete matrix proteins, Growth factors	Diabetic foot ulcers; epidermolysis bullosa	6-mo shelf life when cryopreserved at −70°C; requires rapid time-sensitive thawing and needs to be applied within 30 min after thawing
EZ Derm (Genzyme Corp, Cambridge, Massachusetts)	Cross-linked porcine collagen; available perforated or nonperforated	Partial-thickness burns; venous, diabetic, and pressure ulcers	Long shelf life; immediate availability; potential for immune response; increased amount of exudate
GraftJacket (Wright Medical Technology, Arlington, Tennessee)	Cadaveric acellular dermal matrix	Tendon and lower-extremity wound repair; diabetic ulcers	2-y shelf life; premeshed for ease of application; cryogenic preservation
Hyalomatrix PA (Addmedica Paris, France)	Partial benzyl ester of hyaluronic acid coupled with a thin silicone layer, providing fluid loss control and a microbial barrier; functions as a temporary epidermis	Partial-thickness burns; deep burns in children	No animal or allogeneic human-derived components
Hyalograft 3D (Fidia Advanced Biopolymers Padova, Italy)	Esterified hyaluronic acid matrix seeded with autologous fibroblasts	Full, partial-thickness wounds; scleroderma cutaneous ulcers	May be combined with LaserSkin (TissueTech autograft system, Miami, FL) for treatment of deep wounds
Integra (Integra LifeSciences Corp, Plainsboro, New Jersey)	Temporary acellular silicone epidermal substitute over a dermal scaffold consisting of collagen and chondroitin-6-sulfate	Deep partial-thickness and full-thickness burns; postsurgical wounds; diabetic ulcers	Bilayered; good barrier function; long shelf life; unlikely to cause host immunologic reaction; may be applied over bone; removal of silicone layer and autograft required; possible fluid entrapment beneath construct
OASIS Wound Matrix (Cook Biotech, Lafayette, Indiana)	Porcine small intestine submucosa provides scaffold for growth of new tissue; acellular, but contains collagen/Growth factors	Partial- and full-thickness burns; diabetic, venous/pressure ulcers	1.5-y shelf life; immediate availability; potential host immune response

(continued on next page)

Table 1
(continued)

Products/ Company	Structure/Characteristics	Uses	Advantages/ Disadvantages
TransCyte (Advanced BioHealing, Inc, LaJolla, California)	Nylon mesh of Biobrane seeded with allogeneic human dermal fibroblasts; cryopreserved matrix contains high levels of proteins and growth factors with no viable cells	Full- and partial-thickness burns	1.5-y life frozen; because nylon is not biodegradable, it serves as a temporary wound cover; silicone membrane must be removed
Bilayered Constructs			
Apligraf (Organogenesis, Inc, Canton, Massachusetts)	Comprised of bovine collagen and living human keratinocytes and fibroblasts, derived from human neonatal foreskin; after application, the viable cells may continue to produce matrix proteins and growth factors	Venous, diabetic, and pressure ulcers; epidermolysis bullosa; pyoderma gangrenosum; vasculitic ulcers; scleroderma; donor sites after skin harvesting	Provides living cells to the wound, with potential for temporary stimulation; mimics structure and function of skin; extensive safety record; relatively short shelf life
OrCel (Ortec International, New York)	Allogeneic neonatal fibroblasts and keratinocytes, which are cultured onto opposite sides of a matrix of cross-linked bovine collagen; matrix contains viable cells that secrete growth factors and cytokines to promote healing	Split-thickness donor sites; epidermolysis bullosa; venous and diabetic ulcers	9-mo shelf life if cryopreserved; secretion of cytokines and growth factors; immediate availability; good cosmesis

From Lazic T, Falanga V. Bioengineered skin constructs and their use in wound healing. Plast Reconstr Surg 2011;127(Suppl):75S–90S; with permission.

mesh, potentially allowing placement directly over the bowel.[36] The primary disadvantages of these bioprosthetic meshes are the cost and lack of long-term clinical data. Because products, such as Surgisis (Cook Biotech, West Lafayette, Indiana), Permacol (Covidien, Mansfield, Massachusetts), and AlloDerm (LifeCell Corp, Branchburg, New Jersey), are considerably greater in cost than the synthetic mesh counterparts, the difference in implant cost should be justified for potential indications.

ADMs are currently used in numerous applications for trunk reconstruction, including ventral hernia repair, fascial reconstruction following tumor resection, traumatic loss or infection, reconstruction of open abdominal defects, and TRAM flap donor site repair. They have been particularly useful for reconstructing large ventral hernias and other fascial defects that involve unavoidable placement of mesh over the bowel and neurovascular structures, replacement of infected mesh, placement into contaminated or irradiated fields, or repair of enterocutaneous fistula.[34,36]

Reconstructive and Cosmetic Breast Procedures

In implant-based breast reconstruction, the addition of ADMs has offered many potential advantages relative to traditional techniques and has been widely applied in both primary and secondary reconstruction.[38,39]

Table 2
Available passive dressing types

Type	Description	Indications	Advantage/Disadvantage	Available Products
Alginates	Produced from brown seaweed; fibrous gel is formed when calcium in the dressing exchanges with sodium from the wound; absorbs 20 times of weight; nonocclusive; requires secondary dressing	Moderate to heavy exudate in superficial to deep wounds; autolytic debridement; rope form to pack deep or tunneling wounds; infected wounds	*Advantage:* Conformable and allows gas exchange along with protection from contamination; draws out contaminates and excess exudate in heavily draining wounds *Disadvantage:* May dehydrate wounds with minimal exudate; contraindicated in third-degree burns; need to be changed daily	Algicell Calcium Alginate (Derma Sciences, Princeton, New Jersey); AlgiDERM (Bard Medical, Covington, Georgia); KALTOSTAT (ConvaTec, Skillman, New Jersey); Tegagen (3M, St Paul, Minnesota)
Hydrocolloids	Mixture of materials, such as gelatin, pectin, polycarboxymethyl cellulose, elastomers, bonded to semipermeable film or a foam sheet; highly occlusive and usually waterproof; absorbs moisture slowly; available in sheet form or paste/granules to fill deep wounds	Light to moderate exudate in shallow full-thickness defects; wounds requiring moisture, such as granulation tissue; used under compression dressing; autolytic debridement, especially with necrotic, dry eschar	*Advantage:* Available in ultrathin conformable form; reduce pain; highly occlusive property allows patients to continue daily activity; molds well to wound; some transparent forms allow visualization of wound *Disadvantage:* May leave residue or adhere to wound surfaces; not recommended with heavy exudate, active infection, or sinus tracts; contraindicated in third-degree burns; highly occlusive property can promote anaerobic infection; may promote hypertrophic granulation tissue	Alleyvn (Smith & Nephew, London, United Kingdom); DuoDERM (ConvaTec, Skillman, New Jersey); Hydrocol (Bertek, Rockford, Illinois); Invacare Hydrocolloid (Invacare Supply Group, Elyria, Ohio); Tegasorb (3M, St Paul, Minnesota)
Hydrogels	Glycerin- or water-based cross-linked polymer gels; semipermeable; secondary dressing can provide enhanced absorption and compression; bead-type dressing can absorb microorganisms, exudate, or wound debris	Minimum to moderate exudates in superficial to deep wounds; rehydration of wound bed; gel form can pack deep wounds and conform to wound defects; autolytic debridement, especially with necrotic, dry eschar	*Advantage:* Cooling effect of sheet hydrogels may provide relief in burned or excoriated wounds; can be used with active infection *Disadvantage:* Minimal absorption, desiccates quickly without covering; excess use can cause wound maceration; may promote yeast; sheet dressing requires secondary securement	Amorphous types include Comfeel Triad (Coloplast, Minneapolis, Minnesota), DuoDERM (ConvaTec, Skillman, New Jersey), and Restore Hydrogel (Hollister, Libertyville, Illinois) Sheet types include Aquasite (Dermasciences, Princeton, New Jersey), CarraDres (Carrington Laboratories, Irving, Texas)

From Fan K, Tang J, Escandon J, et al. State of the art in topical wound-healing products. Plast Reconstr Surg 2011;127(Suppl):44S–59S; with permission.

Table 3
Available active dressing types

Type	Descriptions	Indications	Example Products
Antimicrobial	Silver-releasing foam shown to decrease ulcer area, odor, leakages, and maceration; no significance in terms of achieving complete wound healing; greater reduction in chronic, infected, ulcer size with silver-containing foam dressings	Moderate to heavy exudates depending on the passive dressing; may be primary or secondary depending on the dressing chosen	Acticoat (Smith & Nephew, London, United Kingdom); Algicell Ag (Derma Sciences, Princeton, New Jersey); Aquacel Ag (ConvaTec, Skillman, New Jersey); Iodosorb Gel and Iodoflex Pad (Healthpoint, Fort Worth, Texas); Silvercel (Johnson & Johnson, New Brunswick, New Jersey); Silverlon (Silverlon Consumer Products, Geneva, Illinois)
Collagen Dressings	Provides a scaffold for growth of tissue; hydrophilicity allows cell attachment; collagen encourages hemostasis; chemotactic to fibroblasts, granulocytes, macrophage; oxidized regenerated cellulose inactivates excess protease and protects growth factors	Moderate to heavy exudates in superficial to deep wounds; can be use in infected wounds; can be used in skin grafts, donor sites, red or yellow wounds	Promogran wound matrix, Fibracol plus collagen dressing with alginate (Systagenix, North Yorkshire, United Kingdom); Medifill (Human BioSciences, Gaithersburg, Maryland); Oasis (Cook Biotech, Fort Worth, Texas); Colactive (Smith & Nephew, London, United Kingdom); CellerateRX (Wound Care Innovations, Fort Lauderdale, Florida)

From Fan K, Tang J, Escandon J, et al. State of the art in topical wound-healing products. Plast Reconstr Surg 2011;127(Suppl):44S–59S; with permission.

In primary reconstruction, the reported clinical benefits of ADM include[40,41]

1. An increased ability for the surgeon to define placement of both the inframammary fold and the expander/implant position
2. An increased layer of protection between the prosthetic implant and the potentially poorly vascularized mastectomy skin
3. A larger initial submuscular pocket leading to improved use of native mastectomy flaps
4. More rapid expansion and time to complete reconstruction

Other reported advantages include the potential for improved management of the threatened implant and a reduced need for explantation as well as a potential for a reduction in the incidence of capsular contracture, although the data for the latter are currently unknown.[42–45]

In secondary procedures following prosthetic breast reconstruction, these materials have shown to be effective in a variety of situations that include implant displacement, symmastia, capsular contracture, incisional support, and pocket conversion. They can also be placed in the setting of delayed breast reconstruction and to augment nipple projection.[40]

Despite the multitude of potential benefits, the acceptance of techniques using ADM in breast reconstruction has not been universal, which is largely because of the concerns regarding the increased potential for complications. Specifically, there have been reports of an increased risk of seroma and infection with these products.

Table 4
Overview of current injectable soft tissue fillers

Allogenic	Composition	Clinical Characteristics	Advantage/Disadvantage
Cosmoderm/Cosmoplast (Inamed Aesthetics, Santa Barbara, California)	Injectable implants derived from highly purified human collagen; cultured from a single cell line of human dermal fibroblasts, isolated then purified for injection; cell line undergoes extensive testing for viruses, retroviruses, and tumorigenicity	Prepackaged in 1-mL syringe; CosmoDerm is FDA approved for shallow wrinkles or acne scars and is injected into the superficial papillary dermis; CosmoPlast is injected into the mid-dermis to deep dermis for the correction of more pronounced wrinkles or scars. Results typically last 3–6 mo	Advantages include proven decreased hypersensitivity from bovine collagen, thus not need pretreatment skin testing, patients can undergo treatment at initial consultation; disadvantages include contraindication for patients with lidocaine allergies, no proven superiority in volume persistence to its bovine counterpart
Cymetra (LifeCell Corp, Palo Alto, California)	Injectable form of micronized AlloDerm (FDA approved decellularized processed dermal allograft); Epidermis completely removed, followed by removal of dermal cells and stabilization of the dermal matrix, cryofractured into micronized particles into packaged syringes	Viscous consistency after hydration requires a large-caliber needle for introduction; indicated for use in nasolabial folds, lips, and acne and depressed scars; generally avoided in periocular line correction and glabellar contouring to avoid risk of intravascular injection and migration; results typically last 3–9 mo	Advantages include complete absence of immunogenicity; disadvantages include more painful and less smooth injection caused by large particle size, and also limited to subcutaneous space and not allow intradermal injection, again caused by the large size of the particles
Synthetic			
Restylane (Medicis, Scottsdale, Arizona)	Represents fundamental change in injection technology, transitioning from a protein-based material to one of extracellular matrix composition; a highly concentrated stabilized hyaluronic acid gel, the product uses hyaluronan's high capacity for holding water and high viscoelastic properties	FDA approved for mid-dermal applications, such as deeper wrinkle reduction, lip augmentation, nasolabial folds, and glabellar creases; also successfully used in treatment of tear trough deformities; Results typically last 6–12 mo after injection	Advantages include minimal hypersensitivity reactions, easily injected with nice flow through small-gauge needle, long persistence after injection; disadvantages include higher cost, higher incidence of bruising, and potential for severe swelling and pain from lack of anesthetic mixture

Hylaform/Hylaform Plus (Inamed Aesthetics, Santa Barbara, California)	Sterile colorless cross-linked molecules of hyaluronic acid derived from avian source	FDA approved for injection into the mid-dermis to deep dermis for correction of moderate to severe facial wrinkles and folds, but not for lip augmentation; subdermal injection lead to inferior results, and if injected too superficially, it may cause skin discoloration; results typically last 3–4 mo	Advantages include no skin test is necessary, thus can be used at initial consultation; disadvantages include shorter longevity than other hyaluronic acid products; cannot be used in patients with hypersensitivity to avian proteins, most notably eggs
Alloplastic Implants			
Radiesse (BioForm Medical Inc, San Matteo, California)	Mixture of an aqueous based gel carrier blended with spherical particles of synthetic calcium hydroxyapatite; spherical shape and small uniform size of calcium hydroxyapatite particles allows for consistent mechanical action during injection and stability in situ after injection; size allows for limited potential for migration; gel carrier comprised of cellulose, glycerin, and high-purity water, has unique characteristic of being highly viscous and elastic while allowing for shear thinning	Indicated for correction of nasolabial folds, vertical lip lines, acne scars, marionette lines, and restoring volume in and around the cheeks; also being studied for use in treatment of vocal cord insufficiency, radiographic marking, vesicoureteral reflux, stress urinary incontinence, and HIV-associated facial lipoatrophy. The high density and low solubility of the bioceramic particles of calcium hydroxyapatite provide for long-term durability of the implant and excellent biocompatibility, with reported clinical effects of approximately 2 y	Advantages include no risk of antigenic or inflammatory reaction, implants do not calcify and remain soft and flexible, and because of very low particle solubility, volume retention may theoretically persist for years; disadvantages include potential for aggregate of scar contracture around collection of the particles, radiopacity that may interfere with facial radiograph
Scultra (Dermik Laboratories, Berwyn, Pennsylvania)	Comprised of microparticles of poly-L-lactic acid, a biodegradable synthetic polymer that resorbable sutures like Vicryl and Dexon are also made of	FDA approved only for treatment of HIV facial lipoatrophy, but also used in Europe for wrinkles; injected in the deep dermis or subcutaneous space, must be used within 72 h of reconstitution; effects typically last 1–2 y	Advantages include longevity with no necessary skin testing; disadvantages include flow behavior and size that does not allow for intradermal implantation, higher potential for long-term reactions, such as granulomas

(continued on next page)

Table 4
(continued)

Allogenic	Composition	Clinical Characteristics	Advantage/Disadvantage
Juvederm (Allergan, Santa Barbara, California)	Derived from Streptococcus equipment and manufactured by a bacterial fermentation process; use of Hylacross technology (not sized or pushed through a specially sized screen and broken into pieces) Contains unmodified or uncross-linked free Hyaluronic acid which acts as lubricant to help decrease extrusion force and make injection easier; high concentration of Hyaluronic acid	Suitable for use in any wrinkles, moderate or deep, as well as scar correction; approved for nasolabial folds, off-label use for lip augmentation, marionette fold correction, prejugal sulci, and volume filler for atrophy and acne scars; will absorb water after injections and thus slightly expand within 24 h after correction; effects typically lasts 9–12 mo	Advantages include longevity with better initial and sustained correction than bovine filler; disadvantage include more volume injection required, lack anesthetic, thus patients feel pain during injection
ArteCol/ArteFill (Artes Medical, San Diego, California)	Permanent injectable filler comprised of PMMC microspheres suspended in bovine collagen transport solution with lidocaine; Injected subdermally or subcutaneously, microspheres become encapsulated after collagen dissipates within 1–3 mo	FDA clinical trial showed success and satisfying rating superior to Zyderm control in treatment of nasolabial folds and glabellar, upper lip, and corner of the mouth wrinkles; injected into subdermal space and subcutaneous tissue and is evenly massaged to reduce clumping; collagen dissipates within 1–3 mo but smooth microspheres provides lasting results of around 2 y	Advantages include longevity of effect and long clinical history of successful human implantation of PMMC; disadvantages include required skin testing for presence of bovine collagen allergy, size and viscosity of material not allowing dermal implantation, and risk of clumping and localized foreign body reaction, as with all particulated injectable fillers

Abbreviations: HIV, human immunodeficiency virus; PMMC, polymethylmethacrylate.
Data from Refs.[17–33]

Furthermore, some surgeons have been slow to adopt such techniques because of the cost of these materials. Even with the increased number of competing products now available on the market, the cost is not inconsequential.[46]

Currently, there are several commercially available ADM products, including AlloDerm and Strattice (LifeCell Corp, Branchburg, New Jersey); DermaMatrix (Synthes Corp, West Chester, Pennsylvania); AlloMax (Davol, Inc, Warwick, Rhode Island); Permacol (Covidien, Mansfield, Massachusetts); SurgiMend (TEI Biosciences, Boston, Massachusetts); DermACELL (LifeNet Health, Virginia Beach, Virginia); and FlexHD (Ethicon Inc, Somerville, New Jersey). The various proprietary ADM formulations differ in terms of the specific cleansing and purification processes, the amount of collagen cross-linking, and the methods of storage.[46] An overview summary of these products is described in **Table 5**.

Although ADM products have been largely used in breast reconstruction, similar techniques have been applied in cosmetic breast surgery.[35] ADM placement can yield a natural contour for significant irregularities. In addition, significant implant malposition can be corrected with the support of a sling as well as internal support placed to help prevent bottoming out in inferior pedicle breast reduction.[47–49] However, one significant deterrent from widespread application in cosmetic procedures has been cost.[50,51]

NERVE REPAIR

The standard technique for peripheral nerve repair is bridging the defect with an autologous nerve graft between the two nerve stumps. Alternatively, for short nerve defects up to a few centimeters, a nerve guide/conduit can be used. The entubulation model provides an environment for outgrowing axons and growth of Schwann cells that are necessary elements for optimal return of nerve function.[52]

The potential advantages of a nerve guide include no donor site for the nerve graft, prevention of axonal escape at suture lines, and the use in particular locations that are normally difficult to reach. Reconstruction of a nerve using the entubulation technique will also save time compared with conventional grafting techniques.[53]

Although many trials have been done with nerve tubes of different materials in nonclinical models, including both nonbioabsorbable and bioabsorbable conduits, nondegradable nerve guides using materials like silicone, polytetrafluoroethylene, and polyethylene have a relative disadvantage in that they remain in situ as a foreign body and can cause chronic foreign body reactions

with excessive scar tissue formation, eventually compressing the nerve. A second procedure would then be needed to remove the tube, risking damage of the nerve.[54]

There are currently 4 absorbable nerve conduits approved by the FDA that are now available for clinical use: NeuraGen (Integra Neurosciences, Plainsboro, NJ) and NeuroMatrix (Collagen Matrix, Inc, Oakland, NJ), which are both collagen-derived nerve guides, and Neurotube (Synovis, St Paul, MN) and Neurolac (Polyganics BV, Groningen, Netherlands), which are synthetic polyester-based conduits. The availability of clinical published data on these products are currently limited and widely varied.[53]

CRANIOFACIAL REPAIR

Although autologous bone transplantations are still considered the gold standard for craniofacial bone repair, an increasing number of alloplastic materials have been available for application as an alternative. There are obvious restrictions to autologous bone grafting, including limited availability of donor bone as well as the need to remodel the harvested bone into complex shapes.[55] In addition, significant bone resorption using free bone grafts and the enhanced morbidity and risks from harvesting bone grafts cannot be disregarded.[56]

The general advantages of using biomaterials include no donor-site morbidity and shortening of the operative time and potential hospital stay. But infection rates and cost are reported to be higher. Alloplastic materials may be used alone or in combination with bone transplants or osteoinductive cytokines. Ideally, their role in reconstructive procedures is not only simply replacing the missing bone part but also to stimulate osteoconduction by acting as a scaffold for bone regrowth. The implantable materials are also required to be biocompatible, with minimal leukocyte infiltration and fibrosis.[56]

Synthetic Calcium Phosphate

Numerous synthetic calcium phosphate (CaP) biomaterials are currently available commercially and have been classified according to their composition, such as hydroxyapatite, beta-tricalcium phosphate (β-TCP), or biphasic calcium phosphate.[57] They are biocompatible, osteoconductive, and bioactive, developing a direct and adherent bond with bone. Under physiologic conditions, hydroxyapatite is essentially nonresorbable, whereas β-TCP has been shown to degrade within 6 weeks after implantation.[58] Both are brittle materials with low fracture resistance. The dissolution of CaP biomaterials depends on

Table 5
Summary of ADM products

Product	Source	Prep/Soak Details	Orientation	Shelf Life	Advantage/Disadvantage	Calculate Approximate Price Per Square Centimeter ($)
AlloDerm	Human	Prep time: 2 min Rinse in normal saline or lactated ringer	Yes	2 y	Advantage: well studied, recognized by insurance Disadvantage: nonsterile pouch, long rehydration period, antibiotic sensitivity	28.00
Strattice	Porcine	Prep Time: 2 min Room-temp normal saline or lactated ringer	No	18 mo	Advantage: cost, sterile, short prep time, no orientation Disadvantage: nonhuman, nonsterile pouch, short shelf life	24.65 – 30.76
DermaMatrix	Human	Prep time: <3 min Room-temp normal saline or lactated ringer	Yes	3 y	Advantage: short prep time, 4 thicknesses available	28.51 – 31.94
FlexHD	Human	Prep time: None	Yes	3 y	Advantage: ready to use Disadvantage: cost	27.31 – 34.76
Permacol	Porcine	Prep time: None	No	3 y	Advantage: cost, sterile, ready to use, no orientation Disadvantage: Nonhuman, cross-linking, odor, not for breast	21.63
SurgiMend PRS	Fetal bovine	Prep time: 60 s Room-temp saline	No	3 y	Advantage: cost, sterile, fenestrated, short prep time, no orientation Disadvantage: nonhuman	23.00
AlloMax	Human	Prep time: 3 min Room-temp normal saline	No	5 y	Advantage: only sterile human ADM, short prep time, long shelf life, no orientation Disadvantage: cost	32.38
DermACELL	Human	Prep time: None	Yes	2 y	Advantage: ready to use Disadvantage: cost, antibiotic sensitivity	34.00

Abbreviations: Prep, preparation; temp, temperature.
From Cheng A, Saint-Cyr M. Comparison of different ADM materials in breast surgery. Clin Plast Surg 2012;39(2):167–75.

composition (hydroxyapatite vs β-TCP ratio), surface area of the implant, porosity, and crystallinity. Biphasic CaP products contain hydroxyapatite and β-TCP in various ratios aimed at producing grafting material that can degrade within a physiologically optimized time frame while providing mechanical stability until sufficient growth of bone has occurred.[57,58]

CaP cements are also available. These cements combine a dry powder and a liquid component in a setting reaction that occurs under physiologic pH and temperatures.[57] These cements are injectable and able to be molded for variable periods before hardening. They are also described as resorbable, although clinical experience has demonstrated retention of the material over extended periods. Although CaP cements have been successfully used for clinical applications, such as vertebroplasty[59] and cranial defect repair,[60] they are brittle and contraindicated for use in areas of mobility, active infection, or in situations when they directly contact the sinuses or dura.[61] Examples include Norian (Synthes Craniomaxillofacial, West Chester, PA), BoneSource (Stryker Leibinger, Kalamazoo, MI, Germany), and Mimix (Walter Lorenz Surgical, Jacksonville, FL).

Synthetic Polymers

Polymers currently used for oral and maxillofacial osseous reconstruction and augmentation include silicones, poly(lactic acid) (PLA), poly(glycolic acid) (PGA), poly(lactic-co-glycolic acid) (PLGA), poly(ethylene), poly(caprolactone), and poly (methyl methacrylate) (PMMA). Because these materials are biologically inert and do not possess osteogenic, osteoconductive, or osteoinductive properties, none of these materials are currently incorporated into commercial bone grafting products. But the biocompatibility of many synthetic polymers, combined with the ability to reliably reproduce and control their composition, rate of degradation, porosity, ability for cell attachment, and handling properties has made them an attractive material for investigation.[55]

Currently, the most common synthetic absorbable polymers available for oral and maxillofacial applications include the poly(alpha-hydroxy esters), PGA and PLA, and their copolymer PLGA. They have been used as resorbable sutures for years and more recently as degradable plates and screws for bone fixation in craniofacial, orthognathic, and trauma surgery.[62–65] These devices have advantages over traditional titanium plates and screws, such as the elimination of long-term palpable devices, as well as in continued skull growth in the pediatric population.[62]

Nondegradable polymers, on the other hand, have been commercialized for permanent implants in craniofacial augmentation or reconstruction. Solid facial implants made from silicone elastomer have been used for almost 50 years for skeletal augmentation of the malar eminence, zygomatic arch, and chin.[66] Porous high-density polyethylene (MedPor, from Porex Industries, Fairburn, GA) is another customizable prefabricated porous implant available for use as skeletal augmentation material, with indications, such as a space maintainer following globe exenteration and structural support for orbital reconstruction following trauma and tumor resection.[67]

PMMA is another nondegradable polymer commonly used in craniofacial osseous reconstruction, with established biocompatibility and history of clinical use of more than 50 years.[68] Although the exothermic nature of the setting reaction and the leaching of unreacted monomer from the implanted PMMA has been shown to cause bone necrosis and inflammation,[69] PMMA is still considered an aloplastic material of choice for cranioplasty in adults with good soft tissue quality and no frontal sinus exposure or previous history of infection.[68]

Recombinant Growth Factors

The appeal of recombinant growth factor products for bone regeneration include the reduced need for bone harvesting, availability, and inclusion of high concentrations of a purified biologic agent involved in the bone healing process. The implantation of such factors into a bone defect and the controlled release of the factor over time should promote the proliferation and differentiation of osteogenic stem cells within the wound, accelerating the healing process.[55]

Recent commercial availability of recombinant growth factor products has given oral and maxillofacial surgeons an additional option for the reconstruction of bony defects. Recombinant human bone morphogenetic protein-2 in an absorbable collagen sponge carrier (Infuse from Medtronic, Fridley, MN) has been approved for maxillary sinus augmentation and localized alveolar ridge augmentation in oral and maxillofacial surgery. The use of Infuse bone graft in orthopedic procedures includes spinal fusion and open tibia fractures. Platelet-derived growth factor in a β-TCP carrier (GEM 21S from Osteohealth, Shirley, NY) has also been approved in the United States for the treatment of bone defects and gingival tissue recession associated with advanced periodontal disease. The advantages of these products have also led surgeons to find other off-label uses, such as the reconstruction of mandibular continuity defects following tumor resection, grafting of maxillary clefts, and the reconstruction of hard tissue avulsion defects following trauma.[70] However, because clinical experience with such technology is relatively new, long-term effects of implanting materials and potential efficacy have yet to be clearly delineated against their relatively high cost.

DRUG DELIVERY

Delivery of cells and bioactive factors in combination with the placement of a support structure or scaffold is an important strategy that continues to be actively investigated in tissue engineering. Injectable scaffold systems hold great promise in tissue engineering applications because they can potentially deliver water-soluble drugs and growth factors in combination with cells to a tissue defect in a manner that provides an adequate environment for long-term cell survival, proliferation, and differentiation.[55] One of the biggest challenges lies in directing the release of multiple drugs and growth factors at various time intervals from the scaffold to achieve appropriate temporal and spatial delivery.[71] Although various new delivery methods continue to be developed and tested, some of the general concepts underlying many of these systems are discussed.

Degradation/Diffusion-Based Delivery Systems

One of the most common methods of creating controlled release of a drug is to use the physical properties of the scaffold material to regulate the amount of the drug delivered. To create controlled release, the target drug is mixed with the scaffold precursors during fabrication. In such systems, the properties of the scaffold, such as pore size or cross-linking density, regulate release by diffusion. The rate of scaffold degradation can also affect how much drug is released over time.[72] Another method of creating controlled release is to incorporate drugs into microspheres. Microspheres can be fabricated through a variety of techniques, including solvent evaporation and spray freeze-drying. Additional components, such as bovine serum albumin, can be added along with the target drug to help preserve the biologic activity of the drug during the fabrication process. The rate of drug release from microspheres is regulated by diffusion, and the release of kinetics of the target drug can be altered by changing the polymer used, the amount of protein loaded, and the size of the microsphere.[73]

Affinity-Based Delivery Systems

As an alternative to relying on a material's physical properties to regulate release, affinity-based delivery systems use noncovalent interactions between the desired drug and the scaffold to provide controlled release. One of the main examples of an affinity-based delivery system is a heparin-binding delivery system (HBDS), which can be used to deliver any protein drug that binds to heparin. Such delivery systems were initially designed to release basic fibroblast growth factor, but HBDSs have been recently used in conjunction with fibrin scaffolds to treat peripheral and central nervous system injuries.[72]

Immobilized Drug Delivery Systems

A different approach to drug delivery involves covalently attaching the target drug into the scaffold material. In this manner, the drug will not be lost to diffusion and the time course of release would be comparable with the lifetime of the scaffold.

SUMMARY

Increasing the sophistication and diversity of biomaterial products that are available have contributed to their expanding role in various facets of plastic surgery in recent years. In some areas, products of existing concepts continue to be fine tuned for greater ease of use, safety, and efficacy, whereas, in others, innovation for future application are still undergoing active investigation and development. Tailored bioengineered skins for wound-specific coverage continue to improve healing time and quality, whereas superior, longer-lasting ADMs have expanded their roles into wider applications. In drug delivery systems, injectable scaffolds and other delivery methods continue to be explored for more effective temporal and spatial release of drugs.

As new technology and new products continue to emerge, it will be of paramount importance for clinicians to continually look at the available evidence when weighing the risks and benefits of their use, remembering to carefully evaluate the safety, efficacy, and cost consideration individualized to each patient.

REFERENCES

1. Centers for Medicare & Medicaid Services. Guidance to surveyors for long term care facilities. Available at: http://www.cms.hhs.gov. Accessed April 28, 2012.
2. Fan K, Tang J, Escandon J, et al. State of the art in topical wound-healing products. Plast Reconstr Surg 2011;127(Suppl):44S–59S. Available at: http://www.ncbi.nlm.nih.gov/pubmed/21200273. Accessed March 19, 2012.

3. Groeber F, Holeiter M, Hampel M, et al. Skin tissue engineering–in vivo and in vitro applications. Adv Drug Deliv Rev 2011;63(4–5):352–66. Available at: http://www.ncbi.nlm.nih.gov/pubmed/21241756. Accessed March 10, 2012.

4. Lazic T, Falanga V. Bioengineered skin constructs and their use in wound healing. Plast Reconstr Surg 2011;127(Suppl):75S–90S. Available at: http://www.ncbi.nlm.nih.gov/pubmed/21200276. Accessed March 19, 2012.

5. Atiyeh BS, Gunn SW, Hayek SN. State of the art in burn treatment. World J Surg 2005;29(2):131–48. Available at: http://www.ncbi.nlm.nih.gov/pubmed/15654666. Accessed March 16, 2012.

6. Atiyeh BS, Costagliola M. Cultured epithelial autograft (CEA) in burn treatment: three decades later. Burns 2007;33(4):405–13. Available at: http://www.ncbi.nlm.nih.gov/pubmed/17400392. Accessed March 7, 2012.

7. Horch RE, Kopp J, Kneser U, et al. Tissue engineering of cultured skin substitutes. J Cell Mol Med 2005;9(3):592–608. Available at: http://www.ncbi.nlm.nih.gov/pubmed/16202208. Accessed April 28, 2012.

8. Ovington L. The art and science of wound dressings in the twenty-first century. In: Falabella A, Kirsner R, editors. Wound healing. Boca Raton (FL): Taylor & Francis Group; 2005. p. 1–7.

9. Cuzzell J. Choosing a wound dressing. Geriatr Nurs 1997;18(6):260–5. Available at: http://www.ncbi.nlm.nih.gov/pubmed/9469058. Accessed April 28, 2012.

10. Jones V, Grey JE, Harding KG. Wound dressings. BMJ 2006;332(7544):777–80. Available at: http://www.pubmedcentral.nih.gov/articlerender.fcgi?artid=1420733&tool=pmcentrez&rendertype=abstract. Accessed March 19, 2012.

11. Hess CT, Kirsner RS. Orchestrating wound healing: assessing and preparing the wound bed. Adv Skin Wound Care 2003;16(5):246–57 [quiz: 258–9]. Available at: http://www.ncbi.nlm.nih.gov/pubmed/14581817. Accessed April 28, 2012.

12. Hess C. Wound care. 5th edition. Philadelphia: Lippincott Williams & Wilkins; 2005.

13. Vermeulen H, van Hattem JM, Storm-Versloot MN, et al. Topical silver for treating infected wounds. Cochrane Database Syst Rev 2007;(1). CD005486. Available at: http://www.ncbi.nlm.nih.gov/pubmed/17253557. Accessed April 28, 2012.

14. Jørgensen B, Price P, Andersen KE, et al. The silver-releasing foam dressing, Contreet Foam, promotes faster healing of critically colonised venous leg ulcers: a randomised, controlled trial. Int Wound J 2005;2(1):64–73. Available at: http://www.ncbi.nlm.nih.gov/pubmed/16722854. Accessed April 28, 2012.

15. Edwards JV, Bopp AF, Batiste S, et al. Inhibition of elastase by a synthetic cotton-bound serine protease inhibitor: in vitro kinetics and inhibitor release. Wound Repair Regen 1999;7(2):106–18. Available at: http://www.ncbi.nlm.nih.gov/pubmed/10231512. Accessed April 28, 2012.

16. Broder KW, Cohen SR. An overview of permanent and semipermanent fillers. Plast Reconstr Surg 2006;118(Suppl 3):7S–14S. Available at: http://www.ncbi.nlm.nih.gov/pubmed/16936539. Accessed April 5, 2012.

17. Eppley BL, Dadvand B. Injectable soft-tissue fillers: clinical overview. Plast Reconstr Surg 2006;118(4):98e–106e. Available at: http://www.ncbi.nlm.nih.gov/pubmed/16980841. Accessed March 8, 2012.

18. Maloney BP, Murphy BA, Cole HP. Cymetra. Facial Plast Surg 2004;20(2):129–34. Available at: http://www.ncbi.nlm.nih.gov/pubmed/15643579. Accessed April 30, 2012.

19. André P. Evaluation of the safety of a non-animal stabilized hyaluronic acid (NASHA – Q-Medical, Sweden) in European countries: a retrospective study from 1997 to 2001. J Eur Acad Dermatol Venereol 2004;18(4):422–5. Available at: http://www.ncbi.nlm.nih.gov/pubmed/15196154. Accessed April 30, 2012.

20. Narins RS, Brandt F, Leyden J, et al. A randomized, double-blind, multicenter comparison of the efficacy and tolerability of Restylane versus Zyplast for the correction of nasolabial folds. Dermatol Surg 2003;29(6):588–95. Available at: http://www.ncbi.nlm.nih.gov/pubmed/12786700. Accessed April 30, 2012.

21. Manna F, Dentini M, Desideri P, et al. Comparative chemical evaluation of two commercially available derivatives of hyaluronic acid (hylaform from rooster combs and Restylane from streptococcus) used for soft tissue augmentation. J Eur Acad Dermatol Venereol 1999;13(3):183–92. Available at: http://www.ncbi.nlm.nih.gov/pubmed/10642054. Accessed April 30, 2012.

22. Kanchwala SK, Holloway L, Bucky LP. Reliable soft tissue augmentation: a clinical comparison of injectable soft-tissue fillers for facial-volume augmentation. Ann Plast Surg 2005;55(1):30–5 [discussion: 35]. Available at: http://www.ncbi.nlm.nih.gov/pubmed/15985788. Accessed April 30, 2012.

23. Kane MAC. Treatment of tear trough deformity and lower lid bowing with injectable hyaluronic acid. Aesthetic Plast Surg 2005;29(5):363–7. Available at: http://www.ncbi.nlm.nih.gov/pubmed/16151656. Accessed April 30, 2012.

24. Lowe NJ, Maxwell CA, Lowe P, et al. Hyaluronic acid skin fillers: adverse reactions and skin testing. J Am Acad Dermatol 2001;45(6):930–3. Available at: http://www.ncbi.nlm.nih.gov/pubmed/11712042. Accessed April 30, 2012.

25. Lemperle G, Morhenn V, Charrier U. Human histology and persistence of various injectable filler substances for soft tissue augmentation. Aesthetic

Plast Surg 2003;27(5):354–66 [discussion: 367]. Available at: http://www.ncbi.nlm.nih.gov/pubmed/14648064. Accessed April 30, 2012.

26. Friedman PM, Mafong EA, Kauvar AN, et al. Safety data of injectable nonanimal stabilized hyaluronic acid gel for soft tissue augmentation. Dermatol Surg 2002;28(6):491–4. Available at: http://www.ncbi.nlm.nih.gov/pubmed/12081677. Accessed April 30, 2012.

27. Monheit GD. Hylaform: a new hyaluronic acid filler. Facial Plast Surg 2004;20(2):153–5. Available at: http://www.ncbi.nlm.nih.gov/pubmed/15643583. Accessed April 30, 2012.

28. Mayer R, Lightfoot M, Jung I. Preliminary evaluation of calcium hydroxylapatite as a transurethral bulking agent for stress urinary incontinence. Urology 2001; 57(3):434–8. Available at: http://www.ncbi.nlm.nih.gov/pubmed/11248613. Accessed April 30, 2012.

29. Comite SL, Liu JF, Balasubramanian S, et al. Treatment of HIV-associated facial lipoatrophy with Radiance FN (Radiesse). Dermatol Online J 2004;10(2):2. Available at: http://www.ncbi.nlm.nih.gov/pubmed/15530292. Accessed April 30, 2012.

30. Vleggaar D, Bauer U. Facial enhancement and the European experience with Sculptra (poly-l-lactic acid). J Drug Dermatol 2004;3(5):542–7. Available at: http://www.ncbi.nlm.nih.gov/pubmed/15552606. Accessed April 30, 2012.

31. Humble G, Mest D. Soft tissue augmentation using sculptra. Facial Plast Surg 2004;20(2):157–63. Available at: http://www.ncbi.nlm.nih.gov/pubmed/15643584. Accessed April 30, 2012.

32. Cohen SR, Holmes RE. Artecoll: a long-lasting injectable wrinkle filler material: Report of a controlled, randomized, multicenter clinical trial of 251 subjects. Plast Reconstr Surg 2004;114(4):964–76 [discussion: 977–9]. Available at: http://www.ncbi.nlm.nih.gov/pubmed/15468406. Accessed April 30, 2012.

33. Bogdan Allemann I, Baumann L. Hyaluronic acid gel (Juvéderm™) preparations in the treatment of facial wrinkles and folds. Clin Interv Aging 2008;3(4):629. Available at: /pmc/articles/PMC2682392/?report=abstract. Accessed May 8, 2012.

34. Silverman RP. Acellular dermal matrix in abdominal wall reconstruction. Aesthet Surg J 2011;31(Suppl 7):24S–9S. Available at: http://www.ncbi.nlm.nih.gov/pubmed/21908821. Accessed April 28, 2012.

35. Fosnot J, Kovach SJ, Serletti JM. Acellular dermal matrix: general principles for the plastic surgeon. Aesthet Surg J 2011;31(Suppl 7):5S–12S. Available at: http://www.ncbi.nlm.nih.gov/pubmed/21908819. Accessed April 28, 2012.

36. Butler CE. The role of bioprosthetics in abdominal wall reconstruction. Clin Plast Surg 2006;33(2):199–211, v–vi. Available at: http://www.ncbi.nlm.nih.gov/pubmed/16638463. Accessed April 30, 2012.

37. Butler CE, Langstein HN, Kronowitz SJ. Pelvic, abdominal, and chest wall reconstruction with AlloDerm in patients at increased risk for mesh-related complications. Plast Reconstr Surg 2005;116(5):1263–75 [discussion: 1276–7]. Available at: http://www.ncbi.nlm.nih.gov/pubmed/16217466. Accessed April 30, 2012.

38. Gamboa-Bobadilla GM. Implant breast reconstruction using acellular dermal matrix. Ann Plast Surg 2006;56(1):22–5. Available at: http://www.ncbi.nlm.nih.gov/pubmed/16374090. Accessed April 30, 2012.

39. Zienowicz RJ, Karacaoglu E. Implant-based breast reconstruction with allograft. Plast Reconstr Surg 2007;120(2):373–81. Available at: http://www.ncbi.nlm.nih.gov/pubmed/17632337. Accessed April 30, 2012.

40. Nahabedian MY, Spear SL. Acellular dermal matrix for secondary procedures following prosthetic breast reconstruction. Aesthet Surg J 2011;31(Suppl 7):38S–50S. Available at: http://www.ncbi.nlm.nih.gov/pubmed/21908823. Accessed April 28, 2012.

41. Spear SL. Discussion. Acellular dermis-assisted prosthetic breast reconstruction versus complete submuscular coverage: a head-to-head comparison of outcomes. Plast Reconstr Surg 2009;124(6):1741–2. Available at: http://www.ncbi.nlm.nih.gov/pubmed/19952628. Accessed March 19, 2012.

42. Spear SL, Howard MA, Boehmler JH, et al. The infected or exposed breast implant: management and treatment strategies. Plast Reconstr Surg 2004;113(6):1634–44. Available at: http://www.ncbi.nlm.nih.gov/pubmed/15114123. Accessed April 30, 2012.

43. Stump A, Holton LH, Connor J, et al. The use of acellular dermal matrix to prevent capsule formation around implants in a primate model. Plast Reconstr Surg 2009;124(1):82–91. Available at: http://www.ncbi.nlm.nih.gov/pubmed/19568048. Accessed March 19, 2012.

44. Komorowska-Timek E, Oberg KC, Timek TA, et al. The effect of AlloDerm envelopes on periprosthetic capsule formation with and without radiation. Plast Reconstr Surg 2009;123(3):807–16. Available at: http://www.ncbi.nlm.nih.gov/pubmed/19319043. Accessed April 30, 2012.

45. Basu CB, Leong M, Hicks MJ. Acellular cadaveric dermis decreases the inflammatory response in capsule formation in reconstructive breast surgery. Plast Reconstr Surg 2010;126(6):1842–7. Available at: http://www.ncbi.nlm.nih.gov/pubmed/21124125. Accessed March 25, 2012.

46. Sbitany H, Langstein HN. Acellular dermal matrix in primary breast reconstruction. Aesthet Surg J 2011; 31(Suppl 7):30S–7S. Available at: http://www.ncbi.nlm.nih.gov/pubmed/21908822. Accessed April 28, 2012.

47. Brown RH, Izaddoost S, Bullocks JM. Preventing the "bottoming out" and "star-gazing" phenomena in

inferior pedicle breast reduction with an acellular dermal matrix internal brassiere. Aesthetic Plast Surg 2010;34(6):760–7. Available at: http://www.ncbi.nlm.nih.gov/pubmed/20602099. Accessed April 30, 2012.

48. Spear SL, Seruya M, Clemens MW, et al. Acellular dermal matrix for the treatment and prevention of implant-associated breast deformities. Plast Reconstr Surg 2011;127(3):1047–58. Available at: http://www.ncbi.nlm.nih.gov/pubmed/21088648. Accessed March 3, 2012.

49. Maxwell GP, Gabriel A. Use of the acellular dermal matrix in revisionary aesthetic breast surgery. Aesthet Surg J 2009;29(6):485–93. Available at: http://www.ncbi.nlm.nih.gov/pubmed/19944993. Accessed April 30, 2012.

50. Hartzell TL, Taghinia AH, Chang J, et al. The use of human acellular dermal matrix for the correction of secondary deformities after breast augmentation: results and costs. Plast Reconstr Surg 2010;126(5):1711–20. Available at: http://www.ncbi.nlm.nih.gov/pubmed/21042128. Accessed April 30, 2012.

51. Cheng A, Saint-Cyr M. Comparison of different ADM materials in breast surgery. Clin Plast Surg 2012;39(2):167–75. Available at: http://www.ncbi.nlm.nih.gov/pubmed/22482358. Accessed April 30, 2012.

52. Strauch B. Use of nerve conduits in peripheral nerve repair. Hand Clin 2000;16(1):123–30. Available at: http://www.ncbi.nlm.nih.gov/pubmed/10696581. Accessed April 30, 2012.

53. Meek MF, Coert JH. US Food and Drug Administration/Conformit Europe-approved absorbable nerve conduits for clinical repair of peripheral and cranial nerves. Ann Plast Surg 2008;60(1):110–6. Available at: http://www.ncbi.nlm.nih.gov/pubmed/18281807. Accessed March 8, 2012.

54. Meek MF, Coert JH. Clinical use of nerve conduits in peripheral-nerve repair: review of the literature. J Reconstr Microsurg 2002;18(2):97–109. Available at: http://www.ncbi.nlm.nih.gov/pubmed/11823940. Accessed April 25, 2012.

55. Kretlow JD, Young S, Klouda L, et al. Injectable Biomaterials for Regenerating Complex Craniofacial Tissues. NIH Public Access 2009;21(5):3368–93.

56. Neovius E, Engstrand T. Craniofacial reconstruction with bone and biomaterials: review over the last 11 years. J Plast Reconstr Aesthet Surg 2010;63(10):1615–23. Available at: http://www.ncbi.nlm.nih.gov/pubmed/19577527. Accessed April 16, 2012.

57. LeGeros RZ. Properties of osteoconductive biomaterials: calcium phosphates. Clin Orthop Relat Res 2002;(395):81–98. Available at: http://www.ncbi.nlm.nih.gov/pubmed/11937868. Accessed April 30, 2012.

58. Spivak JM, Hasharoni A. Use of hydroxyapatite in spine surgery. Eur Spine J 2001;10(Suppl 2):S197–204.

Available at: http://www.ncbi.nlm.nih.gov/pubmed/11716019. Accessed March 9, 2012.

59. Oner FC, Dhert WJ, Verlaan JJ. Less invasive anterior column reconstruction in thoracolumbar fractures. Injury 2005;36(Suppl 2):B82–9. Available at: http://www.ncbi.nlm.nih.gov/pubmed/15993121. Accessed April 30, 2012.

60. Friedman CD, Costantino PD, Takagi S, et al. BoneSource hydroxyapatite cement: a novel biomaterial for craniofacial skeletal tissue engineering and reconstruction. J Biomed Mater Res 1998;43(4):428–32. Available at: http://www.ncbi.nlm.nih.gov/pubmed/9855201. Accessed April 30, 2012.

61. Cunningham LL. The use of calcium phosphate cements in the maxillofacial region. J Long Term Eff Med Implants 2005;15(6):609–15. Available at: http://www.ncbi.nlm.nih.gov/pubmed/16393129. Accessed April 30, 2012.

62. Sanger C, Soto A, Mussa F, et al. Maximizing results in craniofacial surgery with bioresorbable fixation devices. J Craniofac Surg 2007;18(4):926–30. Available at: http://www.ncbi.nlm.nih.gov/pubmed/17667688. Accessed April 30, 2012.

63. Fedorowicz Z, Nasser M, Newton JT, et al. Cochrane database of systematic reviews. Chichester (United Kingdom): John Wiley & Sons, Ltd; 1996. CD006204. Available at: http://www.ncbi.nlm.nih.gov/pubmed/17443617. Accessed April 30, 2012.

64. Bell RB, Kindsfater CS. The use of biodegradable plates and screws to stabilize facial fractures. J Oral Maxillofac Surg 2006;64(1):31–9. Available at: http://www.ncbi.nlm.nih.gov/pubmed/16360854. Accessed April 18, 2012.

65. Laughlin RM, Block MS, Wilk R, et al. Resorbable plates for the fixation of mandibular fractures: a prospective study. J Oral Maxillofac Surg 2007;65(1):89–96. Available at: http://www.ncbi.nlm.nih.gov/pubmed/17174770. Accessed March 9, 2012.

66. Quatela VC, Chow J. Synthetic facial implants. Facial Plast Surg Clin North Am 2008;16(1):1–10 v. Available at: http://www.ncbi.nlm.nih.gov/pubmed/18063244. Accessed April 30, 2012.

67. Yaremchuk MJ. Facial skeletal reconstruction using porous polyethylene implants. Plast Reconstr Surg 2003;111(6):1818–27. Available at: http://www.ncbi.nlm.nih.gov/pubmed/12711941. Accessed April 5, 2012.

68. Moreira-Gonzalez A, Jackson IT, Miyawaki T, et al. Clinical outcome in cranioplasty: critical review in long-term follow-up. J Craniofac Surg 2003;14(2):144–53. Available at: http://www.ncbi.nlm.nih.gov/pubmed/12621283. Accessed April 30, 2012.

69. Santin M, Motta A, Borzachiello A, et al. Effect of PMMA cement radical polymerisation on the inflammatory response. J Mater Sci Mater Med 2004;15(11):1175–80. Available at: http://www.ncbi.nlm.nih.gov/pubmed/15880924. Accessed April 30, 2012.

70. Herford AS, Boyne PJ, Williams RP. Clinical applications of rhBMP-2 in maxillofacial surgery. J Calif Dent Assoc 2007;35(5):335–41. Available at: http://www.ncbi.nlm.nih.gov/pubmed/17822159. Accessed April 30, 2012.

71. Mikos AG, Herring SW, Ochareon P, et al. Engineering complex tissues. Tissue Eng 2006;12(12):3307–39. Available at: http://www.pubmedcentral.nih.gov/articlerender.fcgi?artid=2821210&tool=pmcentrez&rendertype=abstract. Accessed April 28, 2012.

72. Willerth SM, Sakiyama-Elbert SE. Approaches to neural tissue engineering using scaffolds for drug delivery. Adv Drug Deliv Rev 2007;59(4–5):325–38. Available at: http://www.pubmedcentral.nih.gov/articlerender.fcgi?artid=1976339&tool=pmcentrez&rendertype=abstract. Accessed March 10, 2012.

73. Mahoney MJ, Saltzman WM. Controlled release of proteins to tissue transplants for the treatment of neurodegenerative disorders. J Pharm Sci 1996;85(12):1276–81. Available at: http://www.ncbi.nlm.nih.gov/pubmed/8961138. Accessed April 30, 2012.

Surgical Treatment of Congenital Lymphedema

Corinne Becker, MD[a],*, Lionel Arrive, MD[b],
Anne Saaristo, MD[c], Michel Germain, MD[a],
Paolo Fanzio, MD[a], Bernardo Nogueira Batista, MD[a],
Gael Piquilloud, MD[a]

KEYWORDS

- Lymphedema • Magnetic resonance lymphography • Lymph nodes transplantation • Microsurgery
- VEGF-c • Lymphangiogenesis

KEY POINTS

- The ideal treatment for lymphedema of the limbs must restore function and normal cosmetic appearance.
- Human lymph nodes express high levels of the lymphatic vessel growth factor VEGF-c, which is responsible for stimulating lymphangiogenesis in the treated limb.
- Primary lymphedema can be associated with other organ malformations and genetic disorders: cancer and diseases of the central nervous system, lungs, heart, kidneys, and other organs can accompany lymphedema of sudden onset. The most prevalent hereditary disorders associated with lymphedema are Milroy disease, Meige syndrome, lymphedema-distichiasis, and yellow nail syndrome.
- Patients with hypoplastic forms of lymphedema on MRL are the preferred candidates for autologous lymph nodes transplantation.
- When the lymphedema is not too advanced, complete or near complete recovery is possible.

INTRODUCTION

The ideal treatment for lymphedema of the limbs must restore function and normal cosmetic appearance. Physiotherapy (manual drainages, pressotherapy, compression, bandages) is the usual treatment for chronic lymphedema and is considered by many as the only treatment for long-term management. It is not a curative therapy, but helps to control the evolution of the disease. Chronic lymphedema is a progressive condition, characterized by a degenerative and inflammatory process resulting in diffuse, irreversible tissue fibrosis. Surgical treatment is an alternative method of controlling chronic lymphedema.[1]

Precise diagnosis of lymphedema has achieved major progress: lymphangiography with oil and lymphoscintigraphy were once very useful, but these examinations have important drawbacks (eg, infection, pulmonary embolism). Magnetic resonance lymphangiography (MRL) with T2-weighted imaging has greater sensitivity, and allows complete visualization of the lymphatic system without any injection.[2]

Free autologous lymph node transplantation in hypoplastic forms of lymphedema is a new approach for lymphatic reconstruction, a more anatomic strategy compared with the multiple lymphovenous anastomoses. Recent findings on the growth hormones produced by the lymph nodes permit further understanding of the efficacy of these procedures. Three lymph node flaps can be used, depending on the affected segment and available donor sites. These flaps are located on

[a] Lymphedema Center, Paris, France; [b] Department of Radiology, Hôpital Saint-Antoine, Paris, France; [c] Plastic Surgery Department, Turku University Hospital, Turku, Finland
* Corresponding author. Lymphedema Center, 6 Square Jouvenet, Paris 75016, France.
E-mail address: corinne.becker.md@gmail.com

Clin Plastic Surg 39 (2012) 377–384
http://dx.doi.org/10.1016/j.cps.2012.08.001
0094-1298/12/$ – see front matter © 2012 Elsevier Inc. All rights reserved.

the inguinal, thoracic, or cervical area. The transplanted nodes pump the extracellular liquid responsible for lymphedema formation, and contain germinative cells that improve immune functions (**Figs. 1** and **2**).

Human lymph nodes express high levels of the lymphatic vessel growth factor vascular endothelial growth factor (VEGF)-c. This growth hormone is responsible for stimulating lymphangiogenesis in the treated limb. Saaristo and colleagues[3] compared the production of this growth factor by different tissues of the immune and hematopoietic systems. Lymph nodes expressed the highest levels of VEGF-c among the tissues tested (**Fig. 3**).

Each living node contains a plexus between the lymphatic and venous systems. The transplanted lymph nodes also probably work as a biologic lymphovenous anastomosis (**Fig. 4**).

CLINICAL PRESENTATION

Alterations of lymph drainage induce stasis of the lymph and progressive tissue changes with enlargement of the subcutaneous tissue and thickening of the skin.[4] Secondary infections, immune disorders, and cosmetic and psychosocial impairment can severely affect patients with lymphedema.

Diagnosis of lymphedema is done mainly by clinical assessment. A detailed history, clinical

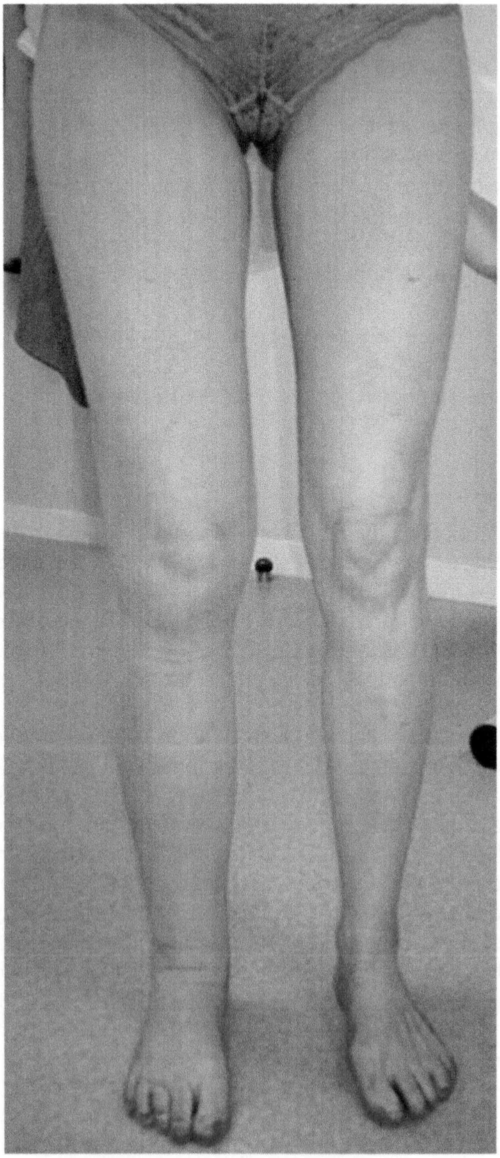

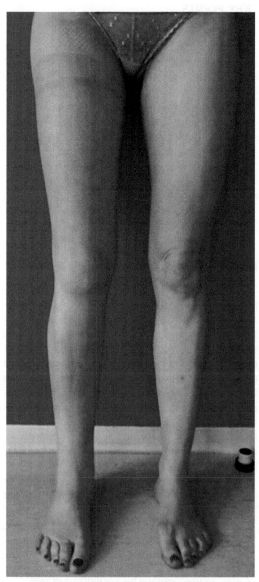

Fig. 1. A 34-year-old woman suffering from lymphedema since puberty, resistant to intensive physiotherapy.

Fig. 2. Patient in **Fig. 1**, 1 year after free node transplantation at the right inguinal region.

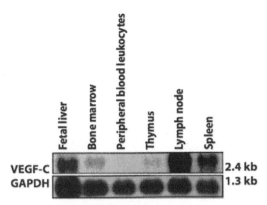

Fig. 3. High expression of VEGF-c by lymph node tissue. (*From* Saaristo AM, Niemi TS, Viitanen TP, et al. Microvascular breast reconstruction and lymph node transfer for postmastectomy lymphedema patients. Ann Surg 2012;255:472; with permission.)

evaluation, and physical examination are necessary. Age of inset, episodes of infections and inflammatory attacks, previous medical treatments, and visits to tropical countries with endemic filariasis should be recorded. Transitory edema of the affected limb and a family history of limb edema should be questioned. Lymphedema is usually painless, but a sensation of heaviness of the affected limb is a common complain. Acute inset or worsening of the lymphedema can produce pain, caused by distention of the aponevrosis around the deep lymphatic system.

In the lower limbs, lymphedema is usually unilateral and, if it is bilateral, it is generally asymmetric. In young adults the lymphedema in the lower limb is unilateral in 70% of cases, and bilateral in the other 30%. The lower body, upper extremities (unilateral or bilateral), the abdomen, genital area, and trunk can be involved. The skin folds at the base of the toes and fingers are broadened. This is caused by excessive skin thickness and fluid accumulation with tissue overgrowth (Stemmer sign).

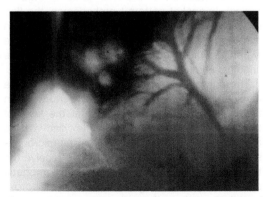

Fig. 4. Anastomotic plexus between veins and lymphatic vessels in the node. (*Courtesy of* S. Godart.)

Skin changes include pinky-red discoloration, hyperkeratosis, papillomatosis, and lymph vesicles. Interdigital mycosis must be treated to prevent secondary infections. Associated venous insufficiency may cause ulcerations of the skin.

Elephantiasis can be observed in hypoplastic and hyperplasic forms, but the disorders of the skin and the multiple folds are very difficult to treat. Evolution into lymphangiosarcoma is rare, but can occur if elephantiasis is not treated.

Perimetry of the limb is an indirect assessment of its volume. It is a traditional tool to evaluate limb changes. Measurements are made at the level of the two distal major joints (knee and ankle in the lower limb), 10 and 20 cm proximal to them.

ASSOCIATED DISEASES

Primary lymphedema can be associated with other organ malformations and genetic disorders. Cancer and diseases in the central nervous system, lungs, heart, kidneys, and other organs can accompany lymphedema of sudden onset. The most prevalent hereditary disorders associated with lymphedema are Milroy disease, Meige syndrome, lymphedema-distichiasis, and yellow nail syndrome.

Milroy Disease

In Milroy disease, there is a mutation of the VEGFR-c encoding gene, located at the 5q35.3 region. This disease is associated with lower and sometimes upper limb edemas. Genital lymphedema can be observed. This hereditary familial lymphedema does not present a macrostructural defect of the lymphatic system. The lymphatic collecting vessels are present, but there is an impairment of absorption of the lymph, reflecting as a functional defect.

Meige Syndrome

This syndrome affects lower limbs and appears during puberty. It is a hereditary form of lymphedema, but the genetic mutation is still unknown.

Lymphedema-Distichiadis

This disorder is associated with cardiac malformation, cleft palate, ptosis, and double eyelashes. In this syndrome, lymphatic collectors lack intraluminal valves, resulting in lymph reflux. The genetic mutation has been identified at the locus q24-3 on the chromosome 16.

Yellow Nail Syndrome

This is a rare syndrome in which lymphedema caused by lymphatic hypoplasia is associated with pleural effusions and yellow distrophic nail. Lymphedema may accompany complex vascular malformations, as seen in Proteus and Klippel-Trénaunay syndromes. In Turner syndrome, it is often present with a characteristic distribution (distal and symmetric, with lymphangiomas).

COMPLEMENTARY INVESTIGATIONS

Today, radiologic evaluation of lymphedema patients can be done through lymphoscintigraphy, MRL, or Photodynamic eye (PDE; Hamamatsu, Japan). Other examinations have historical value or a very specific use during surgery. PDE is useful to access the superficial lymphatic system anatomy through fluoresceine intake from an injection distally to the limb. Lymphoscintigraphy is a good functional examination that studies the ability of the lymphatic system to transport to regional lymph nodes a radioactive marker injected at the toes.

MRL with T2-weighted imaging allows visualization of the lymphatic system anatomy with greater sensitivity than lymphoscintigraphy, without need of any injection (**Figs. 5** and **6**).[2]

SURGICAL TREATMENT BY AUTOLOGOUS LYMPH NODES TRANSPLANTATION

Patients with hypoplastic forms of lymphedema on the MRL are preferred candidates for surgical treatment.[5–7] For some of these patients, long-term physiotherapy, hospitalizations, bandages, compression garments, and other treatments are insufficient to prevent lymphedema. These patients can benefit from autologous lymph node

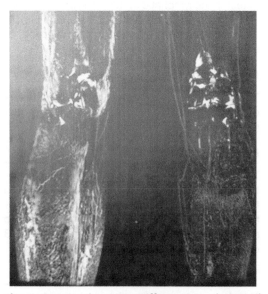

Fig. 5. Preoperative MRL. Diffuse accumulation of liquid in the leg, with hypoplastic ducts.

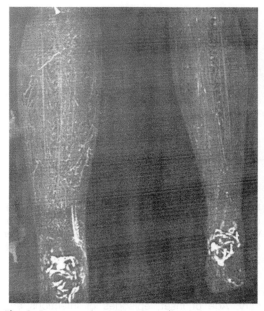

Fig. 6. Postoperative MRL. Normalization.

transplantation: the high concentration of lymphatic growth hormone induces the neoformation of lymphatic vessels improving uptake of lymph by the local lymphatic system.

In hyperplastic cases, high pressure on the lymphatic system can be deviated by lymphovenous bypass. This is the case for patients diagnosed with blockage or absence of the thoracic duct.

In elephantiasis, combination of various techniques is necessary: excisions of the folds; node transplantation; and liposuction at a further stage to excise the remaining lipoedema (hypertrophy of the subcutaneous fat in chronic lymphedema).

Operative Technique

In patients presenting with lymphedema on the entire limb, the flap should be transplanted to the proximal insertion of the limb (axila or inguinal region). In socket-pattern lymphedemas, the flap can be placed at the level of the knee. MRL can help establish the level of the hipoplasy. Large lymphedemas might require two different flaps (inguinal and knee region).

The surgery starts at the recipient site. In the inguinal region, the incision is performed in the inguinal crease. Deeply, just at the level of the inguinal ligament, the circumflex iliac vessels are individualized and prepared for the microanastomosis. A little pocket is created to receive the transplant, at the depth of the deep lymphatic system. At the knee region, an incision of approximately 7 cm is performed at the medial aspect, just above the knee. At the superior medial side of the adductor muscle, the saphenous vessel is the recipient pedicle.

The lymph node flap is usually taken at the thoracic region. An incision of 5 cm is performed in the low axillary region, laterally to the nipple. The lateral edge of the dorsalis muscle is identified and the vessels on its anterior aspect are dissected. The fat tissue located deeply on the lateral thoracic wall and anterior to these vessels contains functional lymph nodes. It can be dissected as a lymph node flap based on small branches of the lateral thoracic vessels or the toracodorsal system. The vessels are prepared with microvascular clamps for identification on the recipient site.

The cervical flap is based on the transverse cervical artery. Incision is performed on the internal part of the clavicle, over the sternocleidomastoidus, which is reflected. The flap is raised as a free-style flap, in the same manner as the thoracic region.

The flap is transferred with microsurgical techniques, under microscope magnification and 10–0 nylon sutures. Skin is closed with multilayer absorbable sutures.

Local excisions of excessive tissue and deep folds are performed on demand. This helps with the prevention of fungal or bacterial infections and allows for optimal physiotherapy postoperatively (**Figs. 7** and **8**).[8]

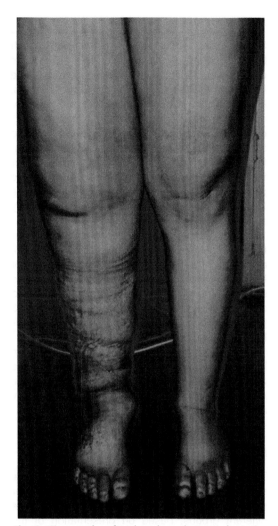

Fig. 8. Six months after lymph node transplantation at the knee level combined with excision of a fold at the ankle region.

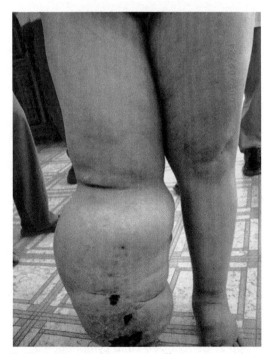

Fig. 7. A 28-year-old woman suffering since puberty from elephantiasis of the right leg, with chronic infections.

Postoperative Management

Patients are normally discharged on the second postoperative day. Physiotherapy with manual drainage and compressive bandages is prescribed for 2 months postoperatively, 3 to 5 days a week in the first month and three times per week in the second month. Continuation of physiotherapy from the third month onward is decided on a case-by-case basis. Compression garments can be used in the first 6 months. Progressively, new lymphatic vessels stimulated by the lymph node–produced growth factor VEGF-c repopulate the limb, replacing progressively the physiotherapy. A total of 20% to 50% of patients can be free of physiotherapy in long-term follow-up.

Evaluating Results

Standardized evaluation of results is difficult because of the great variability of the disease's presentation. Patients with unilateral lymphedema have a contralateral normal limb to compare results. Measurements of the normal side should also be made at follow-up consultations. In cases with bilateral lymphedema, serial measurements of the two affected legs can show the decrease in the circumference of the legs. Results can be compared over time with digital photography. Results in pediatric patients are difficult to objectively quantify, because the child and the leg continue to grow continuously after surgery (**Figs. 9–12**).

Patients are seen for postoperative consultations and follow-up consultations at 6, 12, 18, 24, and 36 months. Repeated lymphoscyntigraphy or MRL can show improvement to the lymphatic system anatomy and function. It can be repeated at follow-up visits once a year after surgery for 3 years (see **Figs. 3** and **4**). Patients have to be followed for recurrent episodes of erysipelas.

Other improvements referred by patients in long-term follow-up are better skin elasticity and texture. Some patients also refer hair growth. Ability to return to work and cease physiotherapy are the two major objectives of this procedure.

RESULTS

The following results are part of a large personal series (C. Becker). It is being analyzed for further publication. Patients were divided into three different groups, based on presentation of the lower limb lymphedema: (1) distal lymphedema, (2) generalized leg lymphedema, and (3) hyperplastic forms.

Group 1: Distal Lymphedema

Serial perimetry of affected and nonaffected limbs was taken postoperative at the level of the ankle and 10 cm and 20 cm proximally (see **Figs. 7** and **8**). All patients in this group showed a reduction of the circumference of the treated limb with normalization in 46%. A total of 88% of the patients had no more infections in the follow-up period. Postoperative lymphoscintigraphy in some of these patients showed the following:

- In 50% of the patients, the transplanted lymph nodes were visualized and new lymph drainage pathways appeared
- In 40% of the patients, lymphangiography improved showing effective lymph drainage pathways

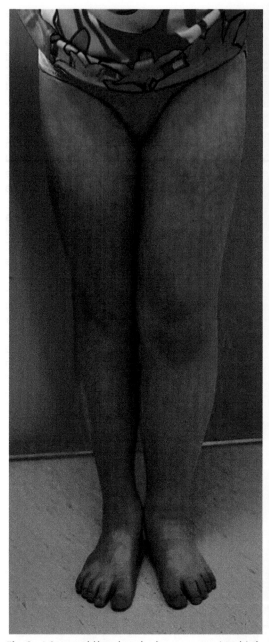

Fig. 9. A 9-year-old boy, lymphedema present since birth.

- In 10% of the patients, no changes at the scintigraphy were seen, even if clinical results were perceived

MRL was particularly able to show new lymphatic pathways (see **Figs. 5** and **6**).

Group 2: Generalized Limb Lymphedema

Although improvements in limb perimetry were present in 98% of the patients, only 20% of them

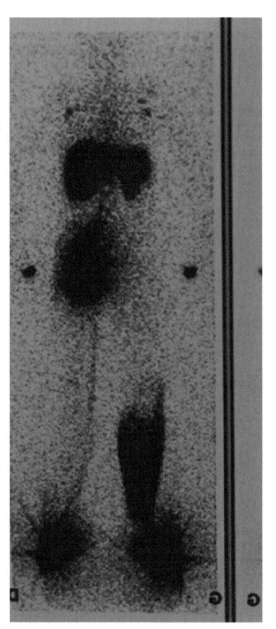

Fig. 10. No drainage of the left leg on lymphoscintygraphy.

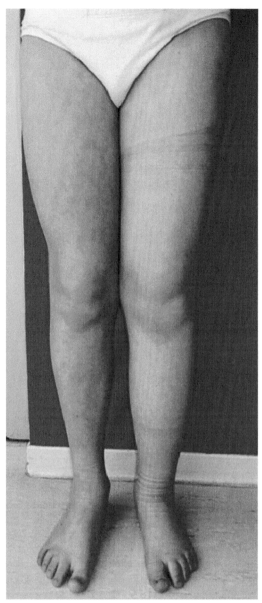

Fig. 11. Results at 18 months after two lymph node transplantations at the left inguinal region and the knee.

achieved complete normalization (see **Figs. 1** and **2**).

In severe and older lymphedemas, a second flap placed at the knee level, at the confluence of the deep and superficial lymphatic pathways further improves the results. The rate of chronic infections decreased from 53% to 4%.

Young patients could go back to work within the 2 postoperative months. In less severe lymphedema, patients returned to work 3 weeks after surgery.

Group 3: Hyperplastic Forms

Hypertrophic forms of primary lymphedema diagnosed through MRL and malformations of the thoracic duct are treated by several lymphovenous anastomoses in the inguinal region. Use of compression garments is mandatory. There seems to be a clinical improvement, with better quality of life and young patients being able to return to work. No radiologic improvement is seen on lymphoscintigraphy or MRL.

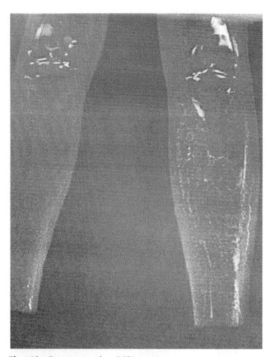

Fig. 12. Postoperative MRL.

SUMMARY

The use of autologous lymph nodes transplantation in hypotrophic forms of primary lymphedema is an innovative and promising treatment. It is a logical approach for the reconstruction of underdeveloped lymph transport system. Recent discoveries regarding VEGF-c lymphangiogenic properties provide a biomolecular explanation for its efficacy. When the lymphedema is not too advanced, complete or near complete recovery is possible.

The use of MRL to visualize lymphatic pathways without contrast injection allows clear differentiation between hypotrophic and hypertrophic forms of the disease, allowing precise indications for surgery.

In hyperplastic forms and lesions of the thoracic duct, lymphovenous anastomoses are indicated, but the presence of patent lymphatic vessels is important. PDE can help identify these vessels, but in late stages of elephantiasis, they can be obstructed. In theses cases, local resections are needed to remove the skin folds and prevent fungal or bacterial infections. Successful management of these difficult patients depends on good collaboration among a multidisciplinary team (eg, radiologists, reconstructive surgeons, and physiotherapists).

REFERENCES

1. Becker C, Assouad J, Riquet M, et al. Postmastectomy lymphedema: long-term results following microsurgical lymph node transplantation. Ann Surg 2006; 243(3):313–5.
2. Arrivé L, Azizi L, Lewin M, et al. MR lymphography of abdominal and retroperitoneal lymphatic vessels. Am J Roentgenol 2007;189(5):1051–8.
3. Saaristo AM, Niemi TS, Viitanen TP, et al. Microvascular breast reconstruction and lymph node transfer for post mastectomy lymphedema patients. Ann Surg 2012;255(3):468–73.
4. Lee BB, Bergan J, Stanley RocksonByung-Boong Lee, et al, editors. Lymphedema. A concise compendium of theory and practice. 1st edition. Springer; 2011.
5. Becker C, Hidden G, Pecking A. Transplantation of lymph nodes: an alternative method for treatment of lymphoedema. Progr Lymphol 1990;4:487–93.
6. Becker C. Les transferts lymphatiques. Ann Chir Plast Esthet 2000.
7. Becker C. Actual treatment of lymphedema. e-Mem Acad Chir 2008;4(1):55–64.
8. Batista BN, Doy A, Modolin ML, et al. Localized massive limphedema in morbidly obese patients. Rev Brás Cir Plast 2009;4(Suppl 3):96.

Microlymphatic Surgery for the Treatment of Iatrogenic Lymphedema

Corinne Becker, MD[a], Julie V. Vasile, MD[b],*,
Joshua L. Levine, MD[b], Bernardo N. Batista, MD[a],
Rebecca M. Studinger, MD[b], Constance M. Chen, MD[b],
Marc Riquet, MD[c]

KEYWORDS

- Lymphedema • Treatment • Autologous lymph node transplantation (ALNT)
- Microsurgical vascularized lymph node transfer • Iatrogenic • Secondary
- Brachial plexus neuropathy • Infection

KEY POINTS

- Autologous lymph node transplant or microsurgical vascularized lymph node transfer (ALNT) is a surgical treatment option for lymphedema, which brings vascularized, VEGF-C producing tissue into the previously operated field to promote lymphangiogenesis and bridge the distal obstructed lymphatic system with the proximal lymphatic system. Additionally, lymph nodes with important immunologic function are brought into the fibrotic and damaged tissue.
- ALNT can cure lymphedema, reduce the risk of infection and cellulitis, and improve brachial plexus neuropathies.
- ALNT can also be combined with breast reconstruction flaps to be an elegant treatment for a breast cancer patient.

OVERVIEW: NATURE OF THE PROBLEM

Lymphedema is a result of disruption to the lymphatic transport system, leading to accumulation of protein-rich lymph fluid in the interstitial space. The accumulation of edematous fluid manifests as soft and pitting edema seen in early lymphedema. Progression to nonpitting and irreversible enlargement of the extremity is thought to be the result of 2 mechanisms:

1. The accumulation of lymph fluid leads to an inflammatory response, which causes increased fibrocyte activation.
2. Fat deposition occurs when malfunctioning lymphatics are unable to transport fat molecules effectively.[1]

Clinically, patients develop firm subcutaneous tissue, progressing to overgrowth and fibrosis.

Lymphedema is a common chronic and progressive condition that can occur after cancer treatment. The reported incidence of lymphedema varies because of varying methods of assessment,[1–3] the long follow-up required for diagnosing lymphedema, and the lack of patient education regarding lymphedema.[4] In one 20-year follow-up of patients with breast cancer treated with mastectomy and axillary node dissection, 49% reported the sensation of arm lymphedema.[5] Of the patients who developed lymphedema, 77% were diagnosed within the 3-year period following breast cancer treatment, and the remaining patients developed arm lymphedema at a rate of about

a Department of Plastic Surgery, Lymphedema Centre, 6 Square Jouvenet, Paris 75016, France; b Department of Plastic Surgery, New York Eye and Ear Infirmary, 310 East 14th Street, New York, NY 10003, USA; c Department of Thoracic Surgery, European Hospital Georges Pompidou, 20 Rue Louis Leblanc, Paris 75908, France
* Corresponding author. 1290 Summer Street, Suite 2200, Stamford, CT 06905.
E-mail address: jvasilemd@gmail.com

Clin Plastic Surg 39 (2012) 385–398
http://dx.doi.org/10.1016/j.cps.2012.08.002

1% per year after the 3 years. Therefore, about a quarter of patients will develop lymphedema years after breast cancer treatment, and a long follow-up is required.

The incidence of lymphedema after breast cancer treatment ranges from 24% to 49% after mastectomy and 4% to 28% after lumpectomy.[1] Patients requiring more extensive breast cancer treatment with axillary node dissection and radiation have the greatest risk for the development of lymphedema. However, even the less extensive lymph dissection in sentinel node biopsy is associated with a 5% to 7% incidence of upper-extremity lymphedema.[6]

The incidence of lymphedema after treatment of other malignancies is reported as follows: 16% with melanoma, 20% with gynecologic cancers, 10% with genitourinary cancers, 4% with head and neck cancers, and 30% with sarcoma. Patients requiring pelvic dissection and radiation therapy for the treatment of non–breast cancer malignancies have a reported lymphedema rate of 22% and 31%, respectively.[3] Risk factors for developing lymphedema after cancer treatment are obesity, infection, and trauma.[1,5]

In addition to the decreased amount of lymph tissue critical to a normal immune response, tissue changes and lymphostasis result in increased susceptibility to infection in the lymphedematous extremity. Clinically, patients may develop cellulitis from minor trauma that would otherwise be insignificant in a normal extremity (**Fig. 1**). Each episode of infection further damages lymphatic channels and perpetuates a vicious cycle. Patients may require lifelong antibiotic prophylaxis.

Lymphedema can also lead to erysipelas, lymphangitis, and even lymphangiosarcoma. Erysipelas is a streptococcal infection of the dermis. Lymphangitis is inflammation of the lymphatic channels as a result of infection at a site distal to the channel, such as a paronychia, an insect bite, or an intradigital web space infection. Lymphangiosarcoma is a rare malignant tumor that occurs in long-standing cases of lymphedema (**Fig. 2**). Stewart-Treves syndrome is angiosarcoma arising from postmastectomy lymphedema and has an extremely poor prognosis, with a median survival of 19 months.[1]

THERAPEUTIC OPTIONS FOR IATROGENIC LYMPHEDEMA
Conservative Treatment

Conservative lymphedema therapy is the backbone for providing symptomatic improvement of lymphedema and may slow the progression of disease. Multiple layers of short-elastic bandages are wrapped circumferentially around the lymphedematous

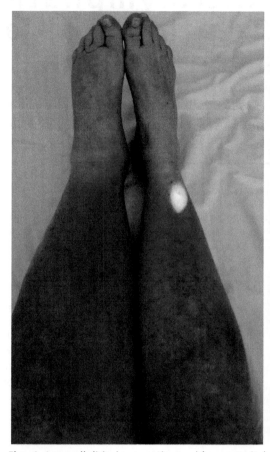

Fig. 1. Leg cellulitis in a patient with congenital lymphedema.

extremity to squeeze edema fluid out of the tissue and push the edema fluid proximally. Customized compression garments are subsequently placed on the extremity to maintain the decreased extremity size. Decongestive lymphatic therapy usually begins with intensive (daily for several weeks) lymphatic massage and bandaging. This therapy is followed by less-frequent maintenance

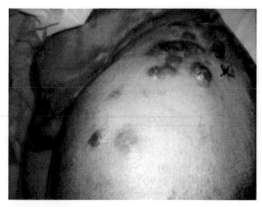

Fig. 2. Lymphangiosarcoma.

lymphatic massage and daily placement of compression garments for the rest of patients' lives. Flare-ups of lymphedema may require repeating the initial intensive daily lymphatic massage with bandaging. Patients with severe lymphedema may require bandaging every night and wearing compression garments everyday.

The major limitation of conservative therapy is that reduction in extremity size is short lived without continual compression; the maintenance of compression (conservative therapy) is difficult to achieve long term because it is time consuming, labor intensive, requires specialized therapists, and requires commitment of patients and patients' support network. Frequently, it is difficult for patients to self-apply bandages. In addition, insurance companies may inadequately cover therapists for bandaging and massage therapy, requiring patients to parcel out therapy sessions. A second major limitation of conservative therapy is that it cannot affect change in extremity girth because of subcutaneous fat deposition and fibrosis. Thus, surgical options for treatment have an important role in the treatment of lymphedema, and a *combination* of treatment modalities may achieve the most improvement.

Surgical Treatment

Surgical options for lymphedema treatment fall into 2 categories: debulking and physiologic.

Debulking procedures may involve elliptical wedge excision of excess skin and subcutaneous tissue from an extremity or liposuction. Wedge excision of tissue can provide immediate symptomatic relief to patients with severe lymphedema. Removal of heavy or hanging bulky tissue from an extremity can improve the function of the extremity[7] and can also improve the application of bandages and compression garments.

Liposuction is another effective modality for removing excess fat deposition as a result of abnormal lymphatic transport. It is helpful as an adjunct to other surgical treatments and can be performed in a second stage of treatment after a first-stage physiologic surgical treatment. Complications of debulking procedures may be chronic wounds, infection, widened scars, hematoma, skin necrosis, potential damage to remaining lymphatics, and worsening of the lymphedema.[3] Compression garments are necessary *lifelong* after debulking methods of treatment.[7,8]

Physiologic procedures seek to reconstruct the lymphatic transport system. Lympholymphatic graft[9] is a procedure that connects an obstructed lymphatic to a healthy lymphatic using a vein or a lymphatic as an interposition graft.[10] The procedure is technically demanding and time consuming because lymphatic channel walls are thin, transparent, and very fragile. In addition, there may be significant donor site morbidity. Lymphovenous anastomosis (LVA) connects an obstructed lymphatic to a vein to shunt the lymph fluid into the venous system and seem to be effective, especially in early stages of lymphedema.[11,12] The LVA remains patent if the lymphatic pressure is higher than the venous pressure. Currently, a subdermal vein is used because it has lower venous pressure. The caliber of subdermal veins is less than a 1 mm, requiring supermicrosurgery with extrafine microsurgical instruments and sutures. Usually, multiple LVAs (3–5)[12,13] are created to a lymphedematous extremity. Although in other centers, an average of 9 LVAs (range of 5–18) are routinely created by teams of surgeons operating with multiple microscopes simultaneously.[14]

Autologous lymph node transplantation (ALNT),[15–17] also called microsurgical vascularized lymph node transfer, is another reconstructive surgical treatment of lymphedema. This article focuses on ALNT and its use in patients with secondary iatrogenic lymphedema. In ALNT, a recipient bed in the lymphedematous extremity is prepared by releasing scar tissue until healthy soft tissue is encountered. Then a small flap containing superficial lymph nodes are harvested from a donor site with an artery and vein and microsurgically anastomosed to an artery and vein at the recipient site.

The ALNT procedure is considered to be physiologic for several reasons. First, scar tissue, which may be blocking lymphatic flow, is released. Second, healthy vascularized tissue in the form of a flap is brought into the previously operated site, which may bridge lymphatic pathways through the scar tissue. Third, the flap contains healthy lymph nodes, which produce vascular endothelial growth factor C (VEGF-C).[18] VEGF-C promotes lymphangiogenesis[19] and is hypothesized to stimulate reconnections in the distal obstructed lymphatic system with the proximal lymphatic system.[20] Fourth, lymph nodes have important immunologic functions, and adding healthy lymph nodes may provide benefit to a lymphedematous extremity predisposed to development of infection.[21] Fifth, lymph nodes themselves are an interface between the lymphatic and venous systems for drainage of lymph into the venous system[22] without surgically created lymphovenous anastomoses distally on the extremity.

INDICATIONS FOR ALNT IN IATROGENIC LYMPHEDEMA

Iatrogenic lymphedema is most commonly associated with the treatment of cancer, such as lymph node dissection and radiation therapy. Alternatively, lymphedema may also be caused by nononcologic procedures, such as saphenous vein removal,[23] hernia repair, liposuction,[24] and thigh lift.[25] When lymphedema is caused by previous surgery, a lymph node flap may be indicated to reconstruct the deficit.

A complete blockage of lymph drainage pathways from removal and/or damage to lymph nodes is an absolute indication for ALNT to replace the missing or damaged lymphatic tissue. This condition can be diagnosed on lymphoscintigraphy as a lack of uptake of a radioactive particle (technetium-99 m) in the inguinal or axillary lymph nodes after distal injection of the particle in the extremity. More recently, magnetic resonance lymphography (MRL) with T2-weighted images,[26] also called lymphatic magnetic resonance imaging (MRI), is being used to visualize the lymphatic system anatomy with greater sensitivity.[27] An absence of lymph nodes and/or lymph channels traversing the surgical site may appear as a black area on MRL (**Fig. 3**).

Other indications for ALNT procedures are lymphedema resistant to conservative treatment, pain or signs of brachial plexus neuropathy,[28] and chronic infections in the lymphedematous extremity. If conservative treatment fails to bring satisfactory long-lasting results and if lymphatic MRI or lymphoscintigraphy demonstrate decreased lymphatic drainage, ALNT is indicated to reconstruct the damaged or missing lymphatic tissue. Release of scar tissue and placement of vascularized, nonirradiated tissue can treat neuromas and stop the progression of brachial plexus neuropathies (**Fig. 4**). Chronic infections are also a main indication for ALNT because of the immunologic function of lymph nodes.

In breast reconstruction patients with lymphedema, it is possible to use a deep inferior epigastric perforator (DIEP) flap or transverse rectus abdominis musculocutaneous flap in continuity with a lymph node flap. This combined flap allows for breast reconstruction with axillary lymphatic reconstruction. However, it is only indicated for breast reconstruction patients with established lymphedema or history of upper-extremity cellulitis. Lymph node transfer is not indicated in breast reconstruction patients without lymphedema because of the risk of inducing an iatrogenic lymphedema by dissecting in a previously operated axilla.

OPERATIVE TECHNIQUE
ALNT for Arm Lymphedema

The dissection always begins at the recipient site, usually the axilla. The scarred fibrotic tissue is incised and, if possible, excised until healthy tissue is reached. During the dissection, thoracodorsal branches are identified and isolated with vessel loops. If a neuroma is encountered or patients have chronic pain or weakness, then external neurolysis of the brachial plexus is done. The release of scar tissue can be challenging, and great care must be taken to avoid injury to the vital structures within the axilla. It is best to work from known to unknown and start dissection from where the anatomy is more normal. When the dissection is complete, the extent of the flap needed can be estimated.

A lymph node flap can be prepared from 3 donor sites: inguinal, thoracic, and cervical. The inguinal lymph node flap harvests superficial lymph nodes based on branches from the superficial circumflex iliac or superficial inferior epigastric vessels. An incision is made along a line between the iliac crest and the pubis bone. The length of the incision depends

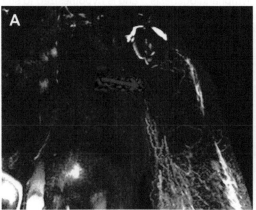 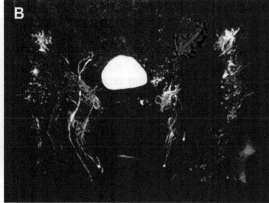

Fig. 3. (*A*) MRL after modified radical mastectomy, axillary node dissection, and radiation treatment. Red arrow points to dark area showing absence of lymph drainage. (*B*) MRL after radical hysterectomy. Red arrow points to dark area showing absence of lymph drainage.

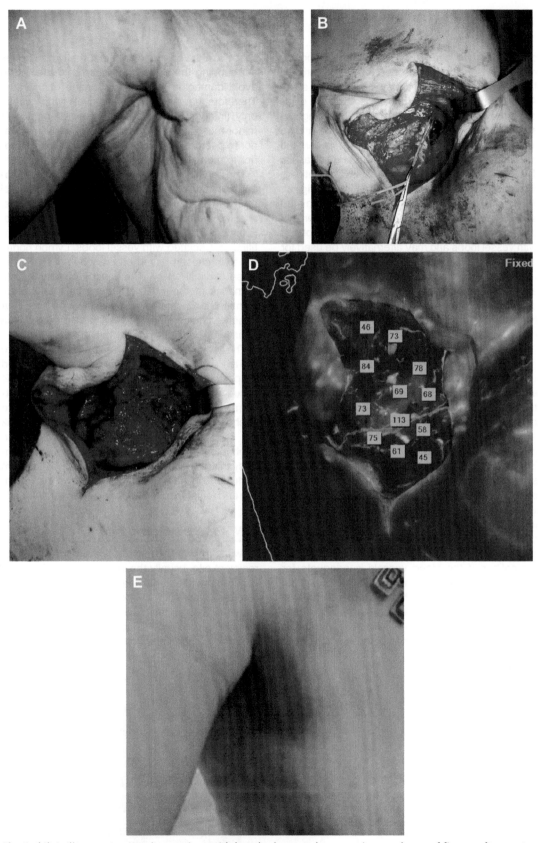

Fig. 4. (*A*) Axillary contraction in a patient with lymphedema and progressive numbness of fingers after mastectomy, axillary node dissection, and radiation. (*B*) Brachial plexus with scar removed. (*C*) Lymph node flap placed in axilla over brachial plexus. (*D*) SPY imaging showing perfusion of lymph node flap. (*E*) Postoperative axillary contraction. Improved sensibility in middle 3 fingers.

on the flap size needed for the defect. Subcutaneous fat is incised to the depth of the cribriform fascia, at the level where superficial veins are seen. At times, there is an unnamed superficial vein diagonally traversing the operative field. This diagonal superficial vein helps to identify the plane and to localize the lymph nodes in the fat between the muscular aponeurosis and the superficial fascia. The superficial circumflex iliac vessels are identified, dissected, and isolated with vessel loops (**Fig. 5**). The lateral part of the flap is elevated to the isolated superficial circumflex iliac vessels. The superficial inferior epigastric vessels are identified and isolated with vessel loops and may alternatively be used for anastomosis. The borders of the dissection are the following: inguinal ligament (caudal), muscular aponeurosis (deep), and cribriform fascia (superficial). It is of paramount importance to not dissect lymph nodes beyond these first two borders to avoid removing the deeper lymph nodes that drain the leg.

The thoracic lymph node flap harvests lymph nodes at the lower axilla based on branches from the thoracodorsal or lateral thoracic vessels. An incision is made on a longitudinal line anterior to the latissimus dorsi muscle and lateral to the breast. The superficial fascia is opened, and thoracodorsal branches are dissected around the main vessel supplying the latissimus muscle, and isolated with vessel loops. A freestyle flap is designed in this region by dissecting vessels and a few nodes. Branches of the lateral thoracic vessels are also identified and isolated with vessel loops (**Fig. 6**). In approximately 60% of cases, branches from the lateral thoracic vessels supply the nodes in the superior portion of the flap. If the caliber of the blood vessels is adequate for microanastomosis, the flap will be based on the branches of the lateral thoracic vessels so that the thoracodorsal branches are left intact. In the remaining 40% of cases, the flap is dissected based on the distal branches of the thoracodorsal

vessels. It is very important that the lymph nodes surrounding the axillary vein are not dissected to avoid damaging lymphatic drainage of the arm. Therefore, harvest is limited to level I lymph nodes only (inferior to the lateral border of pectoralis minor muscle), avoiding the level II nodes (posterior to pectoralis muscle) and level III nodes (superior to medial border of pectoralis minor muscle).

The cervical lymph node flap harvests lymph nodes based on branches from the transverse cervical artery. An incision is made over the medial clavicle, and the sternocleidomastoid muscle is retracted. Branches of the transverse cervical artery are identified and isolated with vessel loops. Lymph nodes are then chosen based on branches of the transverse cervical artery. The venous outflow is from branches of the external jugular vein, which are identified and isolated with vessel loops (**Fig. 7**). A freestyle flap containing a few nodes based on the transverse cervical artery is then dissected.

The lymph node flap is harvested and brought to the axilla for microsurgical anastomosis. It should be placed over the axillary vein, where lymphatic tissue was originally removed for cancer treatment. An absorbable suture may be used to anchor the flap so that it does not shift and kink the vascular pedicle. SPY imaging (Novadaq Technologies, Inc, Mississauga, Ontario) with indocyanine green is then performed to confirm perfusion of the flap. The incisions at the donor site and recipient site are closed over a small drain.

ALNT for Leg Lymphedema

As with arm lymphedema, dissection begins at the recipient site, usually the inguinal region. The scar tissue is released until healthy nonfibrotic tissue is reached. Cephalad to the inguinal ligament, the superficial circumflex iliac vessels are identified and isolated with vessel loops. Just caudal to the inguinal ligament, a space is created for the lymph

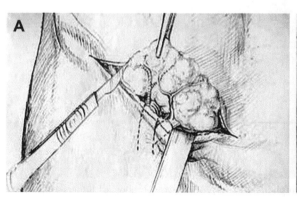
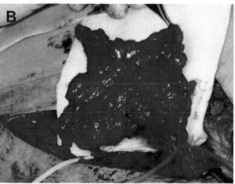

Fig. 5. (*A*) Inguinal lymph node flap. (*B*) Inguinal lymph node flap. Red vessel loop is around superficial circumflex iliac vessel and yellow vessel loop is around superficial inferior epigastric vessel.

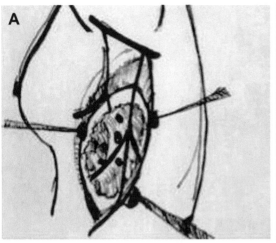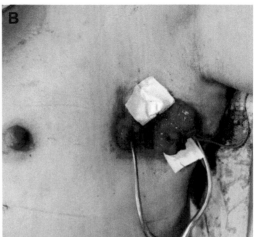

Fig. 6. (*A*) Thoracic lymph node flap. (*B*) Thoracic lymph node flap. Vessel loops are around thoracodorsal and lateral thoracic branches.

node flap. If the flap will be placed at the knee, then a medial incision is made just above the knee. Medial genicular branches or saphenous vessel branches are isolated with vessel loops. Harvest of the donor site (inguinal, thoracic, or cervical lymph node flap) and microsurgical anastomosis proceed in an identical fashion to ALNT for the arm.

ABDOMINAL FLAP IN CONTINUITY WITH LYMPH NODE FLAP

An inguinal lymph node flap may be harvested with an abdominal-based breast reconstruction, such

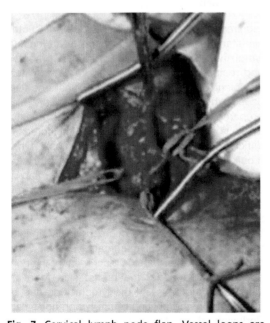

Fig. 7. Cervical lymph node flap. Vessel loops are around transverse cervical arterial and external jugular venous branches.

as the DIEP flap. Because the superficial inguinal lymph nodes used for ALNT are immediately adjacent to the DIEP flap, it is possible to harvest the lymph nodes using the same incision as used in a DIEP flap. Only a few lymph nodes are harvested to minimize any risk of causing iatrogenic leg lymphedema. Superficial lymph nodes may be identified with MRI or computed tomography before surgery.

The DIEP flap dissection proceeds in a standard fashion, except the flap is extended caudally to include 3 to 4 superficial inguinal lymph nodes. The superficial circumflex iliac vessels are identified and isolated with vessel loops. The DIEP flap is completely dissected and its perfusion is isolated to the deep inferior epigastric vessels by temporarily clamping the superficial circumflex iliac vessels. SPY imaging is used to evaluate the perfusion of the lymph node flap. If perfusion of the lymph nodes seems adequate, the DIEP flap pedicle is microsurgically anastomosed to the internal mammary vessels and the lymph node portion of the flap is placed in the prepared axilla. A suture may be used to anchor the lymph node–containing portion of the flap into the axilla. If lymph node perfusion with SPY does not seem adequate, the superficial circumflex iliac vessels may be anastomosed to branches of the lateral thoracic or thoracodorsal vessels (**Fig. 8**). A superficial inferior epigastric artery (SIEA) flap may also be combined with ALNT to reconstruct patients with partial mastectomy or brachial plexus neuropathies.

NONABDOMINAL FLAP WITH LYMPH NODE FLAP

In nonabdominal microsurgical breast reconstruction, the ALNT is always a separate free tissue

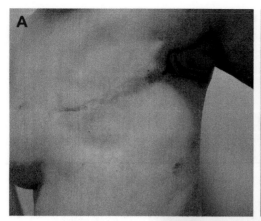
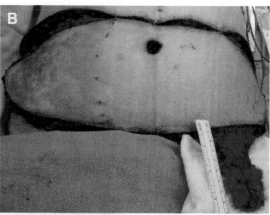
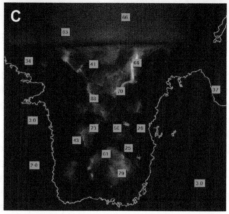

Fig. 8. (*A*) Axillary contraction in a patient with lymphedema after mastectomy and axillary node dissection without radiation therapy. (*B*) DIEP flap with superficial inguinal lymph node flap. The superficial circumflex iliac vessels have been clamped and flap perfusion is isolated to the DIEP pedicle. (*C*) SPY image showing perfusion to the lymph nodes is adequate without superficial circumflex iliac vessels.

transfer. Executing these procedures simultaneously can be complicated, and a team approach is recommended to maximize efficiency. For thoracodorsal artery perforator (TDAP) flap with a lymph node flap, dissection of the pedicled TDAP flap proceeds simultaneously with the dissection of the lymph node flap. To facilitate simultaneous harvest, patients are placed in a lateral decubitus position on a beanbag with the arm prepped in the field, and the ipsilateral inguinal lymph node flap is used. Scar tissue is released at the axilla, and recipient vessels are identified and isolated with vessel loops. Branches off the thoracodorsal vessels may be used for anastomosis with the lymph node flap. The TDAP flap is rotated and secured in position for reconstruction of the breast. Then, the inguinal lymph node flap is harvested, microsurgically anastomosed, and placed in the prepared axilla. SPY imaging is done to confirm perfusion of the lymph node flap (**Fig. 9**).

For a lymph node flap with a nonabdominal free flap, such as a profunda artery perforator flap or gluteal flap, 2 microsurgical anastomoses are required. The nonabdominal flap is dissected simultaneously with the dissection of an inguinal lymph node flap. The scarred axilla is prepared and recipient vessels are identified and isolated. Recipient vessels for the nonabdominal free flap, usually the internal mammary vessels, are also prepared. The inguinal lymph node flap anastomosis is performed first because of the increased difficulty with microsurgical anastomosis when a bulky breast flap reconstruction is present. After anastomosis, the inguinal lymph node flap is placed in the prepared axilla and SPY imaging is done to confirm perfusion. A suture may be used to anchor the lymph node flap in position. Then, the nonabdominal flap is microsurgically anastomosed to the internal mammary vessels. Great care must be taken with the placement of the nonabdominal flap under the breast skin to avoid vascular compromise of the lymph node flap by compression and shifting of the lymph node flap. Perfusion of the lymph node flap is confirmed again after the placement of the nonabdominal flap with SPY imaging.

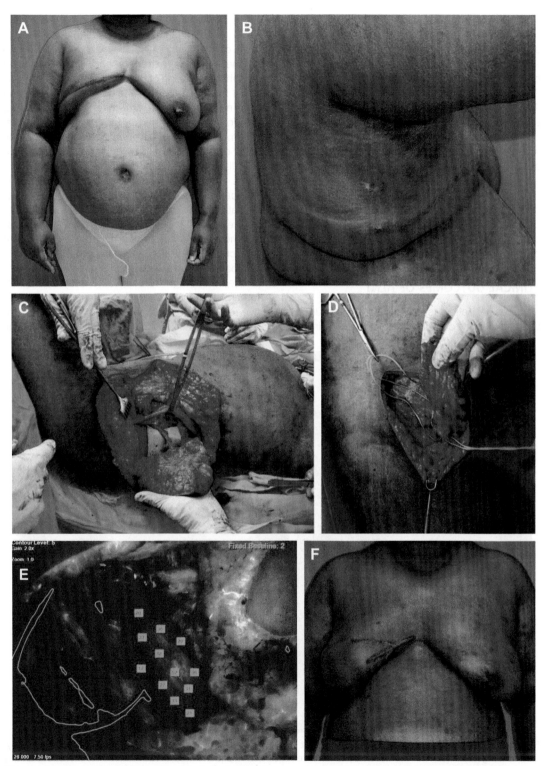

Fig. 9. (*A*) Severely obese (body mass index of 39.6) woman with hypertension and failed implant breast reconstruction with lymphedema after mastectomy and axillary node dissection. (*B*) Lateral thorax, demonstrating ample excess fat. (*C*) TDAP flap isolated on its pedicle. (*D*) Inguinal lymph node flap. Blue vessel loops around superficial circumflex iliac vessels. (*E*) Spy imaging showing adequate perfusion of lymph node flap. (*F*) Postoperative.

ALNT may be combined with other surgical treatments for optimal results. For example, wedge excision may be performed at the same time as ALNT procedures in patients with severe lymphedema. Liposuction is an effective adjunct to ALNT in patients with all stages of lymphedema. After excessive edema fluid is drained from the extremity, excess subcutaneous tissue is still present (lipedema) from long-standing lymphedema and contributes to increased extremity girth. Liposuction may be used in selective regions of the extremity to remove the extra fat. It should be performed carefully by surgeons familiar with lymphedema to avoid further damaging lymphatic channels. Selective liposuction to remove the excess fat deposition may be done parallel to the extremity and in a second stage.

CLINICAL OUTCOMES OF ALNT

Changes in patient symptoms, level of function with activities of daily living, physical examination, and radiological imaging are recorded. After ALNT, most patients report a difference in their level of discomfort and may describe increased lightness of the extremity and improvement in throbbing or aching of the extremity are. Circumferential measurements of the lymphedematous and nonlymphedematous extremity are recorded at the dorsum of the hand or foot, the wrist or ankle, 10 cm above the wrist or ankle, 20 cm above the wrist or ankle, the elbow or knee, 10 cm above the elbow or knee, and 20 cm above the elbow or knee. Postoperative changes are calculated by comparing the difference between the lymphedematous and nonlymphedematous extremity before and after surgery. For example, preoperative measurements (lymphedematous right forearm 26.0 cm - normal left forearm 19.5 cm = 6.5 cm) are compared with postoperative measurements (lymphedematous right forearm 22.0 cm - normal left forearm 19.8 cm = 2.2 cm) to calculate a total relative reduction (6.5 cm − 2.2 cm = 4.3 cm relative reduction). This calculation provides a clinical

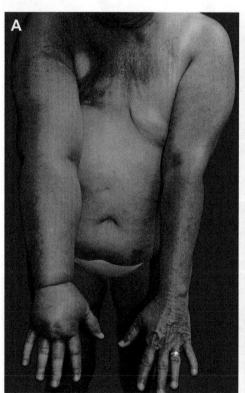
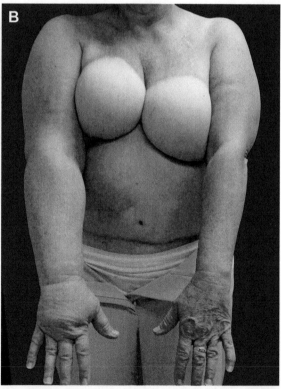

Fig. 10. (A) Patient with 14-year history of right arm lymphedema after mastectomy and radiation therapy, limited range of motion at the shoulder, chronic cellulitis with frequent hospital admissions for infection, taking prescribed daily oral antibiotics. Conservative therapy consisted of maintenance wrapping and compression garments. (B) Three years after ALNT with average circumferential reduction of 1.3 cm for the arm and 3.2 cm at the dorsum of the hand. Full range of motion at the shoulder regained. Continuous oral antibiotic therapy was discontinued, with patient now only having occasional small cellulitis treated with oral antibiotic. Conservative therapy discontinued by the patient (not the physician), and compression garment only used when patient is working outside. Compression garment had not been worn for more than a month at time of photograph.

snapshot of the improvement achieved by ALNT regardless of patient-specific habitus changes throughout time (eg, weight gain or loss, water retention) (**Fig. 10**). Patients with infections before surgery can be monitored for reduction in infection severity, frequency, and need for hospital admission.

In a series of 1500 patients operated over a period of 20 years by the senior author (CB), with stages 1, 2, and 3 of lymphedema (International Society of Lymphology), 98% of the patients had some degree of improvement. Forty percent of the patients with stages 1 or 2 lymphedema had complete normalization (**Fig. 11** and **12**) and did not require additional conservative therapy. In the patients with stage 3 lymphedema, 95% had some degree of improvement. Only 2% had

repeat infection. However, patients with stage 3 lymphedema still required conservative therapy. The minimum follow-up was 3 years. About 10% of the patients had brachial plexus neuropathies. Seventy-five percent of patients with brachial plexus neuropathies had improved symptoms after neurolysis of the nerves and coverage with nonirradiated, well-vascularized tissue (ALNT or other flap). The patients had decreased pain and stabilization of previously progressive symptoms of weakness. Although sensation can recover in the following 2 years after surgery, motor recovery is rare and can only be expected in young patients. Tendon transfers may benefit some of these patients later in their follow-up.

Patients with less severe lymphedema and lymphedema for shorter duration tend to respond better

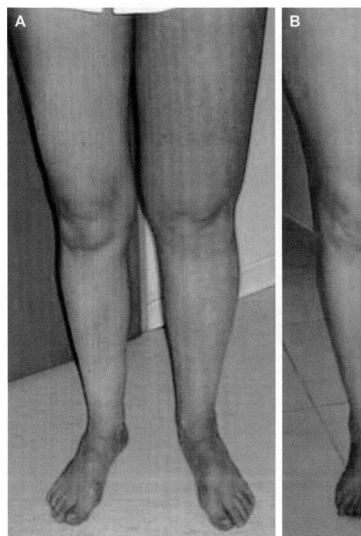
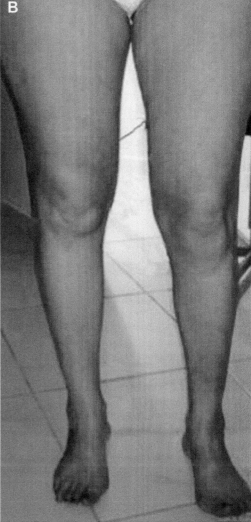

Fig. 11. (*A*) Patient with left leg lymphedema for 8 years after radical hysterectomy 12 years before. (*B*) Two years after ALNT, with complete normalization.

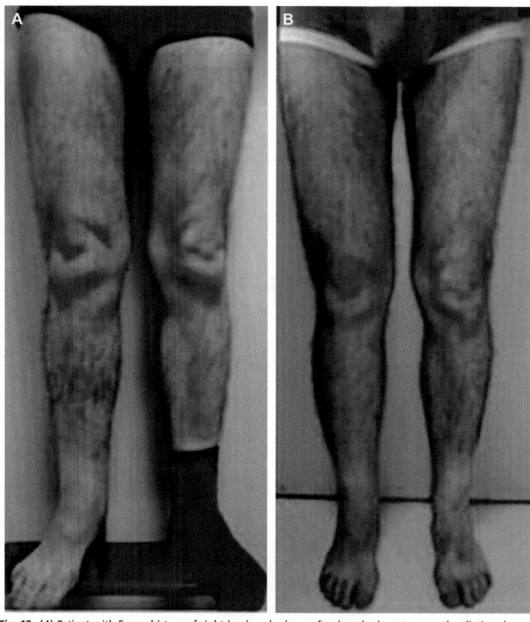

Fig. 12. (*A*) Patient with 5-year history of right leg lymphedema after lymphadenectomy and radiation therapy for Hodgkin lymphoma. (*B*) One year after ALNT, with complete normalization.

to ALNT. In patients with stage 1 and 2 lymphedema, lymphoscintigraphy and MRL can illustrate objective changes with new lymphatic pathways draining the extremity (**Fig. 13** and **14**). Even patients with long-standing lymphedema (more than 15 years) can show improvement with ALNT.

COMPLICATIONS AND CONCERNS ALNT

Lymphocele at the donor site can be avoided with use of a drain postoperatively for the first 24 to 48

hours and local compression. The use of surgical clips on lymphatics leading to the donor lymph nodes during dissection may also help. Deep lymph nodes beyond the inguinal ligament and axillary lymph nodes near the axillary vein should not be disturbed to avoid iatrogenic lymphedema of the extremity. Local infections, hematomas, and delayed wound healing may occur. Flap monitoring is difficult because the lymph node flap is a buried flap. In addition, the vessels are usually small, between 0.5 mm and 1.5 mm, which makes use

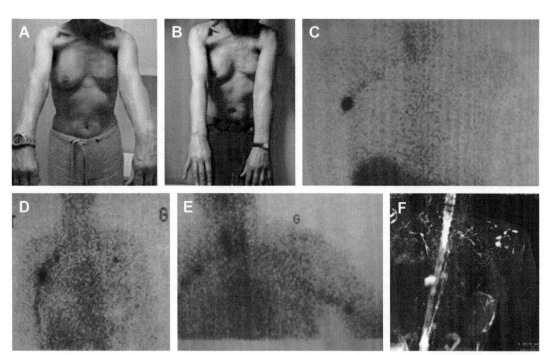

Fig. 13. (*A*) Patient with left arm lymphedema after modified radical mastectomy. (*B*) Patient 8 years after ALNT. (*C*) Preoperative lymphoscintigraphy. Absence of left axillary lymphatic drainage. (*D*) Postoperative lymphoscintigraphy, 1 year after ALNT. Left axillary lymphatic drainage now present. (*E*) Postoperative lymphoscintigraphy, 5 years after ALNT. Further improvement in left axillary lymphatic drainage. (*F*) Postoperative MRL. Red arrow showing lymphatic drainage.

of an internal Doppler probe challenging. Vascular thrombosis is thought to occur in 2% of patients, with no clinical improvement seen. When 2 sets of anastomoses are used in an abdominal flap in continuity with a lymph node flap, the ALNT part of the flap can remain viable if the abdominal flap pedicle thromboses.

SUMMARY ON ALNT

ALNT is an excellent alternative and complementary treatment of secondary iatrogenic lymphedema. It brings vascularized, VEGF-C–producing tissue into the previously operated field to promote lymphangiogenesis and bridge the distal

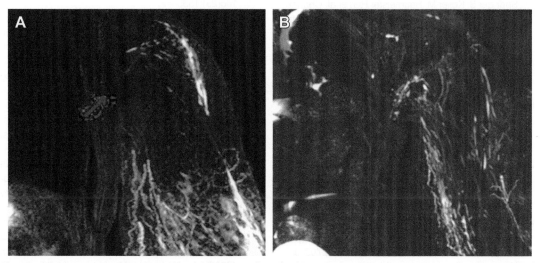

Fig. 14. (*A*) Preoperative MRL in patient with left arm lymphedema. Red arrow pointing to seroma of lymph fluid. (*B*) Postoperative MRL, 1 year after ALNT, showing new lymphatic channels.

obstructed lymphatic system with the proximal lymphatic system. Additionally, lymph nodes with important immunologic function are brought into the fibrotic and damaged tissue. ALNT can improve brachial plexus neuropathies and can be combined with breast reconstruction flaps to be an elegant solution for patients with breast cancer.

REFERENCES

1. Warren AG, Brorson H, Borud LJ, et al. Lymphedema: a comprehensive review. Ann Plast Surg 2007; 59(4):464–72.

2. Asim M, Cham A, Banerjee S, et al. Difficulties with defining lymphoedema after axillary dissection for breast cancer. N Z Med J 2012;125(1351):29–39.

3. Cormier JN, Askew RL, Mungovan KS, et al. Lymphedema beyond breast cancer: a systemic review and meta-analysis of cancer-related secondary lymphedema. Cancer 2010;116(22):5138–49.

4. Ahmed RL, Prizment A, Lazovich D, et al. Lymphedema and quality of life in breast cancer survivors: the Iowa women's health study. J Clin Oncol 2008; 26(35):5689–96.

5. Petrek JA, Senie RT, Peters M, et al. Lymphedema in a cohort of breast carcinoma survivors 20 years after diagnosis. Cancer 2001;92(6):1368–77.

6. McLaughlin SA, Wright MJ, Morris KT, et al. Prevalence of lymphedema in women with breast cancer 5 years after sentinel lymph node biopsy or axillary dissection: objective measurements. J Clin Oncol 2008;26(32):5213–9.

7. Lee BB, Kim YW, Kim DI, et al. Supplemental surgical treatment to end stage (stage IV-V) of chronic lymphedema. Int Angiol 2008;27(5):389–95.

8. Brorson H. From lymph to fat: complete reduction of lymphedema. Phlebology 2010;25(1):s52–63.

9. Springer S, Koller M, Baumeister RG, et al. Changes in quality of life of patients with lymphedema after lymphatic vessel transplantation. Lymphology 2011; 44(2):65–71.

10. Mehrara BJ, Zampell JC, Suami H, et al. Surgical management of lymphedema: past, present, and future. Lymphat Res Biol 2011;9(3):159–67.

11. Mihara M, Murai N, Hayashi Y, et al. Using indocyanine green fluorescent lymphography and lymphatic-venous anastomosis for cancer-related lymphedema. Ann Vasc Surg 2012;26(2):278.e1–6.

12. Demirtas Y, Ozturk N, Yapici O, et al. Supermicrosurgical lymphaticovenular anastomosis and lymphatic venous implantation of treatment of unilateral lower extremity lymphedema. Microsurgery 2009;29(8):609–18.

13. Chang DW. Lymphaticovenular bypass for lymphedema management in breast cancer patients: a prospective study. Plast Reconstr Surg 2010;126(3):752–8.

14. Yamamoto T, Narushima M, Kikuchi K, et al. Lambda-shaped anastomosis with intravascular stenting method for safe and effective lymphaticovenular anastomosis. Plast Reconstr Surg 2011;127(5): 1987–92.

15. Becker C, Hidden G. Transfer of free lymphatic flaps. Microsurgery and anatomical study. J Mal Vasc 1988;13(2):119–22. Available at: http://www. ncbi.nlm.nih.gov/pubmed/3397670.

16. Becker C, Assouad J, Riquet M, et al. Postmastectomy lymphedema: long-term results following microsurgical lymph node transplantation. Ann Surg 2006;243(3):313–5. Available at: http:// wwwncbi.nlm.nih.gov/pubmed/16495693.

17. Assouad J, Becker C, Hidden G, et al. The cutaneolymph node flap of the superficial circumflex artery. Surg Radiol Anat 2002;24(2):87–90. Available at: http://wwwncbi.nlm.nih.gov/pubmed/12197025.

18. Saaristo AM, Niemi TS, Viitanem TP, et al. Microsurgical breast reconstruction and lymph node transfer for postmastectomy lymphedema patients. Ann Surg 2012;255(3):468–73.

19. Lahteenvuo M, Honkonen K, Tervala T, et al. Growth factor therapy and autologous lymph node transfer in lymphedema. Circulation 2011;123(6):613–20.

20. Yan A, Avraham T, Zampell JC, et al. Mechanisms of lymphatic regeneration after tissue transfer. PLoS One 2011;6(2):e17201.

21. Lin CH, Ali R, Chen SC, et al. Vascularized groin lymph node transfer using the wrist as a recipient site for management of postmastectomy upper extremity lymphedema. Plast Reconstr Surg 2009; 123(4):1265–75.

22. Pegu A, Flynn JL, Reinhart TA. Afferent and efferent interfaces of lymph nodes are distinguished by expression of lymphatic endothelial markers and chemokines. Lymphat Res Biol 2007;5(2):91–103.

23. Lahl W, Richter J, Neppach V, et al. Leg edema after surgery of varicose veins. Zentralbl Chir 1981; 106(23):1535–42.

24. Frick A, Hoffman JN, Baumeister RG, et al. Liposuction technique and lymphatic lesions in lower legs: anatomic study to reduce risks. Plast Reconstr Surg 1999;103(7):1868–73.

25. Stadelmann WK. Intraoperative lymphatic mapping to treat groin lymphorrhea complicating an elective medial thigh lift. Ann Plast Surg 2002;48(2):205–8.

26. Arrive L, Azizi L, Lewin M, et al. MR lymphography of abdominal and retroperitoneal lymphatic vessels. AJR Am J Roentgenol 2007;189(5):1051–8.

27. Liu NF, Lu Q, Liu PA, et al. Comparison of radionuclide lymphoscintigraphy and dynamic magnetic resonance lymphangiography for investigating extremity lymphedema. Br J Surg 2010;97(3):359–65.

28. Becker C, Pham DN, Assouad J, et al. Postmastectomy neuropathic pain: results of microsurgical lymph nodes transplantation. Breast 2008;17(5): 472–6. Available at: http://wwwncbi.nlm.nih.gov/ pubmed/18450444.

Tissue Restructuring by Energy-Based Surgical Tools

Marek K. Dobke, MD, PhD[a],*, Thomas Hitchcock, PhD[b],
Lisa Misell, PhD[b], Gordon H. Sasaki, MD[c]

KEYWORDS

- Tissue restructuring • Energy devices • Noninvasive cosmetic surgery • Radiofrequency
- Ultrasound

KEY POINTS

- Advancements in surgical techniques have to the development of many noninvasive concepts or incorporation of existing concepts into plastic surgery armamentarium; stem cells-based therapies, mesotherapy, and energy-based surgical tools such as ultrasonic, radiofrequencies, lasers, cryogenic, hydromechanical, microwave technologies are among the newest developments.
- Clinical outcomes following noninvasive procedures with energy-based devices tend to be much more subtle than those following invasive surgical procedures.
- As with any medical procedure, noninvasive procedures carry some degree of risk of adverse effects as those resulting from non-uniform healing after application of ultrasonic energy, lasers or radiofrequencies in addition to trivial problems such as transient edema, skin erythema, bruises.

OVERVIEW

Various oils, creams, and lotions have been used for skin-quality maintenance and beautification over the centuries. However, the quest for the preservation of youth and beauty has evolved with the introduction of invasive cosmetic plastic surgery procedures, which have been developed and popularized since the beginning of the last century. During the last 2 decades, advancements in surgical techniques have paralleled advancements in dermatologic sciences, leading to the development of many noninvasive concepts (eg, stem cells–based therapies, mesotherapy) and modalities (eg, lasers) and providing new tools for cosmetic surgery and medicine. Energy-based surgical tools, including ultrasonic, radiofrequency (RF), cryogenic, hydromechanical, and microwave technologies with the capability of tissue cutting, sealing, or restructuring, complement these medical concepts well by allowing noninvasive, non–open-access interventions.

Energy-based noninvasive surgical tools can be used for ablative bio-stimulation (eg, collagen production) or tissue restructuring functions (eg, tightening or lifting) and they are the subject of this review. Experience with a laser-therapy device for body contouring (1440 nm wavelength laser for soft tissue sculpting), as an example of laser-based technology applied to body contouring, is reviewed in another article of this issue. Additionally, because the focus of this article is tissue restructuring and its applications in aesthetic surgery, hydromechanical tools (eg, water-jet technology used to cut and emulsify soft tissue) are not featured.

THERAPEUTIC OPTIONS

In general, the application of noninvasive energy-based devices for tissue restructuring can lead to results that are less dramatic than those from surgical procedures.[1–4] However, patients find value in the reduced amount of downtime needed to

[a] Division of Plastic Surgery, University of California San Diego, CA, USA; [b] Ulthera, Inc., 2150 S. Coutry Club Drive, Mesa, AZ 85210, USA; [c] Loma Linda Medical University Center, 800 S. Fairmount Avenue, Pasadena, CA 91105, USA
* Corresponding author. Division of Plastic Surgery, University of California San Diego, 200 West Arbor Drive, San Diego, CA 92103, USA.
E-mail address: mdobke@ucsd.edu

Clin Plastic Surg 39 (2012) 399–408
http://dx.doi.org/10.1016/j.cps.2012.07.008
0094-1298/12/$ – see front matter © 2012 Elsevier Inc. All rights reserved.

recover from noninvasive procedures by energy-based devices. For this reason, the noninvasive energy-based technologies have become popular, even when treatments must be repeated to achieve an optimal result or when approximating the result of an invasive procedure.

The typical 2 tissue-restructuring objectives for currently available energy-based devices are

1. Two-dimensional tissue shrinkage resulting in tissue lifting and/or firming
2. Volume-reducing and body-contouring techniques

Both objectives have energy-based technologies with modalities that are based on controlled thermal damage to the tissue. Therapeutic options for the most common conditions are depicted in **Table 1**. Ultrasound (US), RF, cryolipolysis, laser-assisted therapies, and even soft radiation have found an application in these objectives.

US-BASED DEVICES

US-based devices generate a US beam, which can be focused to a predetermined depth of penetration and placement of energy. After passing innocuously through the skin (or superficial skin layers), focused US waves reach a focal point where alternating waves of compression and rarefaction rapidly heat tissue (ie, thermal coagulation) or mechanically disrupt the target tissue via cavitation. Depending on which tissues are targeted and the degree of tissue disruption, focused US can be used for different purposes. These purposes include the lifting and tightening of the skin and skin-adjacent tissues (ie, microfocused US [MFUS]) or body contouring (ie, high-intensity focused US [HIFUS]).[2–4]

MFUS

MFUS therapy uses US energy (in a low megahertz range) to noninvasively firm, tighten, and shrink the dermis and subdermal tissues producing a lift of soft tissues. There is currently only one commercially available MFUS device approved by the Food and Drug Administration (FDA) (the Ulthera System; Ulthera, Inc, Mesa, Arizona), with another recently available in the Korean market (Doublo System; Hironic Co LTD, Korea), which integrate real-time US imaging with focused US energy. This integration allows the clinician to target the desired treatment depth for the precise delivery of energy below the surface of the skin without affecting the intervening tissues. Multiple removable transducers offer a choice of depths for MFUS penetration (**Fig. 1**). In general, higher-frequency transducers are used for a more superficial tissue effect compared with lower-frequency transducers. For example, a 4-MHz transducer is characterized by a 4.5-mm depth (appropriate for deep dermis or SMAS treatment in facial areas) and a 7-MHz transducer is characterized by a 3.0-mm depth.[3,4] Unlike in focused US ablation therapies (eg, for tumors), which interlace coagulative sonication zones to ensure complete tumor ablation, cosmetic MFUS applications involve

Table 1
Energy-based devices for tissue restructuring: therapeutic options

Technology	Source of Energy	Wavelength or Other Physical Parameter	Tissue Target	Indication
Low-level laser therapy	Red light or near infrared	600–1000 nm	Subcutaneous fat, within a few millimeters range	Desire for focal, noninvasive fat reduction
MFUS	Ultrasound	4–10 MHz	Dermis, SMAS, frontalis, platysma muscles	Excessive skin laxity, need for skin tightening, forehead, brow ptosis
RF	Electromagnetic waves	300 MHz to 3 KHz	Dermis	Excessive skin laxity, mild skin wrinkling
Cryolipolysis	Thermoelectric cooling systems, cold air, contact cold gel panels	−3°C to 7°C	Subcutaneous fat, probably within a few millimeters range	Superficial subcutaneous fat collections, mild tissue ptosis (eg, jowls)
HIFUS	Ultrasound	2 MHz	Subcutaneous fat, up to 30-mm range	Superficial and intermediate fat deposits

Abbreviations: HIFUS, high-intensity focused ultrasound; MFUS, microfocused ultrasound.

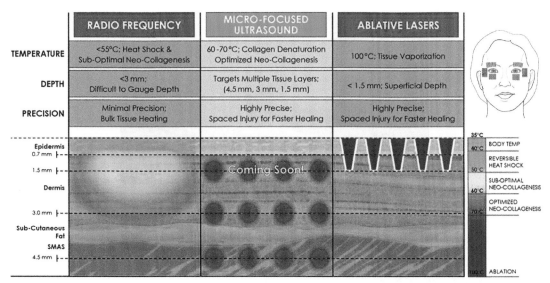

Fig. 1. General characteristics and differences between energy-based modalities for tissue restructuring. (*Courtesy of* Ulthera, Inc, Mesa, Arizona; with permission.)

treatments delivered in lines of small precisely spaced zones of tissue coagulation in the targeted tissues.[3,5] To help track the placement and quantity of the treatment lines delivered, the treatment area is marked using a standardized facial grid (**Fig. 2**). Zones of coagulation placed in the target tissues (eg, SMAS) undergo the wound healing process to produce subcutaneous microscars that contract, resulting in treated tissue firming or an aesthetic unit lift as the result of cumulative linear or gridlike field contracture (**Fig. 3**).

HIFUS

HIFUS generates high-energy US waves (up to 10 000 W/cm^2) for lipolysis. The energy for HIFUS is typically more diffuse, and the focal points converge deeper than MFUS, delivered 10 to 30 mm below the skin level, targeting the subcutaneous adipose tissue. Like MFUS, HIFUS creates a temperature in the range of 56° to 65°C at its focal point, delivering the thermal energy to the targeted fat tissue layer without damaging intervening tissues (overlying and underlying fat). However, because the physical characteristics of HIFUS interaction with tissue predicated in a more diffuse and deeper way (than for skin-tightening devices) but still within a 3-cm reach, for the best possible result skin should contract over decreasing in volume of subcutaneous fat. Truly obese patients with poor skin tone are not good candidates for body contouring using this technology because the skin may not contract or re-drape deeper layers of tissue uniformly (**Fig. 4**).[6,7] Devices that deliver focused US energy

on a 2-MHz wavelength have received much attention recently because they seem to be effective in disrupting adipocyte cell membrane, releasing intracellular content, and initiating triglycerides absorption. The cumulative goals of these treatments are ultimately in tissue volume reduction and contour change for the treated body part (see **Fig. 4**).[6,7]

RF DEVICES

A common mechanism of action for tissue restructuring and body-shaping technologies is through heat generated by tissue impendence to the RF current, resulting in the denaturation of the tissue components and subsequently soft tissue matrix remodeling.[2,7–9] The depth of energy delivered by an RF device depends on several factors, including the configuration of electrodes (monopolar vs bipolar), the conduction medium (type of tissue), parameters, and the frequency of the electrical current applied.[8] The gradient of energy delivered by RF devices is shaped by the position of electrodes. The first device to use monopolar RF for skin tissue tightening was the ThermaCool system (Thermage Inc, Haywood, California). ThermaCool operated in the 6-MHz RF range.[2,7,8] The activation of RF (fixed number of firing in a defined time) produces heat and the homogenous zone of coagulation at the depth depending on RF penetration depending on tip design (see **Fig. 1**b). Heating of the dermal layer causes collagen restructuring; as the healing progresses, the contraction of the collagenous scaffold results in skin firming (**Fig. 5**).

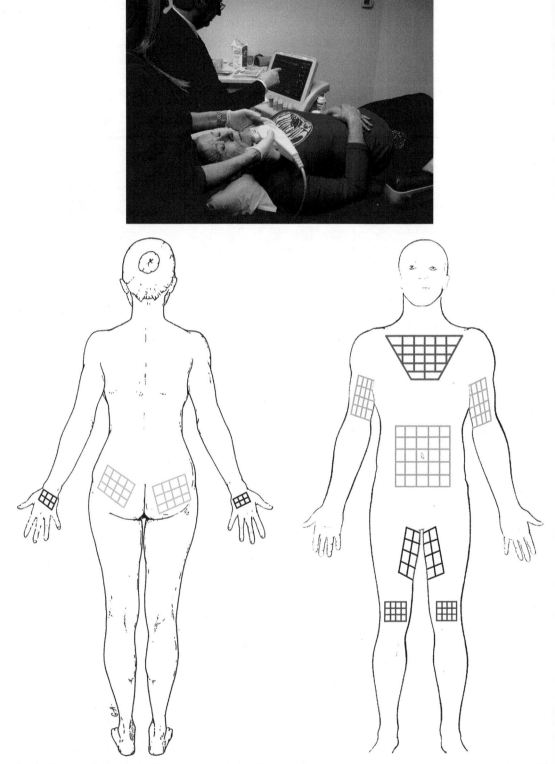

Fig. 2. Focused tissue coagulation is generated with precision of prescribed plane of treatment and healthy intervening tissue between zones of thermal coagulation. Grids and markings of lines of treatments help in positioning of energy delivery (*arrow*).

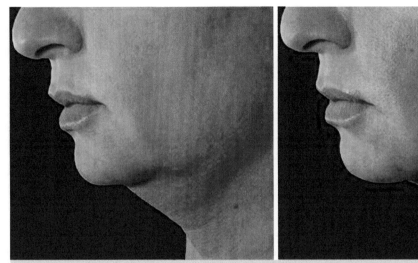

Single treatment – dual plane lower face and neck
Improved jawline definition

Fig. 3. Dual plane (dermis at the level 3 mm) and platysma or SMAS (at the level 4.5 mm) were subjected to focused ultrasound. For enhanced result, treatments are repeated 2 or 3 times in 2-month intervals. (*Courtesy of* Ulthera, Inc, Mesa, Arizona; with permission.)

CRYOLIPOLYSIS

Cryolipolysis energy systems (eg, Lipofreeze, Zeltiq, Pleasanton, California) expose soft tissues to external thermal devices in an attempt to lower temperatures to achieve selective tissue apoptosis. Body contouring by cryolipolysis relies on lowering the temperature of the skin and the underlying subcutaneous fat to the point whereby the lipids within the adipose tissue begin to crystalize

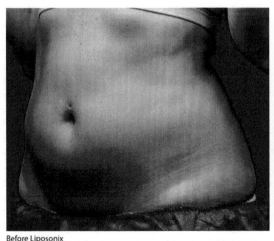
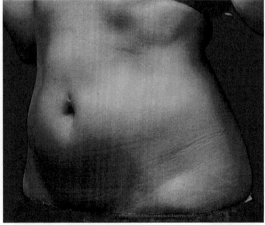

Before Liposonix

8 Weeks Post Treatment
5.0 cm reduction

Photographs courtesy of Solta Medical Aesthetic Center

Fig. 4. HIFUS seems to be particularly effective in nonobese patients with good skin quality. In patients with good skin quality, skin retraction follows thermal ablation of subcutaneous fat producing pleasing aesthetic outcomes. (*Courtesy of* Solta Medical, Inc, Hayward, California; with permission; *Data from* Jewell M, Baxter RA, Cox SE, et al. Randomized sham controlled trial to evaluate the safety and effectiveness of a high intensity focused ultrasound for noninvasive body sculpting. Plast Reconstr Surg 2011;128(1):253–62; and Mulholland RS, Paul MD, Chalfoun C. Noninvasive body contouring with radiofrequency, ultrasound, cryolipolysis, and low-level laser therapy. Clin Plast Surg 2011;38(3):503–20.)

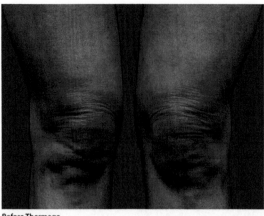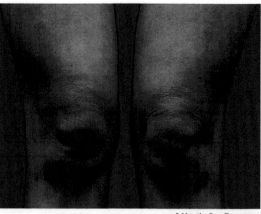

Before Thermage   2 Months Post Treatment

Photographs courtesy of Solta Medical Aesthetic Center

Fig. 5. Nonsurgical skin tightening secondary to radiofrequency treatment (Thermage). Recent modifications of Thermage technologies allow deeper penetration of RF, treatment of deep dermal layers inducing denaturation, and subsequent contraction of the tissue. (*Courtesy of* Solta Medical, Inc, Hayward, California; with permission; *Data from* Hodgkinson DJ. Clinical applications of radiofrequency: nonsurgical skin tightening (Thermage). Clin Plast Surg 2009;36(2):261–8.)

while remaining warm enough to prevent permanent damage to the overlying dermis. This temporary lowering of the surface temperature to approximately −3°C to 6°C does not cause permanent damage to the skin but triggers apoptosis of the adipose tissue and gradual resorption (over the period of weeks) of injured cell contents and lipid remnants, ultimately resulting in the desired loss of volume and skin retraction (**Figs. 6** and **7**). In cryolipolysis, the temperature lowers from the surface (there is no reversed gradient of temperature changes like in MFUS treatments) and the effect depends on the depth of freezing and

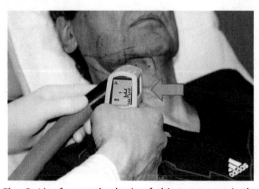

Fig. 6. Lipofreeze: the basis of this treatment is the notion that exposure to specific low temperatures (cold air delivered via hose behind the infrared thermometer) will selectively damage subcutaneous adipose tissue while leaving the skin undamaged. After the targeted freezing of the fat cells, apoptosis and gradual fat resorption begins resulting in a fat layer or deposit volume decrease and body recontouring. Blanching indicated by the arrow.

the different susceptibility of different tissues to freezing.[7,10]

LASER-ASSISTED CONTOURING

Low-level laser therapy (eg, Zerona, Erchonia Medical, McKinney, Texas) has been shown to cause adipocyte content leakage when exposed to laser energy at 635 nm. Research continues to establish the most efficacious specific laser wavelength for this phenomenon. The lasers at this wavelength are thought to stimulate mitochondria to form transitory pores in the bilipid membrane of adipose cells. The pores then allow the cell contents (triglycerides and fatty acids) to leak into the interstitial space. Research has suggested that this is not damaging to the cell but allows for escape of the cell content and assists in the ease in which liposuction might be performed.[7,11,12] There are questions about whether laser-assisted lipolysis alone is sufficient for significant volume reduction. However, technologies that combine laser-assisted liposuction (using laser energy at 1064/1320 nm) may additionally demonstrate a selective capability to induce changes in dermal collagen scaffold and subsequently in dermal tightening, which may be a more promising approach.[11,12] A detailed discussion of laser-assisted tissue sculpting with 1440-nm wavelength devices is presented in another article of this issue.

Indications for Specific Therapeutic Options

As with any procedure, patient selection is key. To ensure reasonable expectations, proper selection

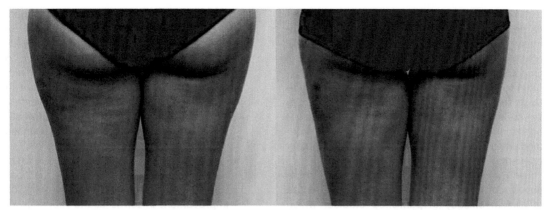

Fig. 7. Before and after Lipofreeze treatments. Repeated treatments resulted in lateral hips tissue firming and reduction of saddlebag fat deposits. (*Courtesy of* Dr Simon Ourian.)

requires explaining to patients that results from noninvasive energy-based procedures will be less dramatic than with invasive methods of rejuvenation (see **Table 1**). Additionally, currently available tissue-tightening devices are not suited for patients with significant loss of tissue tone, with severe laxity, or with structural ptosis (frequently observed in patients with a history of a massive body weight loss). Therefore, unrealistic expectations are obviously a key contraindication for the application of all types of tissue-restructuring modalities. Other considerations involve the treatment of patients with existing medical conditions, which should be handled based on the patients' medical history, what is written of the subject in the medical literature, the practitioner's own clinical experience, and any other clinical information that may be available from the device company. An example of this is the treatment of patients with active inflammatory skin lesions (eg, acne). Such patients should not have affected areas treated with energy-based devices because the energy may lead to the exacerbation of existing problems (**Fig. 8**).

CLINICAL OUTCOMES

Clinical outcomes following noninvasive procedures with energy-based devices tend to be much more subtle than those following surgical procedures. As with any type of procedure, energy-based technologies do not offer guarantees of clinical efficacy, and outcomes will vary between patients depending on factors, such as age, gender, skin type, genetics, and lifestyle. Also, outcomes often vary between devices within each category, and clinical data for certain technologies can be sparse depending on the regulatory requirements. This situation can lead to uncertainty

as to the clinical efficacy and safety of some techniques and devices within each category, especially the "me too"–type devices, which may rely on the clinical data of predecessor technologies for market acceptance and FDA approval. In such cases, clinical experience reports in the medical literature may serve to elucidate the utility of any devices in question.

Some newer modifications of RF- or US-based devices include programs allowing multiple-pass

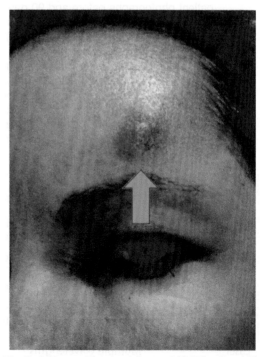

Fig. 8. Patient with preexisting to MFUS forehead lift acne lesion developed eruption of cellulitis around the acne pustule, which subsided with days of topical and oral antibiotics treatments.

techniques for greater efficacy of applied energy.[2] As new energy-based surgical tools proliferated, many of them were modified to enhance their efficacy and additional performance-improving modalities were added (eg, surface cooling capability) to allow more energy to be delivered to the target tissues without safety concerns (eg, burning the superficial tissues). For example, many skin-tightening devices can work in tandem with other modalities in an effort to produce a complementary or even synergistic approach (**Table 2**).

Each of the energy-based technologies mentioned has been shown to produce some degree of clinical efficacy in published studies, which resulted in the FDA approval for at least one device in each category. Notable are the clinical outcomes as defined by the pivotal US studies for the first-in-class devices for each category.

- US
  - MFUS: In a rater-blinded prospective cohort study (n = 35), patients were evaluated after receiving MFUS (Ultherapy, Ulthera Inc, Mesa, Arizona) treatment on the forehead, temples, cheeks, submental region, and the side of the neck using probes targeting tissue at depths of 4.5 mm (both 4 MHz and 7 MHz) and 3.0 mm (7 MHz). Masked assessment of patient photographs before and 90 days after treatment showed clinically significant lifting of the brow (P = .00001), with a mean lift of 1.7 mm.[3,4,13,14]
  - HIFUS: In a multicenter, randomized, sham-controlled, single-blind study, adults with at least a 2.5-cm thick layer of subcutaneous fat were randomized to receive HIFUS treatment (Liposonix, Solta, Hayward, California) of the abdomen

and flanks. Patients received treatment that consisted of 3 passes at 47 J/cm, 59 J/cm, or 0 J/cm (sham control). At week 12, change versus sham was shown to be significant for patients treated with 59-J/cm (-2.44; P = .01) but not with 47 J/cm (-2.06 cm; P = .13). Improvement over sham was also marked by investigator assessment by global aesthetic improvement and patient satisfaction.[6]

- RF: A reduction of facial skin surface in up to a 20% range, compared with the non-treated area and surface characteristics improvement in terms of the reduction of wrinkling, was noted using RF technology.[2] However, a study comparing monopolar RF (Thermage TC-3 System, Solta Medical, Hayward, California) and MFUS, using a split-face brow lift model, revealed no statistically different efficacy between devices.[15] Clinically, cooling systems minimizing patient discomfort are an advantage of modern RF systems. RF systems are contraindicated in patients with a pacemaker, defibrillator, or other implanted electronic devices that could be deprogrammed by RF.[9]

- Cryolipolysis energy devices: Despite the encouraging observations regarding cryolipolysis for body contouring, there are no published long-term safety and efficacy data on humans available in the medical literature to date. One device company has data on file that claims interim data from a multicenter, prospective, non-randomized, bilateral study of 32 patients using cryolipolysis for subcutaneous fat reduction.[16] In this study, patients were given a single treatment on one flank with

Table 2
Examples of commercially available hybrid energy-based skin-tightening devices

Technology	Basic Modality	Performance Modifying Modality	Commercial Example
High-frequency RF	RF	Combination of unipolar and bipolar technology	Accent XL
RF	RF	Continuous cooling of the skin	Exilis
RF	Bipolar RF	Simultaneous vacuum suction	Reaction
RF	Bipolar RF	Infrared light, vacuum, mechanical massage	VelaShape II
Laser	Multiple wavelengths 1064, 1320, 1440 nm	Blend of multiple wavelengths allows simultaneous skin tightening and fat reduction	Smartlipo Triplex

a prototype cryolipolysis device (Zeltiq, Pleasanton, California). It is reported that patients were assessed 4 months following treatment, and 27 out of 32 (84%) showed visible improvement in the treated area, with a mean reduction in the subcutaneous fat (as measured by US) of 22.4%.

- Laser-assisted contouring: A double-blind, randomized, placebo-controlled trial of 67 patients was performed to evaluate the application of a 635-nm low-level laser for use as a noninvasive body-contouring treatment on the waist, hips, and thighs.[17] Study patients received either a low-level laser treatment or a sham treatment 3 times per week for 2 weeks. After 2 weeks, the treatment group saw 62.9% of patients with a circumference reduction of 3.0 in or greater over all body parts, whereas only 6.4% of the sham group showed a reduction of 3.0 in or greater. The mean reduction in circumference at the end of the treatments (week 2) was 3.52 in for the treatment group and 0.62 in for the sham group. However, 2 weeks after the final treatment, the mean circumference for the treatment group increased 0.31 in.

Other technologies using a 900-nm and 1064-nm range also seem efficient in disrupting fat, thus triggering fat deposits resorption. A combination of 1064 nm and 1320 nm seems to be useful for selective fat cell disruption, water vaporization, and demonstrated tissue-tightening potential at the same time.[12,18] Outcomes of clinically promising 1440-nm technology are presented in another article of this issue.

Overall, representative results of focused US, RF, and cryosculpting demonstrate very encouraging overall results (see **Figs. 3–5** and **7**). Further assessment of cryolipolysis and laser-assisted contouring must be made before any true effectiveness can be determined.

COMPLICATIONS AND CONCERNS WITH NONINVASIVE PROCEDURES

With any medical procedure, there is some degree of risk of adverse effects, and there is no exception with noninvasive procedures. Thermally (heat or cold) induced lipolysis raises a concern regarding the release of triglycerides into the lymph and blood. The relatively slow lipolysis process of these technologies probably explains that post-procedure spikes are not significant enough to pose a risk to the general health of patients.[6] In general, both the HIFUS and cryolipolysis

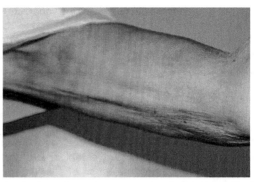

Fig. 9. Some loss of pigmentation (medial arm skin) and linear subcutaneous arm fat atrophy noted in a patient previously treated with RF.

procedures are safe, with no serious adverse effects registered. With many of the energy-based technologies, patients occasionally report transient edema, bruises, and skin erythema.[1,2,8] Arnica topically and orally should facilitate to resolve edema and bruises. Topical and systemic antibiotics may be indicated in case of activation of inflammatory skin conditions (see **Fig. 8**). A short course of steroids, such as oral prednisone, should be reserved for cases with more significant edema with or without signs of nerve impairment (eg, in situations when patients develop asymmetrical animation and presumably some transient neuritis) following RF, HIFUS, or MFUS. However, it should be noted that chronic use of antiinflammatory drugs may impair the efficacy of skin-tightening devices that exploit the body's immune/inflammatory pathways. Linear dyschromia (in the form of hyperpigmentation or hypopigmentation), which is seen rarely and probably in conjunction with the use of more superficially acting RF or US modalities (at the level of papillary dermis), should be protected from ultraviolet by sunblock when outdoors and treated with topical bleaching agents in case of persisting hyperpigmentation.[2,13,14] Skin surface depressions secondary to nonuniform 2- and 3-dimensional recontouring was occasionally observed with monopolar RF devices (**Fig. 9**).[19] These late effects of monopolar RF treatments may resolve spontaneously (or with massage). Scarring of the dermis or fibrous septa of between lobules of subcutaneous fat may require surgical subcision, fat, or synthetic filler administration for contour augmentation.

SUMMARY

Few would dispute that the introduction of energy-based devices to aesthetic surgery and medicine has not been successful. However, the variability in tissue response in terms of restructuring by energy-based devices is rooted in the individual differences in chemical and physical properties, such as tissue stiffness, fat architecture, water content, heat absorption, and many other factors, and may sometimes impact consistency.[11,18,20–22] Although some physically different modalities (eg, use of heat for lipolysis vs use of cool) seem to produce a similar clinical effect, there is no doubt that continued research will establish evidence assisting in the optimal selection of safe energy-based tools that address specific patient objectives for the best possible result.

REFERENCES

1. Alexiades-Armenakas M, Rosenberg D, Renton B, et al. Blinded, randomized, quantitative grading comparison of minimally invasive, fractional radiofrequency and surgical face-lift to treat skin laxity. Arch Dermatol 2010;146(4):396–405.
2. Hodgkinson DJ. Clinical applications of radiofrequency: nonsurgical skin tightening (Thermage). Clin Plast Surg 2009;36(2):261–8.
3. Newman J, Alam M. Ultrasound for fat reduction and body contouring. In: Alam M, Dover JS, editors. Non-surgical skin tightening and lifting. London: Sounders Elsevier; 2009. p. 148–64.
4. Gliklich RE, White WM, Slayton MH, et al. Clinical pilot study of intense ultrasound therapy to deep dermal facial skin and subcutaneous tissues. Arch Facial Plast Surg 2007;9(2):88–95.
5. Brenin DR. Focused ultrasound ablation for the treatment of breast cancer. Ann Surg Oncol 2011;18(11):3088–94.
6. Jewell M, Baxter RA, Cox SE, et al. Randomized sham controlled trial to evaluate the safety and effectiveness of a high intensity focused ultrasound for noninvasive body sculpting. Plast Reconstr Surg 2011;128(1):253–62.
7. Mulholland RS, Paul MD, Chalfoun C. Noninvasive body contouring with radiofrequency, ultrasound, cryolipolysis, and low-level laser therapy. Clin Plast Surg 2011;38(3):503–20.
8. Bogle M. Radiofrequency energy and hybrid devices. In: Alam M, Dover JS, editors. Non-surgical tightening and lifting. London: Saunders Elsevier; 2009. p. 21–32.
9. Polder KD, Bruce S. Radiofrequency: Thermage. Facial Plast Surg Clin North Am 2011;19(2):347–59.
10. Melville NA. Cooling off. Non invasive lipolysis device takes a chilling approach to apoptosis. Cosmet Surg Times 2009;12(6):24–5.
11. DiBernardo B, Reyes J. Evaluation of skin tightening after laser-assisted liposuction. Aesthet Surg J 2009;29(5):400–8.
12. Fakhouri TM, Kader El Tal A, Abrou A, et al. Laser-assisted lipolysis. A review. Dermatol Surg 2012;38(2):155–69.
13. Alam M, Dover JS. Ultrasound tightening of facial and neck skin. In: Alam M, Dover JS, editors. Non-surgical tightening and lifting. London: Saunders Elsevier; 2009. p. 33–9.
14. Alam M. Ultrasound tightening of facial and neck skin: a rater-blinded prospective cohort study. J Am Acad Dermatol 2010;62(2):262–9.
15. Zelickson B. Comparison treatment for laxity with monopolar radiofrequency and focused ultrasound [abstract]. Kissimmee (FL): American Society for Laser in Medicine and Surgery; 2012.
16. Zeltiq, in Data on File.
17. Jackson RF. Low-level laser therapy as a noninvasive approach for body contouring: a randomized, controlled study. Lasers Surg Med 2009;41(10):799–809.
18. Kenkel JM. Commentary. Aesthet Surg J 2009;29(5):407–8.
19. Dawson E, Willey A, Lee K. Adverse events associated with nonablative cutaneous laser, radiofrequency, and light-based devices. Semin Cutan Med Surg 2007;26(1):15–21.
20. Christ C, Brenke R, Sattler G, et al. Improvement in skin elasticity in the treatment of cellulite and connective tissue weakness by means of extracorporeal pulse activation therapy. Aesthet Surg J 2008;28(5):538–44.
21. Dobke MK, DiBernardo B, Thompson R, et al. Assessment of biomechanical skin properties: is cellulitic skin different? Aesthet Surg J 2002;22(3):260–6.
22. Nahm WK, Su TT, Rotunda A, et al. Objective changes in brow position, superior palpebral crease, peak angle of the eyebrow, and jowl surface area after volumetric radiofrequency treatments to half of the face. Dermatol Surg 2004;30(6):922–8.

Early Clinical Experience with the 1440-nm Wavelength Internal Pulsed Laser in Facial Rejuvenation: Two-Year Follow-up

Gordon H. Sasaki, MD

KEYWORDS

- Internal pulsed laser • Facial rejuvenation • Body rejuvenation • Collagen • Lipolysis
- Noninvasive cosmetic surgery

KEY POINTS

- Use of the 1440-nm wavelength has been shown to significantly increase skin thickness and elasticity 6 to 18 months from baseline measurements in the lower third of face and neck.
- The procedure was not recommended for correction of strong and separated bands of the platysma muscle.
- The 1440-nm wavelength produced the highest fat and dermal tissue ablation efficiency, with minimal localization of heat over depth.

INTRODUCTION

The recent adoption of the internal 1440-nm pulsed laser has advanced the safety, efficacy, and versatility of laser lipolysis and tissue tightening in face and body rejuvenation.[1–6] The longer wavelength provides increased localized photothermal and vaporizing effects in front of the fiber on fatty tissue and collagen fibers (water), achieving 20 times more absorption in adipose tissue than the 1064-nm/1320-nm and 40 times more absorption than 924-nm/980-nm wavelengths.[7–11] In recent clinical studies,[4,6] use of the 1440-nm wavelength has been shown to significantly increase skin thickness and elasticity 6 to 18 months from baseline measurements. This article reports the early experience with the 1440-nm wavelength, using a specially designed side-firing fiber in a four-step approach primarily to the lower third of the midface and neck.

LASER DEVICE SYSTEM

The laser workstation delivered the 1440-nm wavelength pulsed laser from a 800-μm side-firing fiber that was enclosed and protruded 2 mm from the tip of a temperature-sensing 1.2-mm cannula. The side-firing fiber distributed about half of its energy perpendicular to the fiber axis and the other half transmitted along the fiber axis (**Fig. 1**). Chevron markings on the handpiece designated the direction of the laser emission perpendicular to the fiber axis. This emission design permitted a more targeted delivery of laser energy to the structures of interest, which included in turn fat, fibrofascial layer of the muscle, and the skin-dermis. During treatment of the fatty tissue and deeper fibrofascial muscle layer, the temperature-sensing cannula acted as a thermal switch by sensing temperatures set between 45°C and 47°C at the immediate laser-delivery point. When the recommended target

Conflict of interest statement: Dr Sasaki is a researcher and training consultant for Cynosure, Inc (the manufacturer of the device discussed in this article). Dr Sasaki received limited funding under an unrestricted research grant for the study. No financial support was provided for the writing of this article.
Loma Linda Medical University Center, Private Practice: 800 S. Fairmount Ave, Ste 319, Pasadena, CA 91105, USA
E-mail address: jgallegos@drsasaki.com

Clin Plastic Surg 39 (2012) 409–417
http://dx.doi.org/10.1016/j.cps.2012.07.009

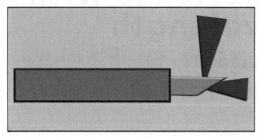

Fig. 1. The side-firing 800-μ fiber delivers about half of its laser energy in the forward direction to the fiber axis and the remainder moves perpendicular to the fiber axis.

temperature was attained, an audible signal was triggered. If the surrounding tissue temperatures exceeded the preset threshold level, a beeping audible signal warned the operator to move to another area to reduce excessive thermal injury. Maintenance of this thermal window distributed laser heat energy evenly to melt fatty tissue and denature collagen in a safe manner. When the laser fiber treated shallow subdermal tissue (5 mm below the dermis), the temperature-sensing cannula was programmed at the same 45°C to 47°C temperature range, which in turn produced a superficial skin temperature between 38°C and 42°C, which was optimal for collagen denaturation and later delayed tissue tightening. An infrared thermal camera (Therma View EHS, FLIR Systems Inc., Niceville, FL) obtained continuous skin temperatures between 38°C and 42°C and ensured a uniform, real-time deliverance of heat by depiction of a confluent orange-red coloration within each treatment site. A hand-held infrared noncontact thermometer (MiniTemp MT6; Raytek Corporation, Santa Cruz, CA) was used simultaneously with the thermal camera to measure rapidly surface skin temperatures by spot-checking to ensure skin safety.

CLINICAL PROTOCOL

Patients were selected for isolated mild to moderate accumulations of fat to the lower third of the face and neck and mild to moderate tissue laxity of the muscle and skin. After review of their medical history, subjects were consented for their office procedure and the usage of local anesthesia. A preoperative physical examination, blood chemistry panels, and electrocardiogram were required from each patient within 2 days of surgery. Before surgery, patients were weighed, photographed by standardized digital imaging, and prescribed a pain medication and antibiotic. In four randomized patients, skin thickness was measured at the same spot three times with a 20-MHz high-frequency ultrasound probe (DermaScan C, Cortex Technology, Hadsund, Denmark) at baseline and 6

months. In one patient, biopsies from opposing sides of the treated neck below the ear lobule were submitted for hematoxylin and eosin staining for assessment of tissues at completion of procedure.

The procedure was not recommended for correction of strong and separated bands of the platysma muscle. Exclusion criteria included pregnancy, uncontrolled diabetes mellitus, collagen disorders, significant cardiovascular diseases, bleeding disorders, smokers, and previous surgical procedures within a year to treatment sites. Aesthetic treatment efficacy from baseline to 6 months was rated by two independent investigators using the Investigator Global Aesthetic Improvement Scale from standardized photographs (0 = no change, 1 = mild improvement, 2 = moderate improvement, and 3 = significant improvement). Patients used a Subject Global Aesthetic Improvement Scale from their baseline to 6 months photographs (0 = no change, 1 = mild improvement, 2 = moderate improvement, and 3 = significant improvement).

PROCEDURE

The procedure was as follows:

- In the sitting position, the patient's treatment sites were marked with one 3 × 5 cm sector lateral to each marionette line and two 5 × 5 cm sectors on each side of the midline of the neck (**Fig. 2**).
- Subjects received an oral sedative 30 minutes before surgery.
- After skin preparation with povidine-iodine antiseptic washes, a 1-cm incision was made behind each ear lobe and also at the transverse submental crease line.
- Twenty to thirty milliliters of tumescent anesthesia mixture (50 mL of 0.5% lidocaine, 1 mg epinephrine per liter of warm saline, and 20 mL of 8.4% sodium bicarbonate) was infused into each sector through the access incisions at the deep and superficial levels of subcutaneous fat.
- After 20 to 30 minutes, the 800-μm side-firing fiber, enclosed in its temperature sensing cannula, was inserted through one of the three access incisions.
- All procedures were performed awake with oximetry and electrocardiogram monitoring without need for external oxygen administration.
- The red-aiming beam from a diode 630-nm laser source visualized the tip of the fiber during the three steps involving the laser with the fiber tip either in the down or up direction. The intensity and distribution of

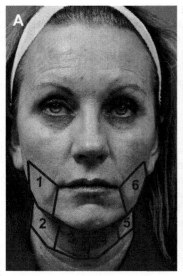
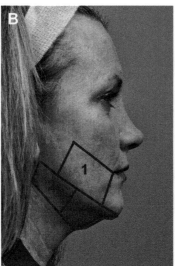
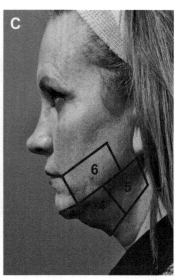

Fig. 2. (A–C) Presurgical markings of the six sectors are outlined with the patient in the sitting position. Sectors 1 and 6 were rectangles (3 × 5 cm) in each lower third of face; sectors 2, 3, 4, and 5 were squares (5 × 5 cm) in the neck.

the red-aiming beam during lasering in a darkened or dimmed room guided the surgeon to position optimally the laser's energy and direction to the mid-level of fat, over the platysma muscle and under the skin-dermis.

Standard laser guidelines, as outlined by the American National Standard for the Safe Use of Lasers in Health Care Facilities, included the use of protective goggles for the patient and staff during phases of laser treatments.

In the first step, the fiber was inserted through one of the access incisions in the down position (**Fig. 3**). Once in place, the activated cannula-

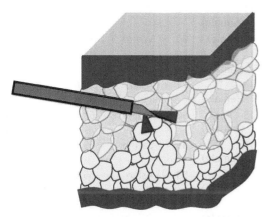

Fig. 3. In the first laser treatment step, the 800-μ side-firing fiber is positioned about 1 cm below the dermis in the down position on activation. Laser energy is released in a forward and down direction to melt excess subcutaneous fat. (*Courtesy of* Margaret Gaston.)

fiber was moved back and forth in a fanlike pattern in the mid-to-deep levels of the subcutaneous fat in each sector. Two sectors on one-half of the neck were treated at a time to optimize laser delivery. The power and pulse frequency settings were set between 6 and 10 W and 25 H, respectively. The endpoints of treatment were determined when the total number of joules delivered ranged between 500 and 700 J/sector, and limited or no tissue resistance to the fiber's passes while the temperature-sensitive cannula maintained a 45°C to 47°C threshold. External skin temperature monitoring was performed with the thermal infrared imaging camera and the hand-held infrared noncontact thermometer.

In the second step, liposuction with a 1.2-mm round two-hole cannula to the lower third of the face and with a 3.2-mm two-hole flat cannula to the neck evacuated the liquefied fat, tumescent solution, and tissue debris under a low vacuum pressure of 350 to 500 mm Hg in the six sectors. Liposuction permitted immediate contour assessment and created an environment with less debris that facilitated more rapid elevation of threshold subdermal temperatures during the subsequent shallow lasering.

In the third step, the activated fiber-cannula was inserted in the down direction (**Fig. 4**), reciprocated in a fanlike motion, and deposited a total of 200 to 300 J on the fibrofascial surface of the platysma muscle in each sector. It was anticipated that the denatured collagen fibers would eventually reorganize and tightened the muscle unit.

In the fourth step, the activated fiber-cannula was turned in the up direction (**Fig. 5**), moved in a

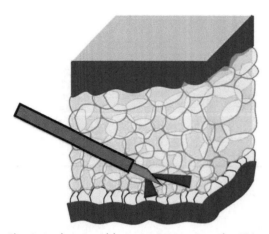

Fig. 4. In the second laser treatment step, the 800-μ side-firing fiber is positioned above the fibrofascial layer of the platysma muscle. On firing, the laser energy is emitted in a down and forward direction to stimulate thermal collagen thickening and tightening of the fascia by remodeling. (*Courtesy of* Margaret Gaston.)

fan-shaped pattern, and delivered about 300 J at 2 to 5 mm below the dermis in each sector. The endpoint of treatment was determined when a total of 200 to 300 J was administered per sector. Cold compresses were applied immediately to hot spots, designated by the infrared thermal camera, to return temperatures to the desired levels.

When laser treatment was completed, the liquefied fat and debris was removed by gentle rolling through the incision sites. Quarter-inch Penrose

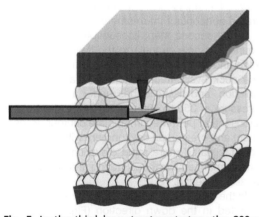

Fig. 5. In the third laser treatment step, the 800-μ side-firing fiber is positioned less than 5 mm below and parallel to the dermis. On activation, its laser energy is released in a forward direction in the subdermal fat and also upward to the undersurface of the reticular dermis to stimulate dermal thickness and tightening by collagen stimulation and remodeling. (*Courtesy of* Margaret Gaston.)

drains were inserted in each postlobule incision site to facilitate further drainage and removed within 24 hours. Compression garments with sponge inserts were applied for 7 to 10 days, after which a series of weekly external ultrasound treatments were given to reduce irregularities and swelling.

RESULTS

Between September 2010 and March 2012, 19 consecutive patients (2 men, 17 women; 41–74 years old, mean age 51.1 years) were indicated for laser lipolysis and tissue lifting for facial rejuvenation (**Table 1**). The mean pretreatment weight was 72 kg (range, 46.6–103.6 kg) with a mean

Table 1
Demographic data of gender, age, ethnicity, weight, and body mass index in 19 patients enrolled in 6-month study

Patient No. (Gender)	Age	Ethnicity	Weight (kg)	Body Mass Index
1 (female)	46	White	73	26.8
2 (female)	56	White	82.1	26
3 (female)	50	Latina	70.3	25.8
4 (male)	65	Asian	87.1	31.9
5 (female)	50	Asian	84.4	32.9
6 (female)	41	Latina	79.9	30.8
7 (female)	53	White	103.6	36.9
8 (female)	74	White	46.6	20.5
9 (female)	60	White	53.5	22.3
10 (female)	42	Latina	80.7	32.6
11 (female)	42	White	88.5	36.8
12 (male)	60	White	95.3	31
13 (female)	48	Asian	54.4	21.2
14 (female)	71	Asian	57.6	24
15 (female)	50	Latina	63	25.4
16 (female)	43	Latina	69.4	28
17 (female)	53	Asian	65.8	23.4
18 (female)	42	Latina	51.3	21.3
19 (female)	43	Latina	61.7	22.6
Mean	51.1		72	27.4

body mass index of 27.4 (range, 20.5–36.9). At the third and sixth month evaluation periods, each patient demonstrated no significant change from baseline weight and body mass index.

An average of 200 mL of tumescent solution (range, 125–280) was infiltrated into the deep and superficial subcutaneous layers within the lower third of face and entire neck. Within the mid-to-deep subcutaneous fat in each sector, the delivered energy ranged from 6 to 10 W at 25 Hz, averaging 695 J/sector (range, 500–700 J/sector). The endpoints of treatment were determined when (1) the average number of joules occurred between 500 and 700 J/sector, (2) the internal temperature consistently obtained varied between 45°C and 47°C, and (3) there was increased ease of passing the firing laser fiber through the tissues (**Fig. 6**).

Depending on preoperative findings, liposuction removed between 50 and 125 mL aspirate, of which about 55%/volume consisted of fat. Heating of the fibrofascial layer of the platysma muscle (**Fig. 7**) averaged about 275 J/sector (range, 200–300 J/sector). Shallow subdermal heating distributed an average of 285 J/sector (range, 250–400 J/sector) at 1 to 5 mm below the dermis. The endpoint of treatment was determined when the total amount of 300 J/sector was delivered and the fiber-cannula passed with minimal resistance.

The achievement of surface temperature skin recordings between 36°C and 42°C is regarded as a secondary endpoint to prevent over-delivery of joules and heat (**Fig. 8**). The total average joules delivered per patient was about 7380 J, which translated to about 1230 J/sector. In patients with moderate skin laxity, the skin was retreated

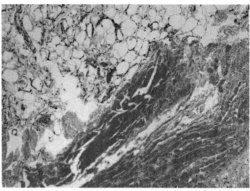

Fig. 7. Moderate coagulation necrosis of fibrofascial layer of the lateral platysma muscle after immediate exposure to the 1440-nm wavelength (8 W, 25 Hz, 250 J at 45°C–47°C) at the completion of the procedure (hematoxylin-eosin, original magnification ×10).

with additional lasing, averaging 150 J/sector, to temperatures between 38°C and 42°C for possible increased tissue tightening based on clinical findings. The surgical time averaged about 1 hour (range, 45–75 minutes) with immediate postoperative recovery time less than 1 hour. Compression garments were continued to another 7 to 10 days to reduce any incidence of exudative or seromatous collections.

In four patients who were randomly selected for DermaScan C measurements, all demonstrated an average of 23% increase in skin thickness compared with baseline at 6 months (**Table 2**). Mean increases were significant (P<.01) at each time point. The ultrasonic images of the dermis at baseline changed to a thicker, more compact dermis at

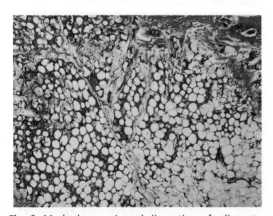

Fig. 6. Marked necrosis and disruption of adipocytes in the subcutaneous fat of the lateral neck were observed down to 10 to 20 mm below dermal-fat junction after immediate exposure to 1440-nm wavelength (8 W, 25 Hz, 700 J at 45°C–47°C) at the completion of the procedure (hematoxylin-eosin, original magnification ×10).

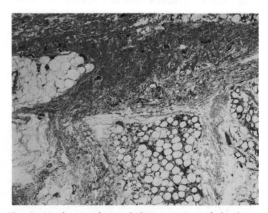

Fig. 8. Moderate thermal denaturation of the lower level of the reticular dermis and collagen fibers within septae at 1 to 3 mm below dermal-fat junction of the lateral neck after immediate exposure to the 1440-nm wavelength (8 W, 25 Hz, 275 J at 45°C–47°C) at the completion of the procedure (hematoxylin-eosin, original magnification ×10).

Table 2
Mean percentage increases in neck skin thickness from baseline during 6-month study period in four patients

Patient	Pretreated	Treated	Increase of Thickness	Percentage of Change
1	0.42 mm	1.88 mm	2.3 mm	22%
2	0.16 mm	1.25 mm	1.41 mm	13%
3	0.40 mm	1.28 mm	1.68 mm	31%
4	0.36 mm	1.46 mm	1.82 mm	25%
Average	0.34 mm	1.47 mm	1.80 mm	23%

6 months, indicating possible enhancement of collagen deposition within the dermis after treatment (**Fig. 9**).

OUTCOMES AND SIDE EFFECTS

Patients were very satisfied with their changes at 6 months, especially in the definition of their mandibular-neck outlines with reduction of the prejowls, marionette folds, and submental fullness (**Figs. 10** and **11**). The incidence of bruising and swelling was low and resolved completely within 2 weeks. No patients developed hematomas, sensory or motor nerve injuries, striations, blisters, or dyschromias after three layers of laser treatment. Three patients developed small fibrous nodules within the subcutaneous fat in the neck that resolved within 6 weeks with postoperative ultrasound treatments. Postoperative discomfort was mild to moderate with patients using analgesic products, such as extra strength acetaminophen or lowest doses of hydrocodone/acetaminophen. Most patients were able to resume normal activities within 2 weeks. There were no unanticipated significant adverse events. Patients experienced about an 80% improvement by 6 months with progressive tissue lifting and contouring thereafter.

Patients and two independent investigators were asked to evaluate global satisfaction results at 3 and 6 months after treatments in the 19 patients on a five-point scale (0 = worse, 1 = no change, 2 = mild, 3 = moderate, and 4 = excellent).

The mean scores at 3 months were 2.75 and 3, respectively, with improvements in contour, fat reduction, and tissue laxity. The mean scores at 6 months were 3 and 3.5, respectively, with continued progressive tissue tightening, contouring, and

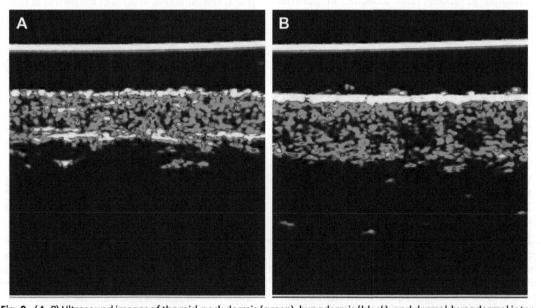

Fig. 9. (*A, B*) Ultrasound images of the mid-neck dermis (*green*), hypodermis (*black*), and dermal-hypodermal interface showing thinner (mean, 0.36 mm) and less compact dermis at baseline (*A*) and 25% thicker (mean, 1.46 mm) and more compact dermis 6 months after treatment (*B*) of patient 4, as listed in **Table 2** and shown in **Fig. 11**.

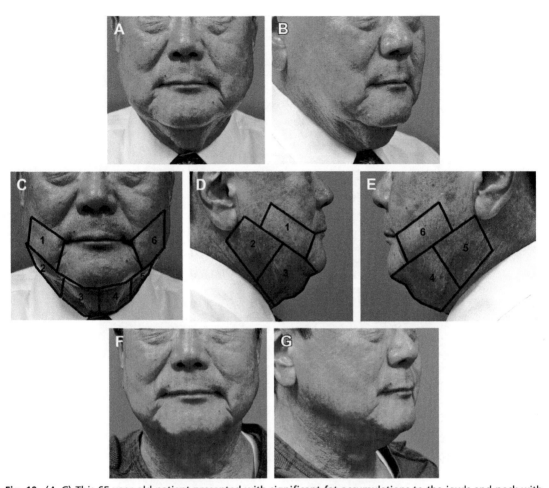

Fig. 10. (A–G) This 65-year-old patient presented with significant fat accumulations to the jowls and neck with marked tissue laxity. Preoperative markings delineate the sectors to be treated (moderate-deep fat, 700 J/sector; superficial musculoaponeurotic system, 350 J/sector; subdermal layer, 280/sector with skin temperature 38°C–39°C; 175 cc lipoaspirate).

definition. All patients would recommend the procedure to others.

DISCUSSION

As demonstrated previously with laser treatments in the 1064- and 1320-nm wavelengths,[12] laser-assisted lipolysis and tissue lifting for facial and neck rejuvenation can be done safely and efficiently using the advantages of the 1440-nm wavelength to produce selective fat destruction and to shorten collagen fibers by denaturation in the fibrofascial layer of the platysma muscle and dermal structures for eventual lifting. Monte Carlo simulation study[9] with three different wavelengths (1064-, 1320-, and 1440-nm) demonstrated that the 1440-nm wavelength produced the highest fat and dermal tissue ablation efficiency, with minimal localization of heat over depth compared with the other two wavelengths. In a randomized, controlled study on the lower half of the abdomen,[5] acute histologic findings with the 1440-nm wavelength energy (1000 J, 55°C) in the deep subcutaneous fatty tissue (10–20 mm below the dermal-fat junction) demonstrated marked immediate fat cell disruption and necrosis and profound collagen fiber denaturation in the reticular dermis and septae. When the 1440-nm wavelength energy was delivered in the shallow depth of the subdermal fatty tissue (<5 mm depth), significant acute denaturation was confined to the collagen fibers in the reticular dermis and septae at skin temperatures between 40°C and 42°C with 10 W (830 J). At the sixth week, progressive collagen fiber fibrosis and reorganization within the reticular dermis and septae were observed histologically and are believed to contribute to delayed optimal tissue lifting at 3 months and thereafter.

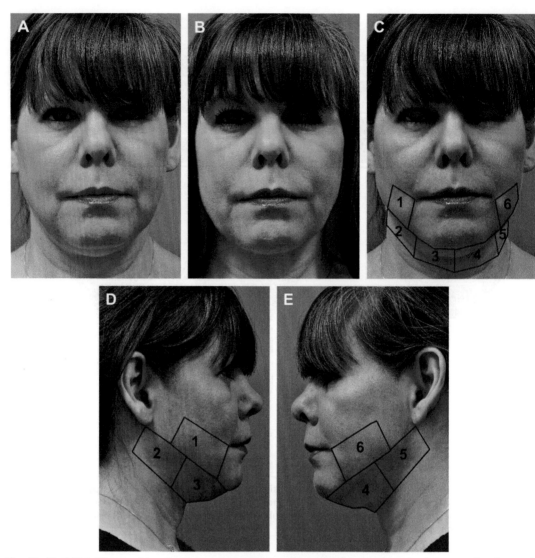

Fig. 11. (*A–E*) This 50-year-old patient presented with significant fullness to the prejowl areas and to her entire neck with moderate degree of tissue laxity. Preoperative markings delineate the six sectors to be treated (moderate-deep, 650 J/sector; superficial musculoaponeurotic system layer, 275 J/sector; subdermal layer, 223 J/sector with skin temperatures 38°C–39°C; 125 mL lipoaspirate).

In this clinical study, controlled lipolysis with the 1440-nm laser in the down and forward directions resulted in a spectrum of adipocyte damage from swelling, rupture of cellular membrane, dispersed lipids, and coagulative necrosis, as demonstrated by previous histologic studies.[2–6] The lipolytic debris was removed by liposuction that contributed to fatty reduction and contouring along with skin accommodation. The present study also delivered heating of collagen fibers with the 1440-nm laser in the down and forward locations in the fibrofascial layer of the platysma muscle to stimulate shortening and tightening of collagen fibers. There were no direct or indirect findings that heating the

superficial musculoaponeurotic system resulted in dysfunctions (paresis, asymmetries, pain, or spasms) after this therapeutic maneuver. Similar clinical findings were observed after focused ultrasonic thermal coagulation points were precisely delivered to the imaged layer of the lower third of face and neck.[13] This small clinical experience also suggested that laser treatments to the reticular dermal layer with the 1440-nm laser in the up position resulted in beneficial tissue-tightening effects beyond that which would be expected from accommodation after liposuction alone, in some of the skin-challenged patients. The stimulation of collagen fiber deposition and remodeling resulted in increased dermal thickness by comparing ultrasonic images at baseline and at 3 and 6 months. Although skin elasticity was not measured, other publications[4,6] for the treatment of cellulite, using the 1440-nm laser, have demonstrated increased skin elasticity and dermal thickness over 6 months to a year. A clinical study,[14] using the 1320- and 1064-nm wavelengths with less affinity to heat water and collagen fibers in the dermis of abdominal skin than that observed with the 1440-nm wavelength, has reported an increase in tissue tightening versus control subjects by three-dimensional vectra analyses over 3 months.

The present clinical experience demonstrated persistence of clinical benefits at 6 months in all patients by objective and subjective analyses. Adverse events were limited to transient swelling and bruising, the severity of which was mild and completely resolved by 2 to 3 weeks. Treatment burns were not observed because the internal and skin temperatures were monitored real time. The treatment endpoint was the number of joules of energy delivered and the skin surface temperature. Limitations of this preliminary study include the small number of patients and short follow-up duration. The encouraging results of the present study warrant more studies in treating larger number of patients of greater severity to optimize the treatment parameters.

SUMMARY

The incorporation of the 1440-nm wavelength offered increased benefits for laser lipolysis and tissue lifting for facial rejuvenation in 19 patients who presented with fat accumulations in the lower third of their faces and neck. Most of these patients exhibited moderate degrees of tissue laxity and sagging. Photographic analyses and subjective responses from Investigator and Patient Global Aesthetic Improvement Scales indicated that the 1440-nm wavelength achieved high thermal absorption within fat and collagen (water) leading to fat reduction and collagen denaturation, and progressive tissue lifting by 3 to 6 months. The combination of the 1440-nm wavelength, side-firing fiber, and the thermal-control systems provided a safe and effective means for facial rejuvenation. Further studies are needed to validate these initial findings.

ACKNOWLEDGMENTS

The author thanks Ana Tevez, RN, Connie Ha, LVN, Erica Lopez Ulloa, CST, and Chelsea Knutson, CST, for surgical assistance and data gathering. The author thanks Margaret Gaston, BS, for statistics, computer assistance, and graphics.

REFERENCES

1. Holcomb JD, Baek JS. Subregional contouring of the face with 1444 nm Nd:YAG lipolysis laser: a novel option for facial rejuvenation. Presented at the Proceedings of the American Academy of Facial Plastic and Reconstructive Surgery. San Diego (CA), October 1–3, 2009.
2. Holcomb JD. 1444 nm pulsed neodymium-YAG laser next generation highly selective lipolysis for facial contouring. Princeton Junction, NJ: Lutronic Corporation; 2009.
3. Sasaki GH, Tevez A, Ha C, et al. Early clinical experience with the 1440-nm wavelength (smartlipo triplex™ work station) for facial rejuvenation. White Paper. Westford (MA): Cynosure; 2011.
4. DiBernardo BE. Treatment of cellulite using a 1440-nm pulsed laser with one-year follow-up. Aesthet Surg J 2011;31(3):328–41.
5. Sasaki GH, Tevez A, Gonzales M. Histological changes after 1440 nm, 1320 nm and 1064 nm wavelength exposures in the deep and superficial layers of human abdominal tissue: acute and delayed findings. White Paper. Westford (MA): Cynosure; 2010.
6. Sasaki GH, Tevez A, Ha C, et al. Treatment of cellulite using a 1440 nm internal laser (18 month follow up). White Paper. Westford (MA): Cynosure; 2012.
7. Duck FA. Physical properties of tissue. San Diego (CA): Academic Press; 1990. p. 320–328.
8. Youn J. Ablation efficiency measurements for laser-assisted lipolysis using optical coherence tomography. Princeton Junction, NJ: Lutronic Corporation; 2009.
9. Youn JA. Comparison of wavelength dependence for laser-assisted lipolysis effect using Monte Carlo simulation. Princeton Junction, NJ: Lutronic Corporation; 2009.
10. Tark KC, Jung JE, Song SY. Superior lipolytic effect of the 1,444 nm Nd:YAG laser: comparison with the 1064 nm Nd:YAG laser. Lasers Surg Med 2009;41:721–7.
11. Roggan A, Friebel M, Dorschel K, et al. Optical properties of circulating human blood in the wavelength range 400-2500 nm. J Biomed Opt 1999;4:36–46.
12. Sasaki GH. Laser-assisted liposuction for facial and body contouring and tissue tightening: a 2 year experience with 75 consecutive patients. Semin Cutan Med Surg 2009;28(4):22.
13. Sasaki GH, Tevez A. Focused imaged ultrasound: clinical efficacy and safety (2 year experience). Aesthet Surg J 2012;32(5):601–12.
14. Sasaki GH. Quantification of human abdominal skin tightening and after component treatments with 1064 nm/1320 nm laser-assisted lipolysis: clinical implications. Aesthet Surg J 2010;30(2):239–45.

Robot-Assisted Plastic Surgery

Aladdin H. Hassanein, MD, MMSc, Brian A. Mailey, MD,
Marek K. Dobke, MD, PhD*

KEYWORDS

- da Vinci • RAMS • Reconstructive • Robot assisted • Robotic • Surgical • TORS

KEY POINTS

- Robot assisted surgery is a technology that is being used frequently among multiple surgical specialties.
- Robot assisted microsurgery (RAMS) and transoral robotic surgery (TORS) are applications relevant to plastic surgery that are being studied and clinically utilized.
- Advantages of RAMS include elimination of tremor and the ability to provide enhanced exposure. TORS facilitates oropharyngeal tumor excision and reconstruction without mandibular splitting.
- High cost and select reconstructive clinical applications require continued substantial innovation to make the surgical robot a prominent part of plastic surgery.

OVERVIEW

The term "robot" derives from the Czech word *robota,* which means "forced labor"; it was first used by the Czech writer Karel Capek in his play *Rossum's Universal Robots* in 1921.[1] The concept of robotics in surgery was promoted by the National Aeronautics and Space Administration (NASA) and the US Army to develop telepresence surgery (operating remotely) because of potential wartime and space applications.[1] The da Vinci Surgical System (Intuitive Surgical, Sunnyvale, CA) emerged as the prominent commercially available robotic system and the first to be approved by the Food and Drug Administration (FDA) in 2000 (**Fig. 1**).[2] The da Vinci system most commonly is being used in cardiothoracic, gastrointestinal, gynecologic, and urological operations; more than 205,000 robot-assisted procedures are performed annually, with a rapidly growing number of hospitals installing systems.[3] Because plastic surgery operations primarily do not involve organ-containing body cavities, technologies, such as laparoscopy, that have revolutionized several surgical subspecialties have not had a major impact in plastic surgery. The surgical robot may have applications in plastic surgery that can provide technical advantages, however, particularly in robot-assisted microsurgery (RAMS) and transoral robotic surgery (TORS). The purpose of this article was to investigate current and potential uses of the surgical robot in plastic surgery, as well as obstacles to its use.

THERAPEUTIC OPTIONS
RAMS

In the mid-1990s, investigators expanded on the previously developed NASA telerobotics systems to create a robot assistant suitable for microsurgery that consisted of a 10-inch-long manipulator with 6° of freedom.[4,5] By 1998, technical feasibility animal studies demonstrated robotic instruments

Disclosure/financial interests: No disclosures of commercial interest related to the content of this article. Dr Dobke is a consultant for Ulthera, Inc.

Division of Plastic Surgery, University of California San Diego, 200 West Arbor Drive, San Diego, California 92103, USA

* Corresponding author. Division of Plastic Surgery, University of California San Diego, 200 West Arbor Drive, San Diego, CA 92103.

E-mail address: mdobke@ucsd.edu

Clin Plastic Surg 39 (2012) 419–424
http://dx.doi.org/10.1016/j.cps.2012.07.010

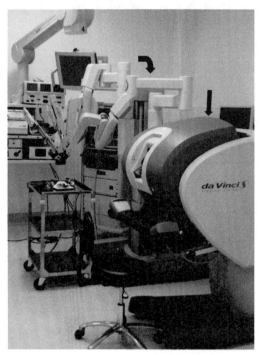

Fig. 1. The da Vinci Surgical System surgical robot. Note the surgeon console (*straight arrow*) and the patient-side cart (*curved arrow*).

to be capable of successfully anastomosing coronary arteries through both open and endoscopic techniques.[6,7] Further efficacy and benefits of the microsurgical robotic system included the ability to perform closed-chest multivessel cardiac bypass and beating heart bypass operations.[6,8] By 2000, the next generation of surgical robots progressed and comprised a robot slave and surgeon-controlled command center; the da Vinci Surgical System was FDA approved for human use.[8] Using 3-dimensional stereoscopic vision and robotic slave arms equipped with instruments, the technology allowed the surgeon to work at a smaller scale than conventional surgery; for microsurgery, this meant potentially greater technical quality and a lower error rate. Comparative studies analyzing microvascular anastomoses concluded that patency and leak rates between traditional microsurgery techniques and robot-enhanced techniques were equivalent; however, the surgical robot group took twice as long.[7,9,10] The robot-enhanced cases had remarkable tremor filtration at a cost of prolonged operating time.[9]

The surgical robot enhances microsurgical precision by suppressing involuntary movements of tremor and low frequency drift.[11,12] The robot standardizes the vascular anastomotic technical skills and may reduce variations in patient outcomes.[11] Furthermore, the robot can limit the affect of fatigue, anxiety, or age-related factors.[13] This occurs owing to scalability of movements up to 1:6 scale, meaning that 6-mm finger movement will result in 1-mm motion of the instrument. Simultaneously available magnification of the operative field and scalability of maneuvers synergistically enhances a microsurgeon's technical capability. RAMS also provides more range of motion and degrees of freedom than the human hand, creating more potential maneuverability during free flaps, replantation, or microneurorrhaphy.

Investigators found that robotic microsurgery skills could be expeditiously learned by residents and practicing surgeons.[14] The da Vinci robot was used to successfully perform a free flap in a porcine model anastomosing a 1.5-mm and 1.3-mm artery and vein, respectively; the authors concluded a similar setup time to the operating microscope and comparable warm ischemia time of the flap.[15] Robotic assistance was used for distal ulnar artery reconstruction with a forearm venous graft in a patient with bilateral hypothenar hammer syndrome.[16] Robotic-assisted microvascular anastomoses are being performed during reconstruction after transoral robotic surgical resection of oropharyngeal tumors by use of a third arm with the da Vinci system.[17–19]

TORS

Traditional open access surgical resection commonly was used for the treatment of oropharyngeal tumors; operations often involved mandibular osteotomy and were associated with patient morbidity and poor functional outcome.[20] Management of these cancers with surgical ablation declined in favor of chemoradiation, which was shown to be effective while preserving anatomy[21–23]; however, complications such as toxicity and dysphagia occur with chemoradiation treatment.[24] TORS is now being used for oropharyngeal tumor resection at some institutions.[25–29] TORS facilitates exposure to the oropharynx, hypopharynx, larynx, and parapharyngeal space without requiring mandibulotomy for tumor excision. Morbidity with TORS is minimized compared with transmandibular or translabial resection; TORS can provide tissue to allow for staging and thus possibly minimize the amount of radiation treatment required.[30]

TORS for head and neck tumor extirpation with the da Vinci system has been FDA approved since 2009. As TORS has become an option for oncological resection, the development of robot-assisted reconstruction following ablative TORS is most relevant to reconstructive surgeons. Selber and colleagues[17] described a preclinical study of

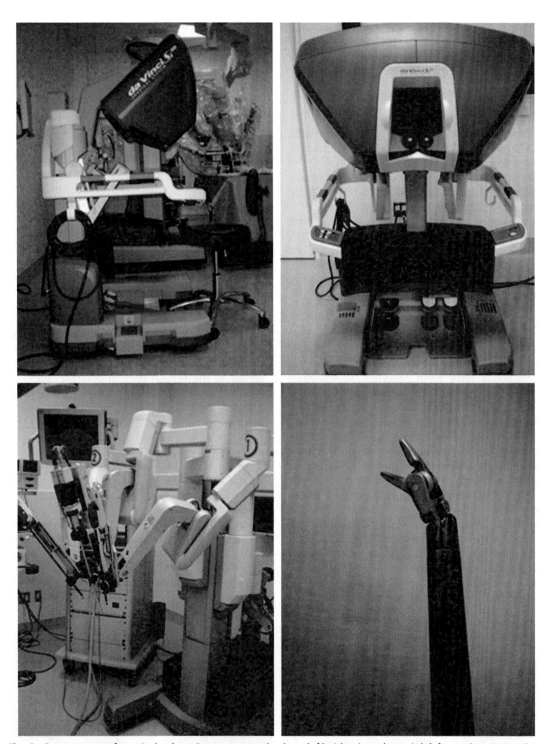

Fig. 2. Components of surgical robot. Surgeon console: (*top left*) side view; (*top right*) front view. Note viewfinder on console for high-resolution visualization. Patient-side cart (*bottom left*). Camera and various instruments fasten to arms (*bottom, right*) Articulating instruments provide 7° of freedom.

TORS reconstruction using cadaveric and porcine models and a case series.[18] These investigators have performed 20 cases of TORS reconstruction, including anterolateral thigh flaps, radial forearm flaps, ulnar artery perforator flaps, facial artery myomucosal flaps, and buccal or pharyngeal transposition flaps; robot assistance was used for microvascular anastomosis.[19] Their preference for selecting TORS for reconstruction is guided by clinical features of the malignancy[19]:

1. Primary site (oropharyngeal)
2. Tumor extent (large)
3. Prior treatment with radiation therapy
4. Patient health (tolerance of long operations).

Other investigators have used reconstructive TORS for local advancement flaps, radial forearm free flaps, and vastus lateralis free flap.[28,31,32] Although long-term outcomes for TORS reconstruction are limited because of the novelty of the procedure, 2 larger series report no flap loss.[19,28] Healing by secondary intention is an acceptable option for small lesions resected by TORS; however, robot assistance is able to provide the ability to precisely inset flaps more easily and prevent lip or mandible splitting in contrast to open reconstruction.[19]

OTHER APPLICATIONS

TORS and RAMS have been the most studied reconstructive uses for the surgical robot; other applications have been reported. Investigators have used the robot for flap harvest. Following preclinical cadaveric dissections, a rectus abdominis muscle free flap was procured robotically for lower extremity wound coverage without complication.[33] Robot-assisted latissimus dorsi muscle harvest was performed in cadavers.[34] Harvesting internal mammary vessels robotically for the recipient free flap breast pedicle in breast reconstruction was described in 22 patients; benefits include minimizing scar and reducing donor site morbidity.[35] Restoration of elbow flexion by donor motor fascicle ulnar nerve transfer to the biceps muscle (Oberlin procedure) using robotic assistance was reported in 4 patients, all of whom regained flexion; the investigators cited increased

precision by elimination of tremor and magnification of the field as advantages of this technique.[36] A case of an oncologic robot-assisted neck dissection using a modified face-lift approach was reported.[37]

TECHNIQUE

The da Vinci system consists of a surgeon console and a 4-armed patient-side cart (**Fig. 2**). The surgeon sits at the console separate from the operating table but typically in the same room. The da Vinci robot operates on a master-slave setup; the system does not function autonomously without direct surgeon input and does not perform automated sequences.[38] The 4-armed patient-side cart allows for changeable instruments in 3 arms and an endoscope. Dual offset cameras feed into viewfinders on the console providing the surgeon with a high-resolution 3-dimensional image of the surgical field (**Fig. 3**). The surgeon's hand motions at the master control are translated to movements of the instruments. Articulation points of the instruments allow for 7° of freedom, similar to the human arm; in contrast, standard laparoscopy provides only 4° of freedom.[2] In addition, hand tremor is eliminated with motion scaling.[18]

LIMITATIONS OF ROBOTIC SURGERY

Cost is a prohibitive factor for widespread adaptation of the surgical robot; the price of the da Vinci systems range from $1.0 to $2.5 million per unit along with high maintenance expenses.[3] The surgical robot has been castigated for the lack of tactile feedback for the surgeon[38]; however, the superior 3-dimensional visualization partially compensates for the absence of haptic perception.[18] In addition, the bulky size of the system can be

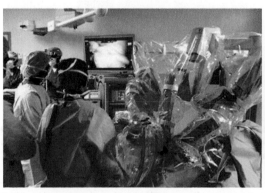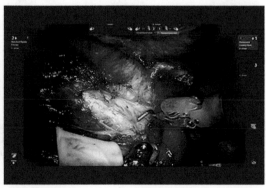

Fig. 3. Intraoperative surgical robot. (*Left*) Patient-side cart draped over surgical field. Assisting surgeons position arms in sterile field as primary surgeon operates remotely on console. (*Right*) Scope image of esophagus. Surgeon views display from console in 3-dimensional high-quality resolution.

cumbersome, particularly in the limited space involved with TORS.[30] The design of the console has been criticized for impeding resident education by removing the operating surgeon directly from the field; a 2-headed mentoring console is available to facilitate training or collaboration with other surgeons.[39]

SUMMARY

The number of robotic-assisted operations with the da Vinci system is expanding across surgical subspecialties. The advantages of the surgical robot (eg, elimination of tremor, field magnification, and the potential to provide enhanced exposure) have facilitated its use for RAMS and TORS, as well as other reconstructive applications. However, the high cost, along with currently limited clinical applications in plastic surgery, make the surgical robot a technology that will require continued substantial innovation to become a prominent tool for the plastic surgeon.

ACKNOWLEDGMENTS

The authors thank the University of California San Diego Center for the Future of Surgery for access to surgical robotic systems.

REFERENCES

1. Satava RM. Surgical robotics: the early chronicles: a personal historical perspective. Surg Laparosc Endosc Percutan Tech 2002;12:6–16.

2. Hanly EJ, Talamini MA. Robotic abdominal surgery. Am J Surg 2004;188:19S–26S.

3. Barbash GI, Glied SA. New technology and health care costs—the case of robot-assisted surgery. N Engl J Med 2010;363:701–4.

4. Das H, Ohm T, Boswell C, et al. "Robot-assisted microsurgery development at JPL". In: Akay M, Marsh A, editors. Information Technologies in Medicine: Rehabilitation and Treatment. Vol 2. New York: John Wiley and Sons; 2001.

5. Saraf S. Role of robot assisted microsurgery in plastic surgery. Indian J Plast Surg 2006;39:57–61.

6. Stephenson ER Jr, Sankholkar S, Ducko CT, et al. Robotically assisted microsurgery for endoscopic coronary artery bypass grafting. Ann Thorac Surg 1998;66:1064–7.

7. Le Roux PD, Das H, Esquenazi S, et al. Robot-assisted microsurgery: a feasibility study in the rat. Neurosurgery 2001;48:584–9.

8. Boyd WD, Kodera K, Stahl KD, et al. Current status and future directions in computer-enhanced video- and robotic-assisted coronary bypass surgery. Semin Thorac Cardiovasc Surg 2002;14:101–9.

9. Knight CG, Lorincz A, Cao A, et al. Computer-assisted, robot-enhanced open microsurgery in an animal model. J Laparoendosc Adv Surg Tech A 2005;15:182–5.

10. Morita A, Sora S, Mitsuishi M, et al. Microsurgical robotic system for the deep surgical field: development of a prototype and feasibility studies in animal and cadaveric models. J Neurosurg 2005;103:320–7.

11. Harada K, Minakawa Y, Baek Y, et al. Microsurgical skill assessment: toward skill-based surgical robotic control. Conf Proc IEEE Eng Med Biol Soc 2011; 2011:6700–3.

12. Elble RJ. Central mechanisms of tremor. J Clin Neurophysiol 1996;13:133–44.

13. Howe RD, Matsuoka Y. Robotics for surgery. Annu Rev Biomed Eng 1999;1:211–40.

14. Karamanoukian RL, Bui T, McConnell MP, et al. Transfer of training in robotic-assisted microvascular surgery. Ann Plast Surg 2006;57:662–5.

15. Katz RD, Taylor JA, Rosson GD, et al. Robotics in plastic and reconstructive surgery: use of a telemanipulator slave robot to perform microvascular anastomoses. J Reconstr Microsurg 2006;22:53–7.

16. Facca S, Liverneaux P. Robotic assisted microsurgery in hypothenar hammer syndrome: a case report. Comput Aided Surg 2010;15:110–4.

17. Selber JC, Robb G, Serletti JM, et al. Transoral robotic free flap reconstruction of oropharyngeal defects: a preclinical investigation. Plast Reconstr Surg 2010; 125:896–900.

18. Selber JC. Transoral robotic reconstruction of oropharyngeal defects: a case series. Plast Reconstr Surg 2010;126:1978–87.

19. Longfield EA, Holsinger FC, Selber JC. Reconstruction after robotic head and neck surgery: when and why. J Reconstr Microsurg 2012. [Epub ahead of print].

20. Machtay M, Perch S, Markiewicz D, et al. Combined surgery and postoperative radiotherapy for carcinoma of the base of radiotherapy for carcinoma of the base of tongue: analysis of treatment outcome and prognostic value of margin status. Head Neck 1997;19:494–9.

21. Forastiere AA, Goepfert H, Maor M, et al. Concurrent chemotherapy and radiotherapy for organ preservation in advanced laryngeal cancer. N Engl J Med 2003;349:2091–8.

22. Induction chemotherapy plus radiation compared with surgery plus radiation in patients with advanced laryngeal cancer. The Department of Veterans Affairs Laryngeal Cancer Study Group. N Engl J Med 1991; 324:1685–90.

23. Pignon JP, Bourhis J, Domenge C, et al. Chemotherapy added to locoregional treatment for head and neck squamous-cell carcinoma: three meta-analyses of updated individual data. MACH-NC Collaborative Group. Meta-analysis of chemotherapy on head and neck cancer. Lancet 2000;355:949–55.

24. Machtay M, Moughan J, Trotti A, et al. Factors associated with severe late toxicity after concurrent chemoradiation for locally advanced head and neck cancer: an RTOG analysis. J Clin Oncol 2008;26:3582–9.

25. Weinstein GS, O'Malley BW Jr, Snyder W, et al. Transoral robotic surgery: supraglottic partial laryngectomy. Ann Otol Rhinol Laryngol 2007;116:19–23.

26. Ozer E, Waltonen J. Transoral robotic nasopharyngectomy: a novel approach for nasopharyngeal lesions. Laryngoscope 2008;118:1613–6.

27. Cognetti DM, Luginbuhl AJ, Nguyen AL, et al. Early adoption of transoral robotic surgical program: preliminary outcomes. Otolaryngol Head Neck Surg 2012. [Epub ahead of print].

28. Genden EM, Desai S, Sung CK. Transoral robotic surgery for the management of head and neck cancer: a preliminary experience. Head Neck 2009;31:283–9.

29. White HN, Moore EJ, Rosenthal EL, et al. Transoral robotic-assisted surgery for head and neck squamous cell carcinoma: one- and 2-year survival analysis. Arch Otolaryngol Head Neck Surg 2010;136:1248–52.

30. de Almeida JR, Genden EM. Robotic surgery for oropharynx cancer: promise, challenges, and future directions. Curr Oncol Rep 2012;14:148–57.

31. Garfein ES, Greaney PJ Jr, Easterlin B, et al. Transoral robotic reconstructive surgery reconstruction of a tongue base defect with a radial forearm flap. Plast Reconstr Surg 2011;127:2352–4.

32. Mukhija VK, Sung CK, Desai SC, et al. Transoral robotic assisted free flap reconstruction. Otolaryngol Head Neck Surg 2009;140:124–5.

33. Patel NV, Pedersen JC. Robotic harvest of the rectus abdominis muscle: a preclinical investigation and case report. J Reconstr Microsurg 2011. [Epub ahead of print].

34. Selber JC. Robotic latissimus dorsi muscle harvest. Plast Reconstr Surg 2011;128:88e–90e.

35. Boyd B, Umansky J, Samson M, et al. Robotic harvest of internal mammary vessels in breast reconstruction. J Reconstr Microsurg 2006;22:261–6.

36. Naito K, Facca S, Lequint T, et al. The Oberlin procedure for restoration of elbow flexion with the da Vinci robot: four cases. Plast Reconstr Surg 2012;129:707–11.

37. Koh YW, Chung WY, Hong HJ, et al. Robot-assisted selective neck dissection via modified face-lift approach for early oral tongue cancer: a video demonstration. Ann Surg Oncol 2012;19:1334–5.

38. Talamini MA, Hanly EJ. Technology in the operating suite. JAMA 2005;293:863–6.

39. Hanly EJ, Miller BE, Kumar R, et al. Mentoring console improves collaboration and teaching in surgical robotics. J Laparoendosc Adv Surg Tech A 2006;16:445–51.

Impact of Reconstructive Transplantation on the Future of Plastic and Reconstructive Surgery

Maria Siemionow, MD, PhD, DSc[a,b,*]

KEYWORDS

- Vascularized composite allografts • Disadvantages of reconstructive transplantation
- Face transplant • Hand transplant • Abdominal wall transplant • Laryngeal transplant
- Tracheal transplant

KEY POINTS

- Complex posttraumatic deficits can be repaired with well-established microsurgical techniques; the tradeoff includes significant donor site morbidity, lack of perfect function restoration, and less-than-optimal esthetic outcomes.
- Reconstructive transplantation includes vascularized composite allotransplants (VCAs), from a human donor, and involves transplantation of tissues derived from ectoderm and mesoderm.
- The major concern in VCA reconstructive transplantation is the need for lifelong immunosuppression to prevent graft rejection.
- The question remains whether reconstructive transplantation should be considered either only after all conventional options have been exhausted or as the first option after traumatic injury causing severe functional and/or esthetic deficits of the human body.

INTRODUCTION OF RECONSTRUCTIVE TRANSPLANTATION INTO PLASTIC SURGERY

The past 2 decades has seen an ongoing search for new reconstructive options to restore functional and esthetic deficits of patients with severe deformities of the face, extremities, hands, and other parts of the body for which application of currently available reconstructive options resulted in less-than-optimal outcomes.

The major problem with reconstruction of complex posttraumatic deficits on the face and extremities was a lack of available tissues that resembled the injured or missing parts, such as the nose, lips, or eyelids in the case of facial deformities, or the lack of spare parts, such as joints, fingers, or hands in cases of extremity injuries involving amputations.

Conventional techniques allowed for staged reconstruction of these deformities, providing coverage, tissue expansion, and functional restoration with borrowed tissues, including free tissue transfers or a combination of all available techniques.

Disclosure/conflict of interest: The author of this manuscript has no financial or commercial associations to disclose.
[a] Cleveland Clinic Lerner College of Medicine of Case Western Reserve University, Cleveland Clinic, 9500 Euclid Avenue, Desk NA-21, Cleveland, OH 44195, USA; [b] Department of Plastic Surgery, Cleveland Clinic, 9500 Euclid Avenue, Desk A-60, Cleveland, OH 44195, USA
* Department of Plastic Surgery, Cleveland Clinic, 9500 Euclid Avenue, Desk A-60, Cleveland, OH 44195.
E-mail address: siemiom@ccf.org

Clin Plastic Surg 39 (2012) 425–434
http://dx.doi.org/10.1016/j.cps.2012.07.011

The well-established microsurgical techniques contributed significantly to the field of reconstructive surgery by introducing procedures such as toe-to-hand transfers, for example, in which missing functions were restored often in one surgical attempt.

The tradeoff, however, included significant donor site morbidity, lack of perfect function restoration, and less-than-optimal esthetic outcomes. In many situations, multiple reconstructive attempts were undertaken, thus limiting sources of available autologous tissues over time, and often leaving patients with the visible stigma of posttraumatic disfigurement.

Autologous free tissue transfers and replantation procedures introduced the idea of tissue transplantation as a method of functional and esthetic restoration. The major advantage of this approach was the fact that autologous transplants did not require immunosuppression to keep the grafts alive. The major disadvantage, however, was the awkward esthetic outcome of single or multiple flaps of varying color and bulkiness used for facial coverage, or the combination of flaps and short toes sticking out from deformed hands.

As a result of the lack of "specialized spare parts" that could be borrowed from the bodies to restore missing functions, the idea of reconstructive transplantation was borne and introduced to plastic surgery. It was based on more than 20 years of experimental and preclinical work testing the technical, functional, and, most importantly, immunologic aspects of reconstructive transplantation.[1–15]

Plastic and reconstructive surgery embraced the new field of reconstructive transplantation using vascularized composite allotransplants (VCAs), such as human hand, face, larynx, trachea, abdominal wall, and lower extremity transplants, and included these into the armamentarium of plastic surgery.

This article discusses the current and future impact of reconstructive transplantation on the field of plastic and reconstructive surgery.

RECONSTRUCTIVE TRANSPLANTATION AS AN ALTERNATIVE SURGICAL OPTION

Reconstructive transplantation includes VCAs and involves transplantation of tissues derived from ectoderm and mesoderm. VCAs typically contain skin, fat, muscle, nerves, lymph nodes, bone, cartilage, ligaments, and bone marrow as opposed to a single tissue organ, which is the case in conventional solid organ transplantation. An example of VCA is limb transplantation, in which the transplanted graft includes skin, muscle, nerve, blood vessels, and bone. The function and immunologic properties of the composite tissue transplant are more difficult to define, because each individual component has its own unique characteristics that ultimately affect the successful outcome of the transplantation. Most applications of VCA predominantly improve quality of life for patients with non–life-threatening conditions and aim to restore anatomic, cosmetic, and functional integrity. The benefits gathered from these procedures must be balanced against the morbidity of the surgical procedure itself, the side effects of lifelong immunosuppression therapy, and the cost of surgery and immunosuppressive medications (**Box 1**).

Advances in VCA transplantation have opened a new era in the field of reconstructive surgery. Since 1998, after the report on the first successful hand transplantation in France, the field of VCA has further developed, opening new alternatives for patients who have lost their extremities and hands.[16]

Box 1
Considerations in reconstructive transplantation

Advantages

- Reconstruction of VCA in a single surgical procedure
- No donor-site morbidity
- Access to the esthetic and functional units and body parts
- Better skin texture, pliability, and color match
- Restoration of form and function with "alike" body parts and components
- Reduced number of surgical procedures and need for general anesthesia
- Reduced number of postsurgery hospitalization days

Disadvantages

- Need for life-long immunosuppressive therapy
- Need for adequate matching between the donor and recipient (age, sex, race)
- Increased risks of comorbidities (viral and bacterial infections, lymphoproliferative disorders, diabetes, avascular necrosis of bones)
- Risk of acute or chronic rejection
- Need for the rescue protocol in the case of VCA rejection
- Social, ethical, and psychological issues
- Significant cost of immunosuppressive therapy

On November 15, 2004, Dr Maria Siemionow at Cleveland Clinic received the world's first Institutional Review Board (IRB) approval to perform face transplantation in humans. This event opened a new era in reconstructive surgery of the human face.

On November 27, 2005, in Amiens, France, a surgical team led by Drs Bernard Devauchelle and Jean-Michel Dubernard announced that they had performed a partial face transplant on a 38-year-old woman whose face had been disfigured by a dog bite.[17] To date, a total of 19 face trans-plantations have been performed worldwide in France, China, the United States, and Spain.[18–32]

The world's first near-total face transplantation was performed in Cleveland in December 2008 by a team led by this author.[23] This procedure was, until now, the most complex face transplant, involving restoration of 3-dimensional craniofacial skeleton with multiple functional units.

To illustrate the approach undertaken by a single surgical procedure of human face reconstructive transplantation, a detailed outline of the sequence

---

Cleveland Clinic Near-Total Face Transplantation Procedure

The patient was a 45-year-old woman who experienced severe facial trauma to her midface from a close-range shotgun blast in September 2004. Her facial deformities included absence of nose, nasal lining, and underlying bone; contracted remnants of the upper lip; loss of orbicularis oris and orbicularis oculi muscle functions; distorted and scarred lower eyelids with ectropion; right-eye enucleation supported by eye prosthesis; and facial nerve deficit manifested by the lack of midface function (**Fig. 1**).

Before face transplantation, the patient had undergone 23 major autologous reconstructive operations that included correction of bone defects with free fibula and split-calvaria/rib grafts; soft-tissue defects with anterolateral free flap, temporalis muscle flap, paramedian forehead flap, and radial forearm free flap; and skin defects with multiple split-thickness skin grafts.

The donor was a brain-dead woman who matched the patient in age, race, and skin complexion. The allo-graft was designed to cover the recipient's anterior craniofacial skeleton, and it included approximately 80% of the surface area of the anterior face. It was based on a Le Fort III composite tissue allograft containing total nose, lower eyelids, upper lip, total infraorbital floor, bilateral zygomas, and anterior maxilla with incisors, and included total alveolus, anterior hard palate, and bilateral parotid glands (**Fig. 2**).[24,25]

The allotransplant inset to the recipient started with the adjustments of a Le Fort III composite allograft to the recipient's skeletal defect. Once bone components of the facial allograft were secured and stable, bilateral microvascular anastomoses of both arteries and veins were performed. Once the craniofacial skeleton was intact, the bilateral facial nerves were connected using standard epineural repair.

First, the donor's vagus nerve, taken as an interpositional graft, was attached to the upper division of the trunk of the right side of the recipient's facial nerve. On the left side, the donor's hypoglossal nerve, used as an interpositional graft, was attached to the upper division of the trunk on the recipient's facial nerve. Both grafts were connected to the main trunk of the donor nerve. Porous polyethylene implants were then used to reconstruct orbital floors. Finally, the lower eyelids, including the recipient's conjunctiva and lash lines, were reconstructed bilaterally using donor eyelid skin. The composite facial allograft inset was completed after skin closure.

Face transplantation requires lifelong immunosuppression to prevent the graft from acute rejection and to support long-term survival. The protocol included induction of immunosuppression with rabbit antithymocyte globulin (1 × 2 mg/kg intravenously once a day for 9 days) in combination with methylprednisolone given as a 1000-mg bolus intravenously on the day of transplant, and rapidly tapered thereafter. The immunosuppressive regimen was maintained with tacrolimus, mycophenolate mofetil, and low-dose oral prednisone.

Functional outcomes improved over time and, after 9 months, sensory discrimination returned to the entire facial skin, as measured with the Pressure-Specified Sensory Device (N K Biotechnical Engineering, Golden Valley, MN), indicating the presence of 2-point sensory discrimination at the area under the lower eyelids, upper lip, and the tip of the nose on both sides of the graft. Motor recovery included improved facial mimetics with asymmetric smile and upper lip occlusion.

The functional recovery of this 3-dimensional facial defect is excellent, with restoration of major functions, such as eating solid food without the need of a gastric tube, drinking from a cup, and reestablishment of intelligible speech after hard palate reconstruction with composite allograft and palatal obturator support.

At 3 years after transplant, the aesthetic outcome has been improved through excision of the redundant skin and subcutaneous tissues (**Fig. 3**). Psychologically, the patient is doing well, without symptoms of depression or posttraumatic stress disorder. Finally, her pain level has been significantly reduced, because the scarred and contracted tissue within her face was removed during face transplantation.[23]

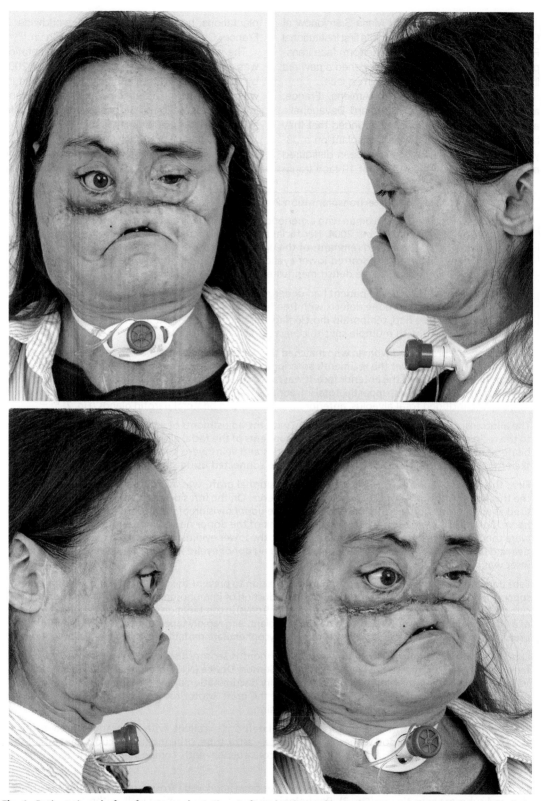

Fig. 1. Patient views before face transplantation. Left and right profiles indicate craniofacial defect with missing nose, upper lip, and lower eyelids contracted by massive scar tissue. (*From* Siemionow MZ, Djohan R, Bernard S, et al. The Cleveland Clinic experience with the first US face transplantation. In: Siemionow MZ, editor. The know-how of face transplantation. London: Springer-Verlag; 2011. p. 343, Fig. 33.1; with permission.)

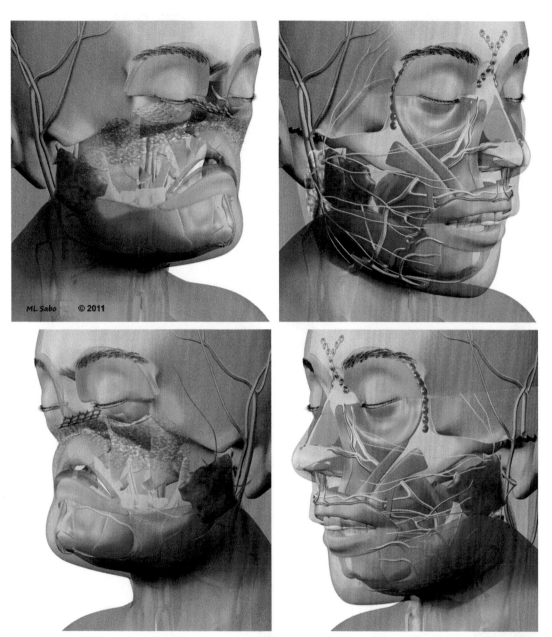

Fig. 2. Schematic illustration of the first U.S. near-total face transplantation (for patient in **Fig. 1**). Figures representing recipient defect before allograft insert (*top left* and *bottom left*) illustrating the need for a 3-dimensional craniofacial reconstruction. This face allograft included more than 535 cm² of facial skin, functional units of full nose with nasal lining and bony skeleton, lower eyelids and upper lip, and underlying muscles and bones, including orbital floor, zygoma, maxilla with teeth, hard palate, parotids and nerves, and arteries and veins (*top right* and *bottom right*). (*Courtesy of* The Cleveland Clinic Education Institute (CCEI) and staff illustrator Mark Sabo, BFA, Cleveland, OH; with permission.)

of events accompanying a reconstructive transplantation case is presented.

The presented summary of conventional approaches to reconstruct severe esthetic and functional defects illustrates the limitations of current conventional techniques and of the body to supply an adequate number and quality of tissues for such complex reconstructions. It is also clear that, despite the surgical efforts undertaken by qualified experts in the field, the outcome

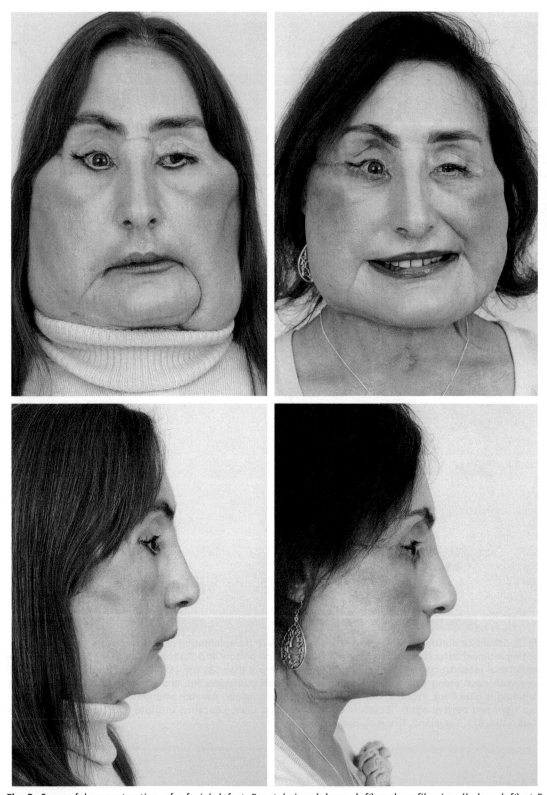

Fig. 3. Successful reconstruction of a facial defect. Frontal view (*above, left*) and profile view (*below, left*) at 5 months after face transplantation, and frontal view (*above, right*) and profile view (*below, right*) at 20 months after face transplantation. (*From* Siemionow MZ, Djohan R, Bernard S, et al. The Cleveland Clinic experience with the first US face transplantation. In: Siemionow MZ, editor. The knowhow of face transplantation. London: Springer-Verlag; 2011. p. 343, Fig. 33.1; with permission.)

was less than optimal and the patient's quality of life did not improve after more than 23 conventional reconstructions.

To overcome these difficulties and introduce innovative approaches to plastic and reconstructive surgery, reconstructive transplantation aims to restore both the esthetic and functional components of the disfigured human face in one surgical procedure. This same approach is taken for other VCA transplants, including extremities, hand, larynx, trachea, and abdominal wall allotransplantation.[16,33–35]

The major difference between conventional reconstruction of complex body deficits and reconstructive transplantation is the privilege of access to human donors, which allows selection of perfect esthetic and functional components (eg, face, hand). Reconstructive transplantation allows compliance with Giles' mantra of replacing "the like with the like" tissues to restore, perfectly, missing parts of the body.

In this aspect, the impact of reconstructive transplantation on the field of plastic and reconstructive surgery is unprecedented and the future development of the field of VCA is guaranteed.

INDICATIONS FOR RECONSTRUCTIVE TRANSPLANTATION

The indications for reconstructive transplantation will obey all general rules applying to solid organ transplantation and will include consideration of medical needs; patient compliance; alcohol and drug dependency; and psychiatric, psychological, and social problems, which are all well defined in IRB-approved protocols.[36] The reconstructive indications will differ based on the type of VCA transplant and the goal of the reconstruction. For hand transplantation, consideration will be given to patients who are not satisfied with current reconstructive options, such as toe-to-hand transfer, or those who are not happy with or not tolerating the use of prosthetic devices. Based on the patient's functional and body image deficits, the indications will include single versus bilateral hand transplants, and will be defined by the level of transplantation (arm vs forearm vs hand).[37–39] For face transplantation, indications will include severe facial deformities after burn or trauma; postcancer deficits in patients who have been cancer-free for at least 5 years; and nonmalignant tumors, such as neurofibromas.[19,20,23,25]

Indications for laryngeal and tracheal transplantation are currently confined to patients with traumatic injuries, because exposure to lifelong immunosuppression is not justified in patients with cancer.[33,34] Current indications for abdominal wall transplants are for patients who are on the waiting list for liver, intestine, or pancreas transplantation and have lost the abdominal domain required for coverage of transplanted organs. Because organ transplant patients are subjected to lifelong immunosuppression, abdominal wall transplantation may thus be justified from an ethical prospective.[35]

Indications clearly will differ among institutions; however, they will always be supported by IRB-approved protocols. Approaches to reconstructive transplantation may change with better understanding of functional, psychological, and social outcomes of these procedures, and justification of the cost involved.

The question remains whether reconstructive transplantation should be considered only after all conventional options have been exhausted or as the first option after traumatic injury causing severe functional or esthetic deficits of the human body.

COMPLICATIONS AND CONCERNS WITH RECONSTRUCTIVE TRANSPLANTATION

The most serious complication reported after VCA transplantation was death. Three patients died after face transplantation. The first was a Chinese recipient of a face transplant who died of immunosuppression-related complications more than 2 years after face transplantation.[18,32] The second was a French recipient of face and bilateral hand transplants who died in Paris a few months after transplant.[29,40,41] The third was a Turkish recipient of face and quadruple extremity transplants who died in the early posttransplant period. No deaths were reported after hand transplantation; however, several patients rejected hands because of either noncompliance with the immunosuppressive protocol or late graft failure. One patient, the recipient of a face and bilateral hand transplant, lost both hands in the early posttransplant period. Considering that only 19 face transplants have been performed worldwide and 3 deaths were reported, this is a significant problem indicating that the inclusion criteria and indications for complex VCA transplants, such as combined extremity and face transplantation, should be carefully monitored and overseen by the hospitals' IRB and ethics committees and should be shared with the medical community to generate open discussion and comments.

The major concern in VCA reconstructive transplantation is the need for lifelong immunosuppression to prevent graft rejection. The immunologic complications remain significant and include severe viral and bacterial infections often requiring hospitalization, as reported for several cases of hand and face transplants.[16,19,23,39]

In addition, new-onset diabetes, avascular bone necrosis, lymphoproliferative disease, and uterine cancer were reported in VCA recipients. These serious complications should be monitored, and thorough evaluation of the pretransplant health status of potential candidates should be considered, because many patients can be presensitized from multiple blood transfusions after trauma and conventional reconstructions. In addition, the posttransplant adjustments of the combined antiviral, antimicrobial, and immunosuppressive therapeutic protocols should be individually tailored based on patients' immunologic competency and responses to these protocols.

A few additional concerns related to VCA transplantation include the functional and cosmetic outcomes and psychological or social reintegration of VCA recipients. The concerns about achievement of good functional outcomes include the need for patient compliance with posttransplant rehabilitation and physical therapy when routine daily exercises and different skill tasks are mandatory. A lack of patient understanding and compliance may result in unsatisfactory outcomes, creating dysfunctional and painful extremities, hands, and faces, and exposing patients to disappointment, frustration, and depression as a result of unrealistic expectations.

Some concerns also exist about VCA "misuse," which pertains mainly to face transplantation, wherein the fear is that some people may consider it a beautifying procedure. Furthermore, with transplants such as larynx, trachea, or abdominal wall, the concern is that, because these areas receive less exposure or visibility in the public eye, their recipients may consequently view them as "less important," which may compromise adherence to lifelong immunosuppressive protocols.

As in any innovative and developing field, many challenges will certainly arise for reconstructive transplant surgeons in the next decade. However, the history of solid organ transplantation has proven that once the idea of a novel therapy or procedure is introduced, the progress is unavoidable.

SUMMARY

The field of reconstructive transplantation involving VCA has emerged over the past 20 years; however, the longest follow-up of the first hand and larynx transplantation reached 14 years, and only 7 years for face transplantation, with most of the VCAs being performed within the past few years. These spectacular surgical procedures undoubtedly have revolutionized the concept of human body reconstruction but, at the same time, have raised many ethical, medical, and societal debates and concerns. As is seen in every new field, reconstructive transplantation is viewed by some as the only approach leading to advancement of plastic surgery, and by others as a trendy, risky, and ethically unjustified field.

Thus, at this developmental stage, the impact of reconstructive transplantation on the future of plastic and reconstructive surgery is still under discussion and surveillance.

Would global change in health reform justify the high cost of these procedures? Would long-term functional and esthetic outcomes counterweigh the occurrence of severe complications, including graft rejection and patient death? Would the benefits of reconstructive transplantation eliminate the need for conventional reconstruction? All of these questions should be raised and discussed when more data are available and true long-term outcomes can be assessed.

Despite these uncertainties and concerns, reconstructive transplantation has marked its presence in plastic and reconstructive surgery, and progress in the field is guaranteed as long as medical, ethical, and societal voices and deliberations are considered.

REFERENCES

1. Siemionow M, Gozel-Ulusal B, Engin Ulusal A, et al. Functional tolerance following face transplantation in the rat. Transplantation 2003;75:1607–9.
2. Siemionow M, Ortak T, Izycki D, et al. Induction of tolerance in composite-tissue allografts. Transplantation 2002;74:1211–7.
3. Gozel-Ulusal B, Ulusal AE, Ozmen S, et al. A new composite facial and scalp transplantation model in rats. Plast Reconstr Surg 2003;112:1302–11.
4. Demir Y, Ozmen S, Klimczak A, et al. Tolerance induction in composite facial allograft transplantation in the rat model. Plast Reconstr Surg 2004;114:1790–801.
5. Siemionow M, Demir Y, Mukherjee A, et al. Development and maintenance of donor-specific chimerism in semi-allogenic and fully major histocompatibility complex mismatched facial allograft transplants. Transplantation 2005;79:558–67.
6. Unal S, Agaoglu G, Zins J, et al. New surgical approach in facial transplantation extends survival of allograft recipients. Ann Plast Surg 2005;55:297–303.
7. Yazici I, Unal S, Siemionow M. Composite hemiface/calvaria transplantation model in rats. Plast Reconstr Surg 2006;118:1321–7.

8. Yazici I, Carnevale K, Klimczak A, et al. A new rat model of maxilla allotransplantation. Ann Plast Surg 2007;58:338–44.

9. Siemionow M, Klimczak A. Advances in the development of experimental composite tissue transplantation models. Transpl Int 2010;23(1):2–13.

10. Kulahci Y, Siemionow M. A new composite hemiface/mandible/tongue transplantation model in rats. Ann Plast Surg 2010;64(1):114–21.

11. Zor F, Bozkurt M, Nair D, et al. A new composite midface allotransplantation model with sensory and motor reinnervation. Transpl Int 2010;23(6): 649–56.

12. Siemionow M, Unal S, Agaoglu G, et al. A cadaver study in preparation for facial allograft transplantation in humans: part I. What are alternative sources for total facial defect coverage? Plast Reconstr Surg 2006;117:864–72 [discussion: 873–5].

13. Siemionow M, Agaoglu G, Unal S. A cadaver study in preparation for facial allograft transplantation in humans: part II. Mock facial transplantation. Plast Reconstr Surg 2006;117:876–85 [discussion: 886–8].

14. Siemionow M, Agaoglu G. The issue of "facial appearance and identity transfer" after mock transplantation: a cadaver study in preparation for facial allograft transplantation in humans. J Reconstr Microsurg 2006;22:329–34.

15. Siemionow M, Papay F, Kulahci Y, et al. Coronalposterior approach for face/scalp flap harvesting in preparation for face transplantation. J Reconstr Microsurg 2006;22:399–405.

16. Dubernard JM, Owen E, Herzberg G, et al. Human hand allograft: report on first 6 months. Lancet 1999;353:1315–20.

17. Devauchelle B, Badet L, Lengelé B, et al. First human face allograft: early report. Lancet 2006; 368:203–9.

18. Guo S, Han Y, Zhang X, et al. Human facial allotransplantation: a 2-year follow-up study. Lancet 2008; 372:631–8.

19. Lantieri L, Meningaud JP, Grimbert P, et al. Repair of the lower and middle parts of the face by composite tissue allotransplantation in a patient with massive plexiform neurofibroma: a 1-year follow-up study. Lancet 2008;372:639–45.

20. Dubernard JM, Lengele B, Morelon E, et al. Outcomes 18 months after the first human partial face transplantation. N Engl J Med 2007;357:2451–60.

21. Meningaud JP, Paraskevas A, Ingallina F, et al. Face transplant graft procurement: a preclinical and clinical study. Plast Reconstr Surg 2008;122:1383–9.

22. Chenggang Y, Yan H, Xudong Z, et al. Some issues in facial transplantation. Am J Transplant 2008;8: 2169–72.

23. Siemionow M, Papay F, Alam D. Near-total human face transplantation for a severely disfigured patient in the USA. Lancet 2009;374:203–9.

24. Alam DS, Papay F, Djohan R, et al. The technical and anatomical aspects of the World's first near-total human face and maxilla transplant. Arch Facial Plast Surg 2009;11(6):369–77.

25. Siemionow MZ, Papay F, Djohan R, et al. First U.S. near-total human face transplantation: a paradigm shift for massive complex injuries. Plast Reconstr Surg 2010;125(1):111–22.

26. World's fifth face transplant: man gets new nose, mouth and chin after shooting accident. The Telegraph Web site. Available at: http://www.telegraph.co.uk/scienceandtechnology/science/sciencenews/5063195/Worlds-fifth-face-transplant-Man-gets-new-nose-mouth-and-chin-after-shooting-accident.html. Accessed June 15, 2009.

27. Surgery News: world's 6th face transplant performed in Paris and 7th in Boston this week: second face transplant in United States. MSNBC Web site. Available at: http://surgery.about.com/b/2009/04/12/surgery-news-worlds-6th-face-transplant-performed-second-face-transplant-inunited-states.htm. Accessed June 18, 2009.

28. Boston Hospital performs face transplant. MSNBC Web site. Available at: http://www.msnbc.msn.com/id/30152143/. Accessed June 15, 2009.

29. Face-and-hands transplant patient dies. MSNBC Web site. Available at: http://www.msnbc.msn.com/id/31367511/. Accessed June 20, 2009.

30. Partial face transplant patient goes public in Spain. USA Today Web site. Available at: http://www.usatoday.com/news/health/2010-05-04-face-transplant_N.htm. Accessed June 11, 2010.

31. First Full-Face transplant claimed in Spain. CBS News Web site. Available at: http://www.cbsnews.com/stories/2010/04/23/health/main6425492.shtml. Accessed June 9, 2010.

32. Chinese face-transplant recipient has died. www.scientificamerican.com web site. Available at: http://www.scientificamerican.com/blog/post.cfm id=chinese-face-transplant-recipient-h-2008-12-22. Accessed August 20, 2012.

33. Knott PD, Hicks D, Braun W, et al. A 12-year perspective on the world's first total laryngeal transplant. Transplantation 2011;91(7):804–5.

34. Delaere P, Vranckx P, Verleden G, et al. Tracheal allotransplantation after withdrawal of immunosuppressive therapy. N Engl J Med 2010;362(2): 138–45.

35. Selvaggi G, Levi DM, Cipriani R, et al. Abdominal wall transplantation: surgical and immunologic aspects. Transplant Proc 2009;41(2):521–2.

36. Morris P, Bradley A, Doyal L, et al. Face transplantation: a review of the technical, immunological, psychological and clinical issues with recommendations for good practice. Transplantation 2007;83:109–28.

37. Gazarian A, Abrahamyan DO, Petruzzo P, et al. Hand allografts: experience from Lyon team. Ann Chir Plast Esthet 2008;144:424–35.

38. Ravindra KV, Buell JF, Kaufman CL, et al. Hand transplantation in the United States: experience with 3 patients. Surgery 2008;144:638–43 [discussion: 643–4].

39. Breidenbach WC, Gonzales NR, Kaufman CL, et al. Outcomes of the first 2 American hand transplants at 8 and 6 years posttransplant. J Hand Surg Am 2008; 33:1037–47.

40. Infection kills face transplant patient. The Washington Times. Available at: http://washingtontimes.com/news/2009/jun/16/infection-kills-face-transplant-patient/. Accessed June 17, 2009.

41. Lantieri L, Hivelin M, Audard V, et al. Feasibility, reproducibility, risks and benefits of face transplantation: a prospective study of outcomes. Am J Transplant 2011;11(2):367–78.

Surgical Advances in Burn and Reconstructive Plastic Surgery
New and Emerging Technologies

Mayer Tenenhaus, MD[a,*], Hans-Oliver Rennekampff, MD[b]

KEYWORDS

- Burn reconstruction • Wound healing • Scars • Epithelialization

KEY POINTS

- Desiccated wounds and wounds exposed to air exhibit a reduced electrical potential. Electrical stimulation mimics the current of injury, in effect restarting or accelerating re-epithelialization and the wound healing process. The use of wireless microcurrent stimulation (WMCS) uses the current-carrying capacity of charged gas molecules, oxygen and nitrogen, to donate electrons to the wound field, transferring a charge to the wound via the air without having to touch or pierce either the wound or surrounding skin.
- The ReCell (Avita Medical, Cambridge, UK) kit is based on well-established laboratory techniques of trypsinization, cell separation, and filtration. Because no cell cultivation is necessary with this technique, the product is available for use in the operating room during the skin transplantation operation (on-site techniques and 1-step individualized regenerative medicine).

INTRODUCTION

Burn and reconstructive plastic surgeons today are faced with an ever-expanding range of life-threatening and complex wound types, each with its own specific pathophysiological features, qualities, and presentations. As experience and expertise evolve, so have new technologies. In this article, the authors introduce and discuss several modalities that are being tested or used in clinical practice to optimize wound bed preparation, effect soft tissue coverage, and improve the quality of the inevitable and resultant scar. Several of these treatment modalities have only recently been introduced to clinical practice and, as such, long-term results may not be available. Every effort has been made to accurately present and reflect these limitations.

WOUND BED PREPARATION
Wireless Microcurrent Stimulation

Although first reported more than 150 years ago, the application of electrical field therapy to facilitate wound healing has, over the past decade, experienced a resurgence of interest. Based on several newer clinical reports and the development of noninvasive and better-engineered hardware, this technology may show promise in wound healing and is currently being tested in Europe. This technology and its potential clinical application are founded on the appreciation of existent electrical currents in both intact as well as wounded skin. Skin, depending on which area of the body is tested, possesses an electrical field of between 10 mV and 60 mV. Cell membranes possess

Conflict of interest statement: None of the authors has any financial interest whatsoever in any of the techniques or instruments mentioned in this article.

[a] Division of Plastic and Reconstructive Surgery, University of California San Diego Medical Center, 200 West, Arbor Drive, #8890, San Diego, CA 92103, USA; [b] Department of Plastic, Hand and Reconstructive Surgery, Hannover Medical School, Carl Neubergstrasse 1, 3025 Hanover, Germany
* Corresponding author.
E-mail address: m.tenenhaus@sbcglobal.net

a membrane potential, a reflection of the electrical potential difference or voltage across the membrane. Cells within intact skin are negatively charged interiorly whereas the exterior of the cell, the extracellular space, is positively charged. The difference in charge arises because cell membranes possess active and passive pumps that move sodium ions out of the cell in exchange for potassium ions, which are pumped into the cell. For the skin, this results in the epidermis being negatively charged relative to the deeper tissues, which carry a positive charge.[1] When wounded and the epidermal barriers are disrupted, the skin battery is short-circuited and an outward current of approximately 30 $\mu A/cm^2$ is generated and can be measured at the wound edge. Since the early 1990s, many reports have described this effect at both the tissue aand cellular levels and applications for wound healing have been proposed.[2–5]

Electrical currents stimulate several cell activities (eg, DNA synthesis, cell proliferation, cell migration, synthesis of the extracellular matrix, collagen, expression of growth factors, and receptors) depending on the cell type.[5,6] When wounding occurs, a weak negatively charged electric field establishes between the skin and underlying tissues, termed the *current of injury*. It is thought that this current persists until the skin defect is repaired and that the healing process is interrupted if the current ceases. Desiccated wounds and wounds that are exposed to air exhibit a reduced electrical potential. Electrical stimulation mimics the current of injury, in effect restarting or accelerating re-epithelialization and the wound healing process.[7]

Electrical stimulation in wound healing is defined as the use of an electrical current to transfer energy to a wound. Studies of stimulation current effects on wound healing using a porcine model identified direct current stimulation as most effective in wound area reduction.[2] Until recently, potential clinical application of these currents required using invasive transcutaneous methods of transferring current through wet electrolytic contact with the external skin surface and the wound bed, 2 electrodes having been required to complete the electric circuit.[2]

A newer method is available that uses the current-carrying capacity of charged gas molecules, oxygen and nitrogen, to donate electrons to the wound field (**Fig. 1**). This method is known as wireless microcurrent stimulation (WMCS). In so doing, a charge can be transferred to the wound via the air without having to touch or pierce either the wound or surrounding skin, resulting in the current of injury measurable by an amp meter. If a weak direct current electric field is applied to

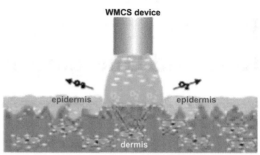

Fig. 1. The unit used to produce the O_2^--induced current in the body is a WMCS device, shown diagrammatically in the figure in a typical exposure situation. The flow of O_2^- molecules from the unit is directed toward the target (the patient), which is isolated from the ground. The target is connected back to the WMCS device through a control box that records the exposure rate and the total exposure or the charge passing through the body.

the atmosphere, the naturally produced N_2^+ and O_2^- move, the former in the direction of the field and the latter in the opposite direction. If the field strength exceeds a certain value, which at atmospheric pressure is approximately 3×10^6 V m^{-1} (3 MV/m, the breakdown field strength), a few free electrons can be accelerated to high velocities and energies, so that they can knock electrons from the oxygen and nitrogen molecules, creating more positive and negative molecules. If an O_2^- molecule lands on a conductive surface (like the skin), it gives up its negative charge, ceases to exist as an O_2^- molecule, and turns into an oxygen molecule and a few water molecules, a process termed *plate-out*. In this process the plated-out O_2^- induces a current in the wound cells and fluids whereas O_2^- never enters the body. In so doing, this novel approach creates a current of injury via a noninvasive electrical field that can potentially cover the total surface area of the wound (see **Fig. 1**).

In the authors' burn center in Germany, WMCS is currently applied in an effort to accelerate the healing of burns wounds. A 1.5-μA current is applied as the present therapeutic basis, and all treatments are performed in sessions of 60 minutes/day per target area (**Fig. 2**). The return path is connected by either a wrist or ankle strap. Preliminarily the authors have found this modality easy to apply and the noninvasive, noncontact mode of application likely minimizes the risk of bacterial contamination and local trauma. Early results with this technology seem to show measurable improvement in the rate of early re-epithelialization in partial-thickness injuries; further study is under way.

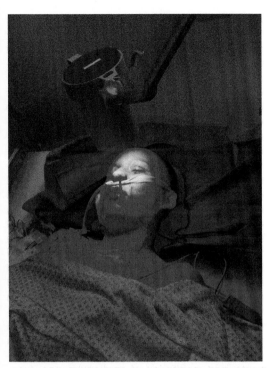

Fig. 2. The Wetland Unit in use for treatment of partial-thickness burn to the face; notice red/orange light, which indicates region of interest.

Extracorporeal Shock Waves for Burn Wound Healing

Over the past several years there has been an increasing body of literature addressing the use of extracorporeal shock waves (ESWs) for healing of a variety of wound types, cellulite, and Dupuytren contracture. Several of these articles describe its use in a subset of burn wounds. In a recent article, the University of Barcelona burn unit prospectively examined its use in the treatment of 15 patients who suffered burn wounds deemed at least deep partial thickness in depth as determined by laser Doppler assessment. Wounds were treated in the emergency department on day 3 and again on day 5 postinjury. Although 1 patient was lost to follow-up and 2 patients required skin grafting, the rest healed well without surgery. Low pain scores were noted during treatment and there was a 5% incidence of hypertrophic scarring.[8] Ottomann and colleagues[9] investigated the effect of ESWs on wound healing in partial-thickness wounds and donor sites. In a prospective randomized trial, a group from Berlin compared time to heal after SWT with 100 impulses/cm^2 at 0.1 mJ/mm^2 to donor sites. The investigators noticed a significantly faster (2 days) healing. In a phase II trial with 50 patients with partial-thickness wounds a similar effect with significantly accelerated wound healing

was noticed.[10] The investigators concluded that a larger phase III trial is warranted.

ESW therapy (ESWT) is based on acoustic wave energy source. The exact mechanism of action of ESWT is at present ill defined.[11] Many hypotheses with regard to mechanisms of action have been reported, ranging from its modulation of free oxygen radical, to decreasing apoptotic rates, and to increasing the expression of heat shock proteins as well as promotion of various growth factors, including transforming growth factor (TGF)-β1 and insulinlike growth factor 1. The latter two effects, the promotion of transforming growth factor (TGF)-β1 and insulin like growth factor 1 perhaps explain the low incidence of problem scar formation noted.[12,13] Experimentally ESWT has been shown to stimulate angiogenesis and increase perfusion to ischemic tissues by increasing vascular endothelial growth factor[14] while diminishing early proinflammatory immune response to deep burn injury in mice.[15] Although promising, this form of therapy is in its infancy. Shock wave therapy is currently being evaluated by the Food and Drug Administration and is in phase III trials for diabetic foot ulcers.

Laser for Wound Bed Preparation

Laser (light amplification by stimulated emission of radiation) modalities have been promoted over the past decades as a method to effect controllable excisional débridement of various wound types with the potential additional benefit of decreasing bacterial burden in the wound. Early attempts using carbon dioxide (CO_2) ablative lasers for burn wound excision and débridement proved slow and costly and incurred a measure of additional thermal injury, significantly limiting its adoption for general use in burn care. A more positive experience, however, was published in 1999 by Dr Robert L. Sheridan and colleagues,[16] who described their experience with the use of laser ablation in the treatment of 21 children who suffered full-thickness burns. The full-thickness wounds were ablated using continuous-wave CO_2 laser system and immediately autografted. The results were compared with controls. Endpoints included engraftment at 7 days and serial Vancouver assessments of scarring. They identified no problems with bleeding and engraftment rates averaged 94.7% ± 3.5% in the control sites and 94.7% ± 3.3% in the study sites ($P = 1.0$). No significant difference was noted in Vancouver Scar Scale scores at an average follow-up of 32.0 ± 5.2 weeks.

Recent publications using animal models of cutaneous chemical injury have also demonstrated efficacy by delivery energy patterns, which incur less residual or surrounding thermal damage. Most promising among them is probably the erbium:yttrium-aluminum-garnet (Er:YAG) laser. Reported benefits are of improved control of depth of excision and/or débridement, allowing differential control to the papillary or upper reticular layers of skin. Accelerated rates of wound healing are suggested but ill defined in several animal studies and thought to result from decreases in bioburden in the wound as well as potential mitogenic effect of low-energy laser stimulation.[17] A clinical case report was published in 2003 by Reynolds N et al in the journal, *Burns*, describes a single case of mixed partial-thickness and full-thickness burns to the foot successfully managed with the use of an Er:YAG laser. It seems likely that with increasing availability and evolving experience, newer forms of laser energy delivery systems may bring this technology to the forefront of clinical practice for use in acute burn wound management.

Hydrotherapy with Carbon Dioxide for Wound Healing

Balneotherapy, derived from the Latin *balneum* (bath), has been advocated for the management of various diseases and wound types since at least biblical times. Near continuous hydrotherapy over days was emphasized by Passavant and von Hebra[18] in the mid-nineteenth century for burn wound treatment and in many centers today hydrotherapy remains a mainstay in burn treatment, with the caveat that meticulous sanitary attention to equipment and microbial surveillance are maintained to prevent infectious colonization and cross-contamination. Hydrotherapy is generally used during the initial cleansing of a patient and facilitates a minimally traumatic débridement of loose necrotic tissue during the wound healing process while affording a measure of pain relief resulting from warm water immersion. Additional therapeutic effects can be expected by the addition of different salts or CO_2 in high concentrations to the water.[19]

Various studies have demonstrated a positive effect of CO_2 on microcirculatory parameters of the skin.[20–22] Karagülle and colleagues[23] reported that immersion into mineral water containing 3500 mg/L CO_2 for 16 minutes increased skin microcirculatory values by 2-fold. Pain threshold levels were unaffected by CO_2 compared with controls.

Further investigations revealed that thermoneutral baths with a CO_2 concentration of greater than 500 mg/L led to a vasodilatation in the skin resulting from precapillary arteriolar dilatation with subsequently improved transcutaneous partial oxygen pressure. A prolonged improvement of the cutaneous microcirculation was recorded for up to 60 minutes post-treatment. A similar effect on the microcirculation of the skin is also observed in dry CO_2 bath where skin areas or extremities are immersed in high concentrations of CO_2 gas (without water). The authors have demonstrated a positive prolonged effect on cutaneous blood flow as measured by laser Doppler imaging. Although the application of CO_2 hydrotherapy has previously been used for the treatment of critically decreased limb perfusion and complex regional pain syndrome,[24] Werner and colleagues[20] investigated the effect of CO_2 on chronic wounds and demonstrated improved healing. Recently, the authors have begun to use this technique in an effort to improve burn wound healing. In the authors' center, a patient's wound is immersed into warm water saturated with 500 mg/L CO_2 for 30 minutes. Extremity wounds can be immersed in water containing CO_2 or, alternatively, invested occlusively in a bag, which is then filled with CO_2 gas for 30 minutes (**Fig. 3**). Caution must be taken with cardiopulmonary unstable patients, and monitoring of cardiopulmonary function is strongly recommended for these patients. The authors hypothesize that the positive effect on microcirculation improves the overall healing process and improves re-epithelialization in skin-grafted wounds, which manifested some measure of graft loss. Preliminary observational evidence suggests that wounds can be improved with this technique. Controlled randomized studies are necessary, however, to demonstrate the positive effect on re-epithelialization of partial-thickness wounds as well as potential salvage of the zone of stasis. In any case, the authors currently consider hydrotherapy with additional CO_2 a helpful adjunct for wound healing.

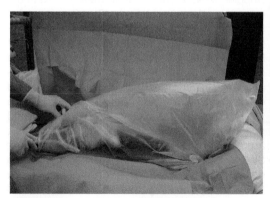

Fig. 3. Lower extremity immersed in high concentrations of CO_2 gas in a sealed plastic bag.

PROMOTION OF EPITHELIALIZATION AND WOUND CLOSURE USING EPIDERMAL CELL SUSPENSION—RECELL

In cases of deep dermal and full-thickness wounds, skin loss is often marked by short-term and long-term complications, such as scar formation, with hypertrophy, contracture, and scar instability. Time to heal classically correlates with the predictability and extent of scar formation. Although conventional split-thickness skin grafts (STSGs) provide wound closure, grafted wound sites often result in unsightly scars, particularly when widely expanded or when the donor skin is procured from texturally and pigmentary dissimilar sites. Anatomically, the skin is made up of 2 layers, the epidermis and the dermis, with its incorporated cell types. The epidermis consists of a cornified epithelium primarily composed of keratinocytes and a significantly (40-times) smaller proportion of melanocytes.

Cultured epithelial autograft sheets (CEAs), first used in the early 1980s for clinically significant burn wounds, were shown to be lifesaving adjuncts at promoting wound closure.[25] Although lifesaving, the use of CEAs is costly and requires lengthy periods of delay whereas biopsies and cell cultures mature and propagate until sufficient product can be made and delivered. Tragically, take rates of these grafts have been variable, and scarring and durability issues remain problematic.

Because re-epithelialization is dependent on the keratinocyte stem cell's ability to form holoclones,[26] it was hypothesized that single cells on a wound would be sufficient for subsequent re-epithelialization. The application of cultured keratinocytes in a fibrin glue suspension is reported by Hundyadi and many other investigators,[27] who documented successful re-epitheliazation of deep partial-thickness and full-thickness wounds. A modification of this application developed by Wood and coworkers[28] in Western Australia has led to a commercially available product that produces a keratinocyte suspension, which can be prepared on site in the operation room (ReCell). The inventor as well as other burn surgeons have presented data that re-epithelialization can be expedited with the use of this technology. Wood and colleagues[28] have shown that a cell suspension obtained with this technology consists of 1.7×10^6 cells/cm^2 harvested skin consisting of approximately 65% keratinocytes, 30% fibroblasts, and 3.5% melanocytes, differentiating itself from standard CEAs, which consist of nearly only keratinocyctes. This difference in content with pigmented cells and fibroblasts cell populations may account for the repigmentation observed with this grafting technology compared with a pure keratinocyte graft. It is also well reported that fibroblasts from the donor area have a strong impact on the final pigmentation.[29] The ReCell technique is currently promoted for both skin re-epithelialization and for the treatment of posttraumatic hypopigmentation.

The ReCell kit is based on well-established laboratory techniques of trypsinization, cell separation, and filtration (**Fig. 4**). Because no cell cultivation is necessary with this technique, the product is available for use in the operating room during the skin transplantation operation (on-site techniques and 1-step individualized regenerative medicine).

To prepare the epidermal cell suspension, a surgeon harvests an STSG with a thickness of 0.2 mm to 0.3 mm. The ratio of area of harvest to treatment area is described as 1:80. One kit produces enough cell suspension to cover approximately a 2% total body surface treatment area. The skin biopsy is placed in a heated trypsinization solution for approximately 20 to 30 minutes. The epidermal cell layer and the dermis are then separated and persistent keratinocytes on the dermis are scraped off while the dermis is discarded. The epidermis is then further minced, the cells separated, and the cell slurry filtered. A cell suspension graft can then be applied to the wound. A spray apparatus with a nozzle supplied in the ReCell kit creates a fine cell suspension spray.

Although other burn surgeons have used this technology in conjunction with STSGs and for expediting donor site healing, the authors have used this technology for deep dermal facial burns and have recently started using ReCell for dyspigmentated burn scars of the face. The authors cover the sprayed wound with either Biobrane or Suprathel, a caprolacton-based material. The authors have previously demonstrated that both materials are noncytotoxic for both keratinocytes and fibroblasts, allowing for good adherence,

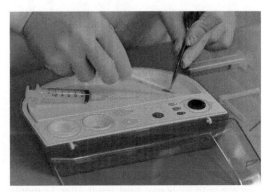

Fig. 4. ReCell kit: separation of STSG after trypsinization.

cellular proliferation, and wound bed protection. The dressing material separates in 10 to 14 days postapplication. The authors have seen favorable results with ReCell application in patients with patch-like acid burns where skin grafts wound have given unsightly results (**Fig. 5**). In these deep wounds, resultant scarring after ReCell treatment was favorable as measured by the Vancouver Scar Scale.

As in every skin grafting operation, complications include donor morbidity as well as wound infection, which can result in complete cell loss. In the authors' hands, results in full-thickness wounds, which were solely treated with a cell

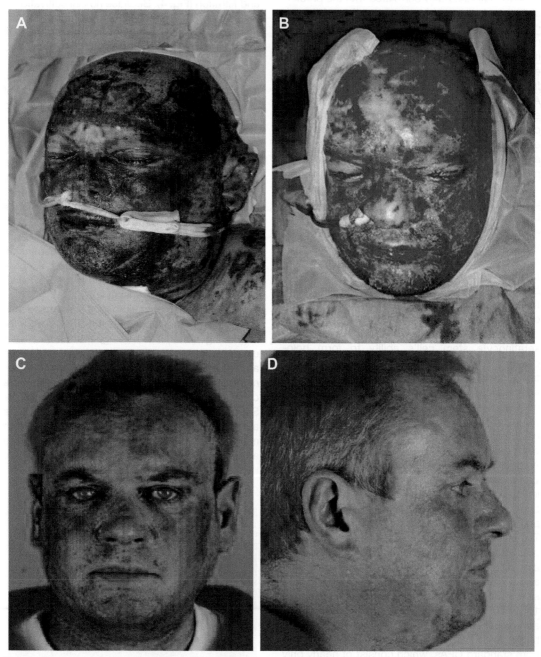

Fig. 5. Severe acid burn to the face (*A*) with subsequent débridement (*B*), ReCell application, and wound coverage with Biobrane; final result after 12 months (*C, D*). (*Data from* Herold J, Busche M, Vogt PM, et al. Autologe nichtkultivierte Keratinozytensuspension in der Verbrennungschirurgie—Indikationen und Anwendungstechniken. GMS Verbrennungsmedizin 2011;4:Doc03.)

suspension, remain disappointing, probably a result of reduced take rates when dermal bonding and integrity are lost. Further experiments are needed to demonstrate and compare early adherence of noncultured cells to culture stimulated keratinocytes, because the latter have different adhesion receptors compared with nonactivated cells.

SCAR MODIFICATION
Medical Needling—Percutaneous Collagen Induction for Scar Improvement

The ideal scar improvement modality would improve dermal matrix fiber orientation and collagen contents and a normalization of the ratio of collagen isotypes. Furthermore, the epidermis should remain intact and epidermal thickness improved. Growth factor release should favor dermal regeneration rather than scar formation. Newer therapeutic interventions have attempted to preserve the epidermis either completely or partially as in nonablative and ablative fractional laser treatment. The same principle of scar improvement applies to a procedure, termed *medical needling* or *collagen induction therapy.*

Percutaneous collagen induction by medical needling results from the natural response to multiple fine wounds in the skin. Ferguson[30] described that such minimal (tattoo) wounding does not lead to a scarring process. Bleeding is minimal and the inflammatory phase moderate. This seems to favor a predominantly TGF-β3 release rather than a strong TGF-β1 and TGF-β2 secretion, the latter associated with scarring. Building on this principle, specialized tools are now commercially available, which use rows of needles ranging in length between 1 mm and 3 mm, to achieve scar penetration (**Fig. 6**).

As in other scar improvement techniques, pretreatment of the skin is initiated. A cocktail of antioxidants and cytoprotectants, such as vitamins A, C, and E or other skin nourishing compounds, are topically applied to the skin and the scar site, pretreated for several weeks. These topical agents can be further propelled intradermally by other means, such as iontophoreses. Medical needling for scar treatment is done under general or local anesthesia with a roller. By rolling backward and forward with some pressure in alternating directions, a ratio of approximately 250 holes/cm^2 is achieved (**Fig. 7**). Postneedling meticulous skin care with washing and application of topical compounds is performed. A bruised appearance is visible for up to 1 week.

Aust and colleagues[31] investigated the results of medical needling in patients with postburn scars.

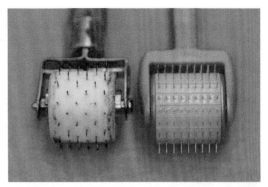

Fig. 6. A variety of devices are available for medical needling with length of needles between 2.2 mm and 3 mm.

The investigators reported a significant improvement in patient satisfaction as measured by the Patient and Observer Scar Assessment Scale. A similar beneficial effect was recently reported by Moortgart and colleagues from Belgium at the International Scar Club Meeting at Montpellier. In the authors' practice, medical needling is performed for those areas where other surgical modalities, like serial excision or skin expansion, with subsequent removal of the scarred area are not possible or when a patient is not willing to consent to such procedures (**Fig. 8**). Medical needling can be repeated after 3 to 4 months as needed. Complications include wound infection and local herpes simplex reactivation.

Laser for Scar Modification

There has been a resurgence of interest in the application of laser modalities for scar modification, no doubt resulting from the wide use and availability of Fraxel laser technology. Fraxel technology removes or addresses fractions of skin,

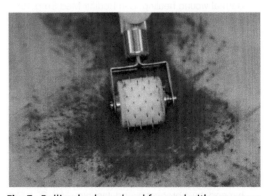

Fig. 7. Rolling backward and forward with some pressure in alternating directions, numerous microholes are made in the scarred tissue. Bleeding and subsequent inflammation are minimal.

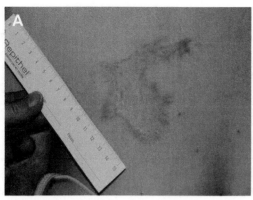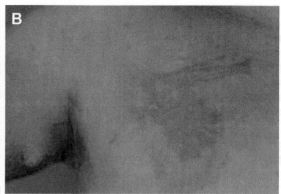

Fig. 8. Medical needling was performed on resultant scar after partial-thickness burn. (*A*) Pre-needling, right 6-month postneedling (*B*).

leaving behind intervening sections of normal skin, which can then repair the adjoining treated areas. In so doing, many of the complications often associated with pure ablative technologies can potentially be minimized.

Combining superficial ablative with nonablative modalities in conjunction with the topical application of cytoprotective and anti-inflammatory agents is showing promise in both evolving studies as well as in clinical practice. The ability to promote organized collagen deposition while facilitating transcutaneous intralesional delivery of medications may prove an ever more efficient therapeutic regimen for treating problem scars.

REFERENCES

1. Jaffe LF, Vanable JW. Electric fields and wounds healing. Clin Dermatol 1984;2:34–44.
2. Bogie KM, Reger SI, Levine SP, et al. Electrical stimulation for pressure sore prevention and wound healing. Assist Technol 2000;12:50–66.
3. Gentzkow GD, Miller KH. Electrical stimulation for dermal wound healing. Clin Podiatr Med Surg 1991; 8:827–41.
4. Kloth LC, McCulloch JM. Promotion of wound healing with electrical stimulation. Adv Wound Care 1996;9:42–5.
5. Biedebach MC. Accelerated healing of skin ulcers by electrical stimulation and the intracellular physiological mechanisms involved. Acupunct Electrother Res 1989;14:43–60.
6. Zhao M, Dick A, Forrester J, et al. Electric field-directed cell motility involves up-regulated expression and asymmetric redistribution of the epidermal growth factor receptors and is enhanced by fibronectin and laminin. Mol Biol Cell 1999;10:1259–76.
7. Fleischli JG, Laughlin TJ. Electrical stimulation in wound healing. J Foot Ankle Surg 1997;36:457–61.
8. Arnó A, Garcia O, Hernan I, et al. Extracorporeal shock waves, a new non-surgical method to treat severe burns. Burns 2010;36:844–9.
9. Ottomann C, Hartmann B, Tyler J, et al. A prospective randomized trial of accelerated re-epithelization of skin graft donor sites using extracorporeal shock wave therapy. J Am Coll Surg 2010;211: 361–7.
10. Ottomann C, Stojadinovic A, Lavin PT, et al. Prospective randomized phase II Trial of accelerated reepithelialization of superficial second-degree burn wounds using extracorporeal shock wave therapy. Ann Surg 2012;255:23–9.
11. Meirer R, Kamelger FS, Huemer GM, et al. Extracorporal shock wave may enhance skin flap survival in an animal model. Br J Plast Surg 2005;58:53–7.
12. Chen YJ, Wang CJ, Yang KD, et al. Extracorporeal shock waves promote healing of collagenase-induced Achilles tendinitis and increase TGF-β1 and IGF-I expression. J Orthop Res 2004;22:854–61.
13. Meirer R, Brunner A, Deibl M, et al. Shock wave therapy reduces necrotic flap zones and induces VEGF expression in animal epigastric skin flap model. J Reconstr Microsurg 2007;23:231–6.
14. Wang CJ, Wang FS, Yang KD, et al. Shock wave therapy induces neovascularization at the tendon-bone junction: a study in rabbits. J Orthop Res 2003;21:984–9.
15. Davis TA, Stojadinovic A, Amare K, et al. Extracorporeal shock wave therapy suppresses the acute early proinflammatory immune response to a severe cutaneous burn injury. Int Wound J 2009;6:11–21.
16. Reynolds N, Cawrse N, Burge T, et al. Debridement of a mixed partial and full thickness burn with an erbium:YAG laser. Burns 2003;29:183–8.
17. Lam DG, Rice P, Brown RF. The treatment of Lewisite burns with laser debridement—"lasablation." Burns 2002;28:19–25.
18. von Hebra CF. Ueber die kontinuierlichen allgemeinen Baeder und deren Anwendung bei der

Behandlung von Verbrennungen. Wiener Med Zeitung 1861;6:351–3.

19. Groenroos M, Pertovaara A. A selective suppression of human pain sensitivity by carbon dioxide: central mechanisms implicated. Eur J Appl Physiol Occup Physiol 1994;68:74–9.

20. Schnizer W, Erdl R, Schoeps P, et al. The effects of external CO_2 application in human skin microcirculation investigated by laser doppler flowmeter. Int J Microcirc Clin Exp 1985;4:343–50.

21. Werner GT, Gadomski M, Wehle F. Kohlensäurebäder in der Behandlung chronischer, schlecht heilender Wunden. Z Phys Med Baln Med Klim 1990; 19:52–6 [in German].

22. Fink M, Heisler C, Candir F, et al. Untersuchungen für die Wirkungen von CO2-Gasbädern von unterschiedlicher Temperatur und Feuchte auf Hautdurchblutung und transkutan gemessenen Sauerstoffpartialdruck. Phys Rehab Kur Med 2001;11: 23–7 [in German].

23. Karaguelle O, Canir F, Kalinin J, et al. Akutwirkung kalter Co2 Teilbäder auf Mikrozirkulation und Schmerzempfindlichkeit. Phys MEd Rehab Kuror 2004;14:13–7 [in German].

24. Hartmann B, Drews B, Kuerten B, et al. Increase in skin microcirculation and oxygen tension and improved venous function in patients with combined arterial and venous circulatory disorders of the leg during and following lower leg immersion in water containing carbon dioxide. Vasa Suppl 1991;32:258–60.

25. Gallico GG, O'Connor NE, Compton CC, et al. Permanent coverage of large burn wounds with autologous cultured human epithelium. N Engl J Med 1984;311:448–51.

26. Barrandon Y, Green H. Three clonal types of keratinocytes with different capacities for multiplication. Proc Natl Acad Sci U S A 1987;84:2302–6.

27. Hundyadi J, Farkas B, Bertenyi C, et al. Keratinocyte grfating:new means of transplantation for full thickness wounds. J Dermatol Surg Oncol 1988;14:75–8.

28. Wood FM, Giles N, Stevenson A, et al. Characterisation of the cell suspension harvested fromm the dermal epidermal junction using a ReCell kit. Burns 2012;38:44–51.

29. Yamaguchi Y, Morita A, Maeda A, et al. Regulation of skin pigmentation and thickness by Dickkopf 1 (DKK1). J Investig Dermatol Symp Proc 2009;14: 73–5.

30. Ferguson MW. Scar-free healing: from embryonic mechanisms to adult therapeutic intervention. Philos Trans R Soc Lond B Biol Sci 2004;359:839–50.

31. Aust MC, Knobloch K, Reimers K, et al. Percutaneous collagen induction therapy: an alternative treatment for burn scars. Burns 2010;36:836–43.

New Concepts and Technologies in Reconstructive Hand Surgery

Taliah Schmitt, MD*, John Talley, MD, James Chang, MD

KEYWORDS

- Hand trauma • Tissue engineering • Microvascular anastomosis • Nerve repair

KEY POINTS

- The induced membrane, or Masquelet technique, has great potential in managing bone defects.
- Tendon tissue engineering is a an innovative solution for repairing extensive tendon deficits.
- Fibrin glue, laser activated chitosan, end-to-side neurorrhaphy, and nerve conduits are used for peripheral nerve repair, along with more novel and untested approaches of nerve regeneration with molecular and cell therapy.
- Sutureless anastomosis, a combination of Food and Drug Administration–approved thermoreversible poloxamer gel and cyanoacrylate glue is in use for microvascular anastomosis.
- Botulinum toxin may become a promising treatment of Raynaud syndrome.
- A dynamic stress-shielding polymer device is effective in reducing scar formation.

INTRODUCTION

In 1944, the pioneer hand surgeon, Sterling Bunnell, described the specialty in these words, "As the problem in hand surgery is composite, the surgeon must also be. There is no shortcut. The surgeon must face the situation and equip himself to handle any and all of the tissues in a limb."[1] Nearly 70 years later, this principle remains the same, but innovations in all composite tissues of the hand have given the hand surgeon advantages that did not previously exist. Concepts and technologies in reconstructive hand surgery continue to evolve, improving patient outcome and surgeon ease. Intelligently designed devices, bioengineered tissues, allografts, and tissue substitutes will soon be available. The systematic method by which perform finger replantation is performed, from bony fixation to skin closure, provides a platform for discussion of the newest innovations available to reconstructive hand surgeons.

BONE

Problem: Bone Reconstruction in Severely Mutilated Digits or Septic Conditions

High-energy trauma or osteomyelitis can lead to complex composite defects in fingers with extensive bone loss. When the finger can be salvaged, bone stabilization becomes the first step of the reconstruction. However, there is often a deficit of bone tissue required for adequate reconstruction. Classic solutions include the use of bone grafts or vascularized bone grafts to fill the bone defect. However, these procedures are not

Funding: No external funding was used in the preparation of this article manuscript.
Disclosure: The authors have no financial interests or conflicts to disclose.
Division of Plastic & Reconstructive Surgery, Department of Surgery, Stanford University Hospital & Clinics, 770 Welch Road, Suite 400, Palo Alto, CA 94304, USA
* Corresponding author.
E-mail address: DrTSchmitt@gmail.com

Clin Plastic Surg 39 (2012) 445–451
http://dx.doi.org/10.1016/j.cps.2012.07.013
0094-1298/12/$ – see front matter © 2012 Elsevier Inc. All rights reserved.

practical in the context of emergency hand situations in which salvage is the primary goal.

Innovative Solution

Initially described by Masquelet and Begue[2] for large diaphyseal bone defects caused by tumor resection, trauma, or osteoarthritis, the induced membrane technique is a two-stage procedure allowing bone reconstruction. The concept is to place space-maintaining material in the region of the defect. This leads to a foreign body reaction, which creates a membrane mimicking the periosteum. Once this is formed, bone graft can be placed in the periosteal sleeve. Recently, Flamans and colleagues[3] applied the Masquelet technique to the hand with promising results.

The first stage involves soft tissue and bone debridement followed by implantation of a polymethyl methacrylate cement spacer in the area of the bone deficit and/or defect. Bone stabilization is then provided with internal and/or external fixation. Soft tissue defects may need to be addressed with free flap coverage.

The second stage is performed 2 months later. The periosteal membrane is incised and the spacer is removed. Autologous cancellous bone graft is placed within the membrane.

The results in the hand are from studies with small numbers but are promising. There are over 15 other studies investigating this technique in bone reconstruction outside the hand.[4–7]

Clinical results in the literature
For clinical results in the literature, see **Table 1**.

Advantages
The membrane induced by the Masquelet technique has been shown to secrete vascular endothelial growth factor, transforming growth factor beta-1, and bone morphogenetic protein-2. Therefore, it has more than a mechanical role—it induces angiogenesis and proliferation of osteoblasts and chondrocytes. Bone graft substitutes, such as hydroxyapatite or tricalcium phosphate, can be used instead or in addition to autologous cancellous bone grafts to increase osteoconduction.

Complications
Nonunion and infections have been noted. However, it is not clear at this time whether this technique has an increased rate of complications over other techniques of reconstruction in these complex cases. Loss of function and finger stiffness is also a risk, but this is often inherently due to the infection or trauma. Overall, the technique is simple and easy to perform. This technique can be used for reconstructive problems of the hand in which vascularized bone graft and flaps are not viable options.

TENDONS
Problem: the Need for More Tendon Graft Material

Tendons are essential to hand function and are frequently involved in hand injuries. When tendon deficits exist, the current solution is to harvest expendable autologous tendon grafts (ie, palmaris, plantaris) or use tendon allograft. However, the extrasynovial nature of these tendons increases the resulting adhesions at the repair sites and often leads to a suboptimal functional outcome.[8]

Innovative Solution

Tendon tissue engineering may be a future solution in cases requiring extensive tendon reconstruction. Neotendons would ideally have the capacity to reduce adhesions and have adequate tensile strength, allowing early active rehabilitation and normal mobility.

Bioengineered tendon constructs first consist of a scaffold—natural or synthetic.[9] Some hand surgeons choose to follow Gillies' reconstructive principle of replacing "like with like" and use decellularized human tendon scaffolds[10] from a donor bank. Other surgeons choose collagen derivatives,[11] polysaccharides, small intestine submucosa,[12] or human umbilical veins[13] as natural scaffolds; whereas the synthetic scaffold uses polymers such as poly(a-hydroxyl acid)s, polylactic acid,[14] or polypropylene. The ideal candidate remains to be decided. Natural scaffolds have the advantage of a high affinity to host cells

Table 1
Summary of the available clinical results of the Masquelet technique in hand surgery

Study	N	Cause of Bone Defect	Results	Complications
Flamans et al[3]	11	Trauma (n = 8) Infection (n = 3)	Bone union rate 82%	2 Nonunion
Proubasta et al[49]	1	Osteomyelitis	Bone union	None

allowing tissue ingrowth, but they theoretically are associated with potential risks such as disease transmission. Synthetic scaffolds have the advantage of being free of disease transmission and are easier to manufacture on a large scale. Being synthetic, however, results in less binding with the host's cells and, therefore, less tissue proliferation. In addition, both types of scaffolds are subject to rejection (immunologic or foreign body reaction). Considerable research is underway, dedicated to creating the ideal tendon scaffold to meet the requirements of biodegradability, biocompatibility, superior mechanical properties, and optimal processing.

The second aspect of tissue-engineered tendon constructs is the addition of cells with regenerative and differentiation potential that can be used to seed these scaffolds. Several lines of cells have been studied, such as tenocytes,[15,16] adipose-derived stem cells,[17] bone marrow stromal cells,[18,19] and fibroblasts. No significant differences were found between these four cell types in their ability to populate the scaffold.[20] To date, it is unclear whether reseeding improves the biomechanical properties of these constructs.

The third area of focus includes strategies to further enhance in vivo regeneration and incorporation of tissue-engineered tendons. The most promising concepts include growth factor supplementation,[21,22] mechanical stimuli,[17,23,24] and contact guidance.

NERVE
Problem: Peripheral Nerve Repair

Peripheral nerve injuries are common and 60% of these are reported to occur in the upper extremities.[25] The current gold standard procedure for managing such injuries is a tensionless end-to-end nerve repair. When the defect is so great that an end-to-end suture will create tension, an autologous nerve graft is performed, creating donor site morbidity and uncertain outcomes depending on the host site vascularization and the level at which the injury occurs. The need for peripheral nerve repair and regeneration strategies is, therefore, high on the priority list in research.

Innovative Solutions

Many strategies have been tested, such as sutureless nerve repair using fibrin glue,[26] laser activated chitosan,[27] and end-to-side neurorrhaphy.[28] Nerve conduits are also a popular solution for segmental nerve defects of up to 3 cm[29] and have been studied since as early as the late nineteenth century. Different types of conduits exist from biologic (eg, vein, arteries) to synthetic materials (eg, collagen, caprolactone, polyglycolic acid), giving promising results in small series studies. However, randomized studies of a larger scale are needed. Brooks and colleagues[30] report the clinical outcome of 132 nerve injuries in a multicenter study for processed nerve allografts with recovery and safety comparable to autografts and better than nerve conduits.

The latest development in nerve regeneration is molecular and cell therapy. The goal is to augment allografts or conduits by adding cells to lower immunogenicity and increase nerve regeneration. Several types of constructs combining allografts or synthetic conduits with cells have been tested, such as adipose-derived stem cells,[31] bone marrow–derived stem cells, Schwann cells, or (more recently) dorsal root ganglion cells.[32] However, all of these combinations are still in the early stages of experimentation.

VESSELS
Problem: the Tedium of Multiple Microvascular Anastomoses

Since Carrel pioneered vascular surgery in the early twentieth century, many techniques have been described to allow suturing of increasingly smaller vessels in a minimal amount of time. Although patency and reliability are indispensable and still achieved in technically challenging anastomoses using round-bodied needles and fine monofilament nylon sutures, the need for increased efficiency and minimal manipulation of small vessels continues to stimulate new technologies.

Several devices are currently used as alternatives to classic sutures, such as couplers (Unilink-3M [3M Healthcare, St. Paul, MN]) or clips (VCS [VCS; LeMaitre Vascular, Boston, MA], U-clip [Medtronic, Inc, Minneapolis, MN]) with outcomes evidence supporting their use.[33] Although these devices reduce the time of the procedure considerably, they remain traumatic for the vessels and can cause foreign body reactions. Their use in digits can also cause the specific problem of foreign body sensation. Other technologies, such as adhesive (eg, cyanoacrylate, fibrin glue) or laser and photochemical bonding, have been tested. However, none of them has proven superior to hand-sewn anastomosis in terms of reliability.

An ideal microvascular anastomotic technique should be fast, atraumatic for the vessel, and easily reproducible in even the smallest vessels. A new sutureless technique described by the Gurtner laboratory[34] may be a promising solution to this common microsurgical problem.

Innovative Solution

A new technique, sutureless anastomosis, uses the combination of Food and Drug Administration–approved thermoreversible poloxamer gel and cyanoacrylate glue.

Indications
Indications include:

- Microvascular anastomosis on vessels as small as 0.5 mm
- End-to-end or end-to-side anastomosis.

Surgical technique
The surgical technique is:

- The poloxamer gel is introduced into the lumens of both ends of the vessel.
- A heating source is then used to create a temperature of 40°C, at which point the gel becomes solid.
- Vessels are approximated and cyanoacrylate applied at the junction to perform the sutureless anastomosis.
- The heating source is removed, allowing the poloxamer to return to its liquid phase and dissolve, leaving the vessel patent.

Clinical results in the literature
Clinical results in the literature include:

- 2-year follow-up, control group of hand-sewn anastomoses in rat model only
- Equivalent patency, flow and burst strength
- Sutureless anastomoses were performed five times faster than hand-sewn anastomoses
- Decreased inflammation and fibrosis at 2 years
- Efficient in small vessels smaller than 1 mm.

Advantages
This technique is reproducible, more efficient, and seems to have less long-term inflammation than the gold standard hand-sewn anastomoses. In addition, it allows patent reconstruction of smaller vessels making it particularly valuable in hand surgery.

Complications
The main disadvantage is the initial foreign body reaction caused by the use of cyanoacrylate glue. However, the inflammation does not seem to be persistent.

Another potential complication is the transmission of diseases through the albumin-based poloxamer; however, albumin-free gels with the same properties are currently being developed.

This innovation awaits translation to human clinical cases.

Problem: Distal Ischemia Caused by Raynaud Phenomenon

Plastic surgeons are occasionally confronted by Raynaud phenomenon in extremities. A variety of vasospastic disorders, including connective tissue or autoimmune diseases, are responsible for this problem. A myriad of medical treatments have been tested to ease the intolerable pain or reduce the vasospasm of these ischemic digits without great success. Surgical techniques are limited to wound management of distal ulceration, sympathectomy and/or adventiectomy, distal vascular bypass, and, finally, amputation of necrotic fingers.

Innovative Solution: Botulinum Toxin A Injections

A few studies in the literature have evaluated the use of botulinum toxin[35–41] for the treatment of Raynaud syndrome with the aim of reducing vasocclusive pain, improving vascular inflow, and healing ulcers in Raynaud fingers. Even though these studies lack controls and include a wide variety of patients (ie, different underlying diseases, variable severity), they all suggest that botulinum toxin may become a promising treatment of these disorders. As summarized by Mannava and colleagues,[36] "Based on preclinical data and limited case series, the palmar injection of botulinum toxins has been described to treat refractory Raynaud phenomenon with nonhealing ulcers or pre-gangrene."

The mechanism through which the toxin improves the finger's perfusion and alleviates pain is still unexplained and is likely more complex than just the expected induced vasodilatation. The need for better clinical trials including standardized injection procedures and controls is necessary.

Indication
The indication is ischemic digits.

Surgical procedure
No standardized procedure has been reported yet, but the technique usually involves:

- Targeted injection around each neurovascular bundle and superficial palmar arch
- Average of 100 units per hand
- Evaluation of tissue perfusion with Doppler.

Clinical results in the literature
For clinical results in the literature, see **Table 2**.

Table 2
Summary of available clinical results of botulinum toxin injections in ischemic digits

Study	N	Type	Volume Injected	Results	Complications (Temporary)
Sycha et al[38]	2	Prospective	1–10 U per digit	Pain improved Stiffness improved	None
Van Beek et al[40]	11	Prospective	100 U per hand	Pain 100% improved Ulcers 100% healed	Intrinsic weakness
Fregene et al[35]	26	Retrospective	10–100 U per hand	Pain 75% improved Color 56% improved Ulcer 48% healed	Intrinsic weakness dysesthesia
Neumeister et al[39]	19	Retrospective	50–100 U per hand	Pain 84% improved Ulcer 100% improved	Intrinsic weakness
Neumeister[37]	33	Retrospective	100 U per hand	Pain 85% improved Ulcers 100% improved	Intrinsic weakness
Smith et al[50]	1	Case report	100 U per hand	Pain improved Ulcers 88% improved	Thenar weakness

Advantages

This nonsurgical treatment holds great potential for patients suffering from vasocclusive pain and recurrent ulcers. It is noninvasive and represents an attempt to salvage severely ischemic fingers otherwise at risk for necrosis and amputation.

SKIN
Problem: Postoperative Scar Management

Wound healing can result in hypertrophic scar or keloid formation, including after hand trauma and elective hand surgery. The result of the scarring can be more problematic in hands because it has the potential to compromise range of motion and resulting hand function. Any incision made in the hand, even if it is made in a manner to release or prevent scar contracture, has the potential to still create functional impairment if scar formation is excessive.

Many technologies are already commercially available to reduce postoperative scarring, such as silicone, tapes, or ointments; however, none of these have been proven in outcomes studies to be truly effective.[42–44]

Innovative Solution

Gurtner and colleagues[45] recently hypothesized that scar formation was directly correlated to its mechanical environment. This group designed a new device to reduce the mechanical stress on healing wounds and, therefore, prevent pathologic scarring. This dynamic stress-shielding device is a flexible transparent sheet of polymer that adheres to the outer layer of the wounded skin. The sheet is prestrained and contracts when applied on the skin, producing a 20% compressive stress shielding effect.

Indication

The indication is postoperative incisions.

Surgical technique

The surgical technique is: application of the prestrained polymer sheet on the closed wound in the fashion of a dressing.

Clinical results in the literature

Although there are no series in hand surgery, a Phase 1 study has been completed in a series of subjects who have undergone elective abdominoplasty. In this study, half of each postoperative scar was treated with the new stress-shielding device. The results of the trial show significantly reduced scarring of the area treated with the polymer sheet, which confirmed similar results of a recent study in swine.

Advantages

Ease of use and versatility are the main assets of the stress-shielding device, which could revolutionize postoperative wound care. The cost-effectiveness of the device remains to be determined.

Complications

No complications were described in the Phase 1 study.

SUMMARY

Hand surgery is a demanding discipline requiring significant technical expertise and the ability to work effectively with the many different component tissues. The concepts and innovations presented here are in addition to recent efforts in hand allotransplantation,[46] novel neural interfaces,[47] and composite tissue regeneration[48] that have been discussed elsewhere. Researchers continue to discover new concepts and technologies that have the potential to repair, regenerate, and restore the hand. These current advances may lead to even more innovations in the dynamic field of hand surgery.

REFERENCES

1. Bunnell S. Bunnell's surgery of the hand. Philadelphia, PA, U.S.A: J. B. Lippincott Company; 1970.
2. Masquelet AC, Begue T. The concept of induced membrane for reconstruction of long bone defects. Orthop Clin North Am 2010;41(1):27–37 table of contents.
3. Flamans B, Pauchot J, Petite H, et al. Use of the induced membrane technique for the treatment of bone defects in the hand or wrist, in emergency. Chir Main 2010;29(5):307–14 [in French].
4. Powerski M, Maier B, Frank J, et al. Treatment of severe osteitis after elastic intramedullary nailing of a radial bone shaft fracture by using cancellous bone graft in Masquelet technique in a 13-year-old adolescent girl. J Pediatr Surg 2009;44(8):e17–9.
5. Apard T, Bigorre N, Cronier P, et al. Two-stage reconstruction of post-traumatic segmental tibia bone loss with nailing. Orthop Traumatol Surg Res 2010;96(5):549–53.
6. Largey A, Faline A, Hebrard W, et al. Management of massive traumatic compound defects of the foot. Orthop Traumatol Surg Res 2009;95(4):301–4.
7. Gouron R, Deroussen F, Juvet M, et al. Early resection of congenital pseudarthrosis of the tibia and successful reconstruction using the Masquelet technique. J Bone Joint Surg Br 2011;93(4):552–4.
8. Seiler JG 3rd, Chu CR, Amiel D, et al. The Marshall R. Urist Young Investigator Award. Autogenous flexor tendon grafts. Biologic mechanisms for incorporation. Clin Orthop Relat Res 1997;(345):239–47.
9. Longo UG, Lamberti A, Petrillo S, et al. Scaffolds in tendon tissue engineering. Stem Cells Int 2012; 2012:1–12.
10. Pridgen BC, Woon CY, Kim M, et al. Flexor tendon tissue engineering: acellularization of human flexor tendons with preservation of biomechanical properties and biocompatibility. Tissue Eng Part C Methods 2011;17(8):819–28.
11. Caliari SR, Ramirez MA, Harley BA. The development of collagen-GAG scaffold-membrane composites for tendon tissue engineering. Biomaterials 2011;32(34):8990–8.
12. Murphy KD, Mushkudiani IA, Kao D, et al. Successful incorporation of tissue-engineered porcine small-intestinal submucosa as substitute flexor tendon graft is mediated by elevated TGF-beta1 expression in the rabbit. J Hand Surg Am 2008;33(7):1168–78.
13. Abousleiman RI, Reyes Y, McFetridge P, et al. Tendon tissue engineering using cell-seeded umbilical veins cultured in a mechanical stimulator. Tissue Eng Part A 2009;15(4):787–95.
14. Vaquette C, Slimani S, Kahn CJF, et al. A poly(lactic-co-glycolic acid) knitted scaffold for tendon tissue engineering: an in vitro and in vivo study. J Biomater Sci Polym Ed 2010;21(13):1737–60.
15. Zhang AY, Bates SJ, Morrow E, et al. Tissue-engineered intrasynovial tendons: optimization of acellularization and seeding. J Rehabil Res Dev 2009; 46(4):489–98.
16. Chong AK, Riboh J, Smith RL, et al. Flexor tendon tissue engineering: acellularized and reseeded tendon constructs. Plast Reconstr Surg 2009; 123(6):1759–66.
17. Angelidis IK, Thorfinn J, Connolly ID, et al. Tissue engineering of flexor tendons: the effect of a tissue bioreactor on adipoderived stem cell-seeded and fibroblast-seeded tendon constructs. J Hand Surg Am 2010;35(9):1466–72.
18. Omae H, Zhao C, Sun YL, et al. Multilayer tendon slices seeded with bone marrow stromal cells: a novel composite for tendon engineering. J Orthop Res 2009;27(7):937–42.
19. Yokoya S, Mochizuki Y, Natsu K, et al. Rotator cuff regeneration using a bioabsorbable material with bone marrow-derived mesenchymal stem cells in a rabbit model. Am J Sports Med 2012 Jun;40(6): 1259–68.
20. Kryger GS, Chong AK, Costa M, et al. A comparison of tenocytes and mesenchymal stem cells for use in flexor tendon tissue engineering. J Hand Surg Am 2007;32(5):597–605.
21. Costa MA, Wu C, Pham BV, et al. Tissue engineering of flexor tendons: optimization of tenocyte proliferation using growth factor supplementation. Tissue Eng 2006;12(7):1937–43.
22. Raghavan SS, Woon CY, Kraus A, et al. Optimization of human tendon tissue engineering: synergistic effects of growth factors for use in tendon scaffold repopulation. Plast Reconstr Surg 2012;129(2): 479–89.
23. Woon CY, Kraus A, Raghavan SS, et al. Three-dimensional-construct bioreactor conditioning in human tendon tissue engineering. Tissue Eng Part A 2011;17(19–20):2561–72.
24. Riboh J, Chong AK, Pham H, et al. Optimization of flexor tendon tissue engineering with a cyclic strain bioreactor. J Hand Surg Am 2008;33(8): 1388–96.
25. Chimutengwende Gordon M, Khan W. Recent advances and developments in neural repair and regeneration for hand surgery. Open Orthop J 2012;6:103–7.

26. Moy OJ, Peimer CA, Koniuch MP, et al. Fibrin seal adhesive, versus nonabsorbable microsuture in peripheral nerve repair. J Hand Surg Am 1988; 13(2):273–8.

27. Lauto A, Foster LJ, Avolio A, et al. Sutureless nerve repair with laser-activated chitosan adhesive: a pilot in vivo study. Photomed Laser Surg 2008;26(3):227–34.

28. Fernandez E, Lauretti L, Tufo T, et al. End-to-side nerve neurorrhaphy: critical appraisal of experimental and clinical data. Acta Neurochir Suppl 2007;100:77–84.

29. Deal DN, Griffin JW, Hogan MV. Nerve conduits for nerve repair or reconstruction. J Am Acad Orthop Surg 2012;20(2):63–8.

30. Brooks DN, Weber RV, Chao JD, et al. Processed nerve allografts for peripheral nerve reconstruction: a multicenter study of utilization and outcomes in sensory, mixed, and motor nerve reconstructions, processed nerve allografts for peripheral nerve reconstruction: a multicenter study of utilization and outcomes in sensory, mixed, and motor nerve reconstructions. Microsurgery 2012;32(1):1–14.

31. Wang Y, Zhao Z, Ren Z, et al. Recellularized nerve allografts with differentiated mesenchymal stem cells promote peripheral nerve regeneration. Neurosci Lett 2012;514(1):96–101.

32. Liu W, Ren Y, Bossert A, et al. Allotransplanted neurons used to repair peripheral nerve injury do not elicit overt immunogenicity. PLoS One 2012;7(2):e31675.

33. Pratt GF, Rozen WM, Westwood A, et al. Technology-assisted and sutureless microvascular anastomoses: evidence for current techniques. Microsurgery 2012; 32(1):68–76.

34. Chang EI, Galvez MG, Glotzbach JP, et al. Vascular anastomosis using controlled phase transitions in poloxamer gels. Nat Med 2011;17(9):1147–52.

35. Fregene A, Ditmars D, Siddiqui A. Botulinum toxin type A: a treatment option for digital ischemia in patients with Raynaud's phenomenon. J Hand Surg Am 2009;34(3):446–52.

36. Mannava S, Plate JF, Stone AV, et al. Recent advances for the management of Raynaud phenomenon using botulinum neurotoxin A. J Hand Surg Am 2011;36(10):1708–10.

37. Neumeister MW. Botulinum toxin type A in the treatment of Raynaud's phenomenon. J Hand Surg Am 2010;35(12):2085–92.

38. Sycha T, Graninger M, Auff E, et al. Botulinum toxin in the treatment of Raynaud's phenomenon: a pilot study. Eur J Clin Invest 2004;34(4):312–3.

39. Neumeister MW, Chambers CB, Herron MS, et al. Botox therapy for ischemic digits. Plast Reconstr Surg 2009;124(1):191–201.

40. Van Beek AL, Lim PK, Gear AJ, et al. Management of vasospastic disorders with botulinum toxin A. Plast Reconstr Surg 2007;119(1):217–26.

41. Iorio ML, Masden DL, Higgins JP. Botulinum toxin A treatment of Raynaud's phenomenon: a review. Semin Arthritis Rheum 2012;41(4):599–603.

42. Tollefson TT, Kamangar F, Aminpour S, et al. Comparison of effectiveness of silicone gel sheeting with microporous paper tape in the prevention of hypertrophic scarring in a rabbit model. Arch Facial Plast Surg 2011;14(1):45–51.

43. Tziotzios C, Profyris C, Sterling J. Cutaneous scarring: pathophysiology, molecular mechanisms, and scar reduction therapeutics: part II. Strategies to reduce scar formation after dermatologic procedures. J Am Acad Dermatol 2012;66(1):13–24.

44. Morganroth P, Wilmot AC, Miller C. Over-the-counter scar products for postsurgical patients: disparities between online advertised benefits and evidence regarding efficacy. J Am Acad Dermatol 2009; 61(6):e31–47.

45. Gurtner GC, Dauskardt RH, Wong VW, et al. Improving cutaneous scar formation by controlling the mechanical environment: large animal and phase I studies. Ann Surg 2011;254(2):217–25.

46. Shores JT, Imbriglia JE, Lee WP. The current state of hand transplantation. J Hand Surg Am 2011;36(11): 1862–7.

47. O'Doherty JE, Lebedev MA, Ifft PJ, et al. Active tactile exploration using a brain-machine-brain interface. Nature 2011;479(7372):228–31.

48. Rinkevich Y, Lindau P, Ueno H, et al. Germ-layer and lineage-restricted stem/progenitors regenerate the mouse digit tip. Nature 2011;476(7361):409–13.

49. Proubasta IR, Itarte JP, Lamas CG, et al. The spacer block technique in osteomyelitis of the phalangeal bones of the hand. Acta Orthop Belg 2004;70(2): 162–5.

50. Smith L, Polsky D, Franks AG. Botulinum toxin-A for the treatment of Raynaud syndrome. Arch Dermatol 2012;148(4):426–8.

Adipocyte-Derived Stem and Regenerative Cells in Facial Rejuvenation

Steven R. Cohen, MD[a,b,c,*], Brian Mailey, MD[a]

KEYWORDS

- Adipocyte • Stem cells • Regenerative • Facial aging • Fat graft • Revolumization

KEY POINTS

- Current methods of producing cell-enriched fat include isolating adipose-derived regenerative cells (ADRC) using a commercial collagenase enzymatic digestive system and then recombining the isolated cells with traditional lipoaspirated fat.
- Cell-enriched fat should be delivered in small concentrated aliquots of fat per unit area of native tissue to optimize engraftment. Initial reports using these methods demonstrate promising results for multiple applications.
- A key to optimizing engraftment includes concentrating the fat per unit volume of graft delivered per area of native tissue in the correct proportions to maximize the surface area of grafted fat and prevent large clumpy deposits.
- The exact fate and regenerative effects of autotransplanted ADRC are still unknown and much work still needs to be done.

OVERVIEW: NATURE OF THE PROBLEM

Autologous fat grafting is a minimally invasive technique for multiple applications in facial aesthetic and reconstructive surgery.[1–3] Fat has been described as the ideal filler.[2] It is biocompatible, versatile, long lasting, and has a natural appearance. Since the first use of fat for soft tissue augmentation in 1893 by Neuber,[4] investigators have noted the variable long-term outcomes. In 1950, Peer and colleagues[5] histologically evaluated fat grafts and found approximately 45% volume survival at 1 year after implantation. More recent investigators report up to 70% of the initial fat-filling tissue volume being reabsorbed.[6,7]

Today, fat grafting is part of the plastic surgeon's repertoire and is considered a primary technique in facial aesthetic, aesthetic breast, and reconstructive surgery.[2,8–11] Meticulous technique greatly influences outcomes, as exact attention to detail is crucial.[2] A key to optimizing engraftment includes concentrating the fat per unit volume of graft delivered per area of native tissue in the correct proportions. This maximizes the surface area of grafted fat and prevents large clumpy deposits. Other techniques to maximize host tissue surface area and provide maximum nutritional support to the implanted graft include

1. using methods that ensure harvested cells are viable
2. processing away the debris of fat, such as blood and fatty acids
3. using a microdroplet delivery technique

Disclosures: Dr Cohen serves as a consultant and advisor for Cytori Therapeutics, Inc and as consultant for Sound Surgical, Inc He and his family have no stock in any of these companies.
[a] Division of Plastic and Reconstructive Surgery, Department of Surgery, University of California, 200 W. Arbor Drive, San Diego, CA 92103, USA; [b] Craniofacial Surgery, Rady Children's Hospital, 3020 Childrens Way, San Diego, CA 92123, USA; [c] Private Practice, FACES+ Plastic Surgery, Skin and Laser, 4510 Executive Drive, San Diego, CA 92121, USA
* Corresponding author. Suite 200, FACS 4510 Executive Drive, San Diego, CA 92121, USA.
E-mail address: scohen@facesplus.com

plasticsurgery.theclinics.com

These techniques provide a blood supply to the fat cells and are important components of successful fat grafting.

A recent paradigm shift in facial plastic surgery and breast surgery occurred to include large-volume fat grafting.[12,13] The introduction of large-volume grafting provided a new independent option for total facial rejuvenation or breast augmentation. Similar to other descriptions, our preferred techniques have evolved from injection of discrete wrinkles and filling folds to using fat for total facial revolumization; fat is clay in the plastic surgeon's hands and can be used in virtually any application.

The recent surge in popularity is not the first time that fat has appeared as a natural all-purpose filler.[1] For many surgeons, fat has cycled in popularity. Some found fat frustrating to use with extremely variable outcomes causing many to completely abandon the technique.[1] However, innovators such as Sydney Coleman and Mel Bircholl persisted in using fat transfer as a primary surgical tool to treat many types of aesthetic and reconstructive cases and developed methods to achieve consistent success.[2,3]

Recent evidence demonstrating an abundance of stem and regenerative cells in adult human fat, which can be segregated and used for a wide variety of disease conditions, reinvigorated the field of fat grafting.[14,15] As with many new technologies and approaches, the use of stem and regenerative cells has been controversial for many reasons, with a lack of properly conducted scientific experiments.[16,17] The concept of harnessing our own cells and using them to fight disease or increase blood supply is a complex issue. Further complicating the issue, many have muddied the waters by publicizing the miracle of stem cell facelifts or breast augmentation. At present, the authors cannot validate the exact contribution of adding stem and regenerative cells to traditional fat grafting in relation to final outcomes.

As clinical applications using adipose-derived regenerative cells (ADRC) have been increasingly reported, there has been valid skepticism and concern about the true additive value of combining additional stem and regenerative cells with fat for use in plastic surgery. Fat alone may be sufficient as a vehicle to transports cells and the addition of ADRCs may do little to help the graft or regenerate tissues. To address concerns, the American Society of Plastic Surgeons and the American Society for Aesthetic Plastic Surgery published a joint position statement concerning stem cells.[18–20] They concluded that scientific evidence was limited with regard to both safety and efficacy. At present, it is still unknown if increasing the concentration of stem cells further amplifies the effects of traditional fat grafting. However, early indications in clinical trials[21,22] do show a tendency for increased fat survival with increased ADRC counts.[21,22] There is increasing anecdotal evidence that ADRCs perform best in hostile environments, such as radiation wounds, burns, and ischemia.

INDICATIONS FOR THERAPEUTIC OPTIONS

Applications for ADRC regenerative therapy are organized into 2 areas[20]:

1. Skin and soft tissue applications (plastic surgery)
2. Other medical specialties (cardiac, urology, and so forth)

Specific indications and clinical uses in plastic surgery range from aesthetics using cell-enriched fat transfer (CEFT) for facial rejuvenation and breast augmentation to reconstructive surgery with wound healing in chronic and radiated wounds. Other specialties, including regenerative medicine applications, consist of potential uses in many disparate fields of medicine including inflammatory bowel disease, diabetes, chronic obstructive pulmonary disease (COPD), neurologic disorders (eg, Parkinson disease, multiple sclerosis, stroke, and others), and cardiac myocyte or urothelial cell regeneration, to name a few.[11,13,23,24] A recent review published in June 2011 reported 18 ongoing clinical trials on the use of ADRCs in regenerative medicine.[23,25] One year later in July 2012, a search on www.clinicaltrials.gov for open recruiting studies with the term "adipose-derived stem cells" or "adipose-derived regenerative cells" revealed 27 trials that were actively recruiting.

Despite intense interest, there are many questions regarding the use of ADRCs in plastic surgery. Foremost, we need to know about safety. Initial studies, including the RESTORE-2 trial have demonstrated no difference in complications using cell-enriched fat versus traditional fat grafting.[26] Other reports in the literature or various commentaries have raised concerns with oncologic safety. However, to date we are unaware of any proven oncologic risk.[20] Equally important, it needs to be determined if stem cells make a true clinical difference and, if so, under what conditions? For instance, it seems ADRCs and cell-enriched fat work best in hostile environments such as radiation wounds and ischemia.[23] However, are soft tissue benefits also observed in healthy tissue when used for facial aging? Is photodamage a reversible ischemic condition induced by capillary loss and replenished by stem cells? Do ADRCs have an effect on elastin regeneration or on apoptosis? Do ADRCs regenerate tissue and increase the survival of fat grafts? Are ADRCs an amplifier for fat grafting? Are there conditions that could be treated solely with ADRCs? What might they be? The purpose of this article is to review traditional fat grafting methods and the use of fat as clay to refine the results of aesthetic and reconstructive surgery, and discuss the rationale and potential applications of adipocyte-derived stem and regenerative cells in facial surgery.

THERAPEUTIC OPTIONS
Traditional Fat Grafting Techniques

The goal of lipoharvesting is to collect small parcels of adipose tissue and/or adipose cell clusters without disturbing cell viability. Each step of the fat grafting process should be optimized. Harvesting, processing, delivery, and storage should each be evaluated on their own merits. Even then, the host and the effect of the host environment are critical determinants of success in traditional fat grafting. Once the fat has been harvested, processing is aimed at creating the purest graft possible by clearing the harvest of blood and tumescent fluid with minimal damage to fat tissue (**Fig. 1**). It is also important to control graft hydration because the residual graft fluid will be a factor when calculating the volume to be grafted resulting in less graft material delivered per unit volume. Fat grafting must minimize inflammation and promote healing.

The presence of blood, fatty acids, and other debris is believed to stimulate an inflammatory response and contribute to graft degradation.[2,3,8] Current methods of processing include centrifugation, decanting, straining, and filtration.[27] Centrifugation is the most common, but may not necessarily be the best technique. Adipocytes may be damaged by exposure to the open air; 50% cell lysis has been shown.[28,29] There are also volume/time limitations. Home-brew approaches, cheesecloth, hand cranks, float, and pluck are highly variable. Most of these are open systems and are not easily performed in a sterile field. Tissue filtration to process fat is performed in a closed system within the sterile field. It results in the least extraneous graft material and allows the user to adjust graft hydration. Decanting the fat or gravity drainage has many advocates, but does not eliminate lipid or inflammatory cells or other systems.

Delivery is performed via a Byron cannula attached to a Celbrush. The Celbrush permits small threads of fat graft to be deposited in a retrograde fashion (**Fig. 2**). For facial fat grafting, an 18-gauge needle is used to make a needle puncture in key areas such as the temporal region and lateral eyebrow, the malar region, the upper and lower eyelid, the nasolabial fold, the marionette basin, the labiomental groove, the prejowl region, the lips, the buccal fat pad, and the mandibular border (**Fig. 3**). During facelift surgery, the skin and Superficial muscular aponeurotic system (SMAS) are elevated and a transbuccal approach can be used for fat transfer. The range of total amount of

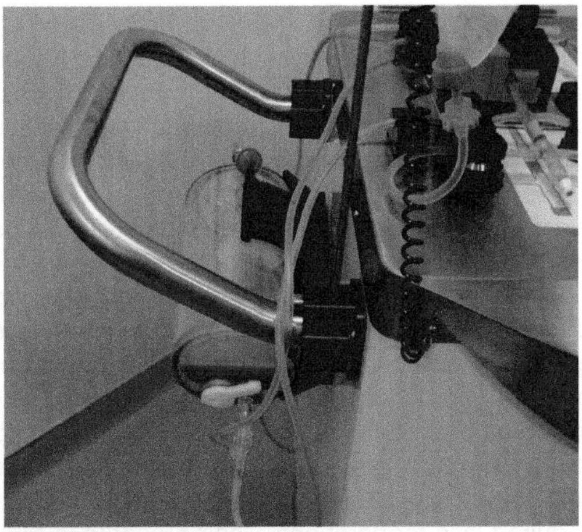

Fig. 1. Lipoharvesting is performed using a device that collects fat under sterile condition for separation and transfer without disturbing cell viability. Once the fat has been harvested, processing is aimed at creating the purest graft possible by clearing the harvest of blood and tumescent fluid with minimal damage to the fat tissue.

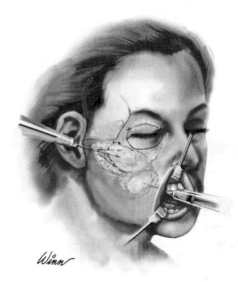

Winn

Fig. 2. Fat graft delivery is performed via a Byron cannula attached to a Celbrush. The Celbrush permits small threads of fat graft to be deposited in a retrograde fashion.

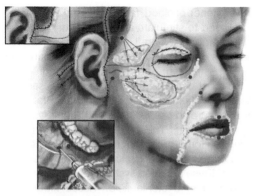

Fig. 3. An 18-gauge needle is used to make needle punctures in key areas, such as the temporal region and lateral eyebrow, the malar region, the upper and lower eyelid, the nasolabial fold, the marionette basin, the labiomental groove, the prejowl region, the lips, the buccal fat pad, and the mandibular border.

fat grafted is from about 20 mL to 200 mL in the face at a single setting.

For many surgeons, the Coleman technique of structural fat grafting, which involves centrifugation, placement of microdroplet grafts delivered by a retrograde injection technique, remains the gold standard (**Fig. 4.**).[30] Other techniques that permit larger volumes of fat to be processed such as bilaminar filtration, which shows a reduction in lipid content and inflammatory cells with excellent control of the degree of hydration, may evolve to be techniques of choice.

CEFT

Since the identification of ADRCs in fat tissue,[14] many scientists and surgeons have begun to use these cells to supplement or enrich fat grafts.[17] In

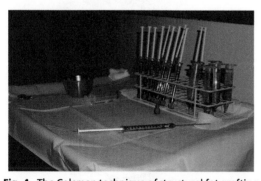

Fig. 4. The Coleman technique of structural fat grafting involves harvesting fat with a 10-mL syringe attached to a 2-hole Coleman harvesting cannula. After centrifugation and refinement, the fat is transferred to 3-mL syringes. Blunt infiltration cannulas are used to place microdroplet grafts in a retrograde fashion through 2-mm incisions. Only blunt cannulas are used, which allows for more dispersion of grafted tissue in small aliquots and reduces the chance of intravascular injection.

addition to their ability to undergo multipotent differentiation, ADRCs have been shown in vitro to express and secrete growth factors, cytokines, chemokines, and extracellular matrix molecules that are important for neovascularization, regulation of apoptosis, modulation of immune response, and extracellular matrix remodeling, and even chemokines responsible for recruitment of endogenous stem and regenerative cells.[31]

As preclinical studies of ADRCs were performed, 2 important aspects were found. First, the host environment seemed to be an important determinant of the behavior and effectiveness of ADRCs.[31] Second, the capacity of stem cells to develop in the host tissue into which they were introduced has little correlation with the functional improvement observed.[31]

ADRCs are the nonbuoyant cellular fraction derived from enzymatic digestion of adipose tissue, and include ADRCs, preadipocytes, and vessel-forming cells. It is believed that ADRCs contribute to graft survival by directly or indirectly aiding in vascularization of the graft. Preclinical work indicates improved graft survival and quality with the addition of ADRCs.[22,32] Early clinical work has not yet formally documented improved long-term graft survival. In breast surgery, ADRCs combined with fat grafting have demonstrated a low incidence of calcification and radiologic abnormalities.[33,34] Recently published studies found that cell-enriched fat grafts had better retention and more normal histology compared with traditional fat grafts.[34,35] Yoshimura and colleagues[36] found cell-enriched fat grafting for breast augmentation to be superior to the conventional techniques they had previously used.[37] Other workers in the field such as Delay and Khouri have had similar outcomes with conventional fat grafting. We have positive anecdotal experiences combining CEFT with surgical rejuvenation procedures (**Fig. 5**). This combination has become a preferred technique for us when treating patients with severe effects of photodamage.

In facial fat grafting, little data are available to determine whether CEFT is important. There is growing evidence at this point, but it is limited to a few studies. Steriodimas and colleagues[22] published an important prospective study comparing cell-enriched fat grafts with conventional fat grafts and found that patients with cell-enriched grafts required less reoperations. Their procedures took place at the same clinic and were performed by the same lead surgeon. They randomly divided 20 patients with congenital or acquired facial soft tissue defects into 2 groups: 10 were treated with autologous fat transplantation (group A; 12 to 165 mL per session, mean 78.5 mL), and the other 10

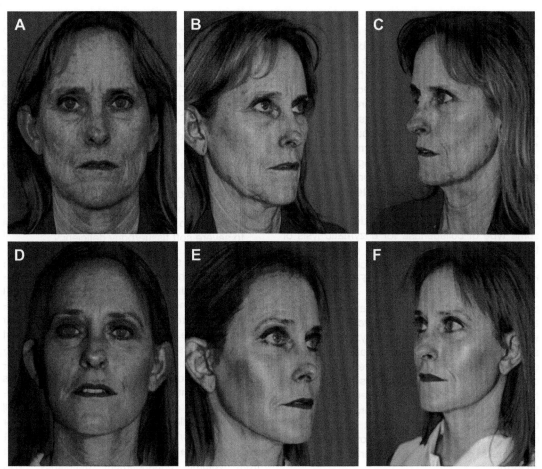

Fig. 5. An example of a patient with severe photodamage treated with a combination of cell-enriched fat grafting and surgical rejuvenation procedures. Preoperative (*A, B, C*) and 1-year postoperative photographs (*D, E, F*) after an endoscopic brow lift, upper and lower blepharoplasties, full SMAS facelift, and cell-enriched fat grafting to the cheeks, temporal regions, lips, buccal space (via transbuccal approach), and marionette basins. ADRCs were extracted from 150-mL of fat and then combined with unenriched, cleaned fat; a total of 64-mL of fat was used for injection.

were treated with ADRC-enriched lipografts (ie, CEFT) (group B; 8 to 155 mL per session, mean 74.3 mL). In group A, 30 to 400 mL of fat (mean 180 mL) were lipoaspirated; 60 to 800 mL (average 380 mL) were aspirated in group B. The patient groups were similar with regard to age, body mass index (calculated as weight in kilograms divided by the square of height in meters), smoking, and comorbidities. Patients were followed up at 6, 12, and 18 months after the initial treatment session and were asked to rate their overall satisfaction with their posttreatment facial appearance on a validated 5-point scale (1 = poor, 2 = fair, 3 = good, 4 = very good, 5 = excellent).

- In group A, 3 patients achieved aesthetically acceptable results after a single treatment, but the remaining 7 required additional sessions of autologous fat grafting; 3 had 1 additional session and 4 needed 2 additional sessions. The volume of fat graft transplanted in these extra sessions ranged from 12 to 75 mL.
- All patients in group B required only 1 treatment session.
- There was only 1 infection among the patients in group A, which was treated with 7 days of oral cefuroxime.
- Analysis of patient satisfaction in the first 6 months clearly demonstrated better results in group B. However, by the 18-month evaluation, there was no statistical difference between the 2 groups in terms of patient satisfaction.

A study performed by Peter Rubin's laboratory demonstrated a tendency for increased fat graft survival on computed tomography scans with increasing numbers of ADRCs. This work was presented at the Cell Society's Annul Meeting (Coronado, CA, 2012), but has not yet been published. Similarly, work from our group has shown positive effects using cell- enriched fat grafts. Specifically, we demonstrated patient-reported improvement in skin pigmentation and texture for patients receiving cell-enriched fat grafts during facial aesthetic surgery. No patients in our conventional fat transfer group reported any improvements in pigmentation. This unique finding has directed additional future research efforts for our laboratory.

Presently, several laboratory techniques and devices (laboratory in a box) are available for obtaining ADRCs. All current devices require some type of collagenase for enzymatic lysis of the covalent bonds that attach cells to blood vessels in the stromal vascular fraction. No device has been approved by the US Food and Drug Administration (FDA) at present. Thousands of procedures using collagenase have been done around the world for various medical applications without a single report of the enzyme causing an adverse issue. Because cell viability and cell counts are highly variable and depend not only on the type of processing but also on the host, the harvest technique, and delivery. It is critical to compare the device and laboratory yields to determine the many factors that may influence outcomes (eg, total cell count, not including red blood cells; cell function; cell performance; and so forth).

TECHNIQUES
Large-Volume Fat Augmentation During Facelift Surgery

Our preoperative patient assessment includes a facial component analysis, which evaluates skin laxity and soft tissue/bony elements. This process categorizes patients into 4 types (**Fig. 6**):

1. None to mild skin laxity and mild to severe soft tissue/bony deficiency
2. Moderate to severe facial laxity and normal soft tissue/bony volume
3. Moderate to severe facial laxity and mild to moderate soft tissue/bony deficiency
4. Moderate to severe facial laxity and moderate to severe soft tissue/bony deficiency

Patients are selected for facelifts with fat grafting only if they have appreciable facial volume deficiency, in addition to thinned cervicofacial soft tissues that show signs of downward displacement. Therefore, patients of type 3 are ideal for this procedure. Patients of type 4 may benefit from this procedure, but may also require additional alloplastic implants or osseous advancements, depending on the severity of osseous atrophy. Patients of type 2 will benefit from a facelift through fat grafting (with or without stem cell enrichment), fillers, and/or alloplastic implants, or bony framework remodeling. Patients of type 1 will not require a facelift but would likely benefit from volume enhancement deficiency. This

Type	Components Affected/Skin Laxity	Components Affected ST/ Bony Deficiency	Treatment Plan
1	None - Mild	Mild - Severe	Volume enhancement alone: Volume fillers (i.e. Sculptra, Radiesse); Fat grafting (+/- CEFT); Osseous advancement or alloplastic implants
2	Moderate - Severe	Normal	Facelift alone (mini-SMAS)
3	Moderate - Severe	Mild - Moderate	Facelift (mini, SMAS) + fat grafting (+/- CEFT)
4	Moderate - Severe	Moderate - Severe	Facelift (mini, SMAS) + fat grafting (+/- CEFT) and/or osseous advancement or alloplastic implants

Fig. 6. Our preoperative patient assessment includes a facial component analysis, which classifies patients based on skin laxity and soft tissue/bony elements. This process categorizes patients into 4 types: (1) none to mild skin laxity and mild to severe soft tissue/bony deficiency; (2) moderate to severe facial laxity and normal soft tissue/ bony volume; (3) moderate to severe facial laxity and mild to moderate soft tissue/bony deficiency; (4) moderate to severe facial laxity and moderate to severe soft tissue/bony deficiency. This system assists us in determining the combination of surgical and fat grafting procedures to provide the best results.

preoperative evaluation requires the patient to be sitting in a well-lit room where all angles of the face can be visualized. Specific areas that must be evaluated are: the forehead, brow, temporal region, upper and lower eyelids, malar, cheek (including nasojugal and nasolabial folds), angle of the mouth, upper and lower lips, chin (including marionette lines), mandibular contour, and neck. Facial symmetry should also be carefully evaluated. Based on the appearance of these areas and the junctions between them, decisions can be made for different parts of the face on whether to lift through undermining and redraping or to aim for volume enhancement through fat grafting.

In the operating room, the patient is placed in a supine position and the areas undergoing liposuction for harvesting the fat grafts are tumesced. The facelift and stab incisions for fat grafting are strategically planned in concealed places of skin rhytids or redundancy and then injected with local anesthetic. Liposuction is commenced using a 3-mm cannula and 60-mL Toomey syringe with a Johnny Lock mechanism to help maintain constant and appropriate suction pressure. If the patient elected for CEFT, part of the fat is transferred to a laboratory device that permits separation of ADRCs, for which a minimum of 100 to 120 mL of fat is required. The remaining lipoaspirate (or the full amount if the patient opted not to have the stem cell component) is then transferred to the bilaminar filtration system. This Puregraft system (Cytori Therapeutics, San Diego, CA), is a dialysis-type technique known to preserve the viability of cells through multiple wash cycles and filtrations by removing blood, free lipids, and tumescence solution. The cleansed fat is then combined with the stem cell–containing solution to create the final cell-enriched fat graft (**Fig. 7**). Nursing and operating room personnel can carry out the cleansing and combining steps while the facelift segment of the surgery is taking place. After the facelift incision is made, the skin flap is elevated with customized subcutaneous undermining, being careful not to undermine into areas that will receive fat grafts. These areas should not be undermined so that the fat can be transplanted into undisturbed tissue to ensure maximum vascularity and graft survival.

Complimentary orbitomalar suspension and surgical correction of SMAS and platysma laxity is then performed to reposition underlying tissues. The degree of SMAS undermining depends on the preoperative evaluation and planned location of fat grafting. For patients with small amounts of cheek inferior migration but significant volume loss, the SMAS may be undermined only to the level of planned fat grafting. However, in patients with significant cheek inferior migration, the SMAS and skin can be elevated in 1 unit, allowing the plane between the skin and SMAS to be left untouched and accept fat grafts (**Fig. 8**). Once the SMAS work is complete, the skin is redraped and excess tissue excised accordingly. The contralateral side is addressed in the same fashion. Finally, attention is returned to the initial side, hemostasis is ensured, and drain insertion and closure performed; this is repeated for the contralateral side.

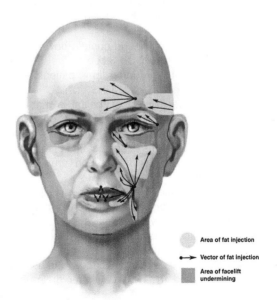

Fig. 8. The areas of surgical SMAS undermining (*purple*) and the areas left preserved for facial fat grafting (*yellow*). Areas of puncture are depicted with black dots and the vectors for cannula insertion are represented by arrows; injection is performed in a retrograde fashion.

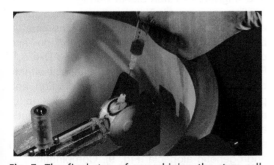

Fig. 7. The final step of recombining the stem cell–containing solution with the other fraction of cleansed lipoaspirate using a closed device. A minimum of 100–120 mL of fat is required for ADRC extraction. The remaining lipoaspirate was cleansed using a bilaminar filtration system while preserving the viability of the cells.

Fat grafting procedure

- The fat grafting part of the procedure commences with injection of local anesthetic into areas receiving fat grafts.
- Fat delivery is performed with a Celbrush instrument (Cytori Therapeutics, Inc, San Diego, CA), permitting precise placement of small aliquots of fat.
- Entry points are made with an 11-blade or an 18-gauge needle puncture and strategically positioned to permit access to various fat grafting regions and maximize the amount of fat injected through each point. The entry points are usually a few millimeters away from the border of the fat injection zone so that fat can be deposited equally throughout the zone, including at the border proximal to the injection site. Key entry points are (see **Fig. 3**)
  1. Lateral to forehead fat graft zone
  2. Lateral to temporal area fat graft zone
  3. Lateral to lateral upper eyelid fat graft zone
  4. Lateral to medial lower eyelid fat graft zone
  5. Inferior to malar/buccal fat graft zone
  6. Lateral to the corner of the mouth to access the nasolabial fold, marionette line, and corner of mouth fat graft zones
  7. In the corner of the mouth (within the vermillion) to access the upper and lower lips
  8. In the lip midline in cupid's bow (within the vermillion) to access the central portion of the upper lip in patients with long lips.
- Retrograde delivery of the fat is made in a fan-shaped pattern while withdrawing the needle (see **Fig. 2**). The amount of fat delivered and the exact location of the graft placement depend on each area being treated.
- Once the amount of fat required is injected, gentle massaging of the area is done to smooth out any irregularities.
- After each area of fat grafting is complete, a loose head dressing is applied.
- Patients are admitted overnight and usually discharged the next day after drains are gently removed.
- Postoperative care involves careful serial reevaluations, the use of arnica gel and oral arnica, and a tapering steroid dose pack if considered necessary by the treating surgeon. Lymphatic massage can be carried out.

The total volume of fat injected has ranged from 20 to 70 mL. When ADRCs are used, they are mixed with the filtered fat in at least a 1:1 ratio (for every 150 mL of fat used to process cells, 150 mL of fat are filtered). Because processing for cells may take up to 1.5 hours, lipoharvesting is performed early to ensure that the cells are ready by the time the facelift is completed.

Mesotherapeutic Applications

Mesotherapy is considered a noninvasive or minimally invasive injection of biologically active materials into the subcutaneous or subdermal tissues for skin health, rejuvenation, and fat reduction.[38,39] This technique has been long used by cosmetic practitioners in Europe and Asia, however the evidence to support its practice has not been performed. Recent studies by Kythera, the manufacturer of ATA-101, a propriety synthetic formulation of sodium deoxycholate, a well-characterized component of human bile that occurs naturally and promotes the breakdown of dietary fat are in phase III studies. Lithera, another startup company, has developed a family of mesotherapeutic agents also targeted at minimally invasive fat reduction. Lithera is entering later phase studies that might lead to FDA approval.

Mesobotox has been popularized by several clinicians to treat enlarged pores and fine wrinkles. Theoretically, the toxin works on relaxing the contraction of the muscles associated with fine lines but also in blocking neural excitation of secretory cells and the contractile components that express the secretion from halocrine glands.

The use of ADRCs may be a potential mesotherapy agent for stimulating collagen synthesis and migration of fibroblasts during the wound-healing process.[40] These effects have been evaluated in a porcine model, demonstrated by measuring growth factor production and collagen synthesis after injection of ADRCs.[40] Potentially, ADRCs may exert beneficial effects on angiogenesis and collagen production and potentially reduce aging and accumulation of abnormal elastin. In addition, mesotherapeutic applications of ADRCs have been anecdotally shown to improve hair growth in women with androgenetic alopecia (**Fig. 9**). Combinations of mesotherapeutic applications of ADRCs and lasers may prove to be beneficial in rejuvenation of skin. In addition, mesotherapeutic applications of ADRCs in scar treatment and other conditions such as periodontal disease have shown benefits.

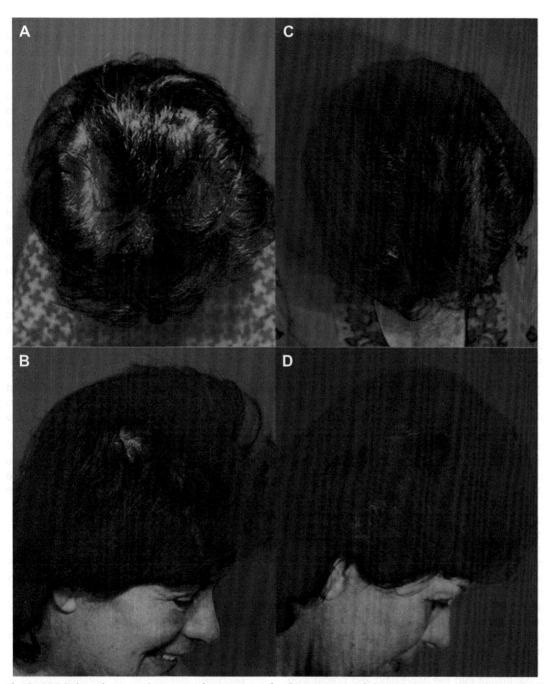

Fig. 9. ADRC's have been used as a mesotherapy agent for the treatment of alopecia. Perioperative pictures (*A, B*) of our patient before mesotherapy using ADRCs extracted from 120 mL of fat and 12-weeks postoperatively (*C, D*). In this patient, alopecia eventually recurred; this anecdotal experience requires additional investigation. ADRCs may exert beneficial effects on angiogenesis and/or collagen production. They may potentially reduce effects of aging and accumulation of abnormal elastin.

COMPLICATIONS AND CONCERNS

Complications are rare after conventional or CEFT. Fat necrosis with loss of fat graft volume can occur. Transient neuropraxia from inadvertent injury to a motor nerve has also been reported. The most common complication after fat injection to the face is clumping, especially with periocular injections. In our experience, we know of 1 instance of a severe local skin reaction from a stem cell facelift exacerbated by a mycobacterial infection. This patient suffered severe facial scarring. No systemic effects have been observed in any patient having CEFT. The immunologic and angiogenic properties of ADRC raise a potential concern that these cells may promote cancer. Anecdotal reports and some animal studies using nude mice suggest these cells could promote tumor growth.[41–45] Conversely, other reports suggest a tumor-suppressive effect of ADRCs.[46,47] Ultimately, the influence of transplanted ADRCs on tumor cells, if any exists, is still unknown.

SUMMARY

Aspirated adipose tissue consists of 2 components[24]:

1. Lipid inclusion containing adipocytes
2. Stromal cells containing a cellular compartment

Since the identification of multilineage stem cells in adult human fat was first published by Zuk and colleagues[14,15] in 2001, the stromal cells of fat have been considered to explain the differences in final graft survival.[17,36,48] However, this fact is still inconclusive. Fat stem cells maintain the ability to undergo cellular differentiation and regeneration.[24] In particular, ADRCs have the potential to differentiate into tissue types of mesenchymal origin, namely adipocytes, chondrocytes, osteoblasts, and myoblasts, depending on environmental influences.[49] The therapeutic potential of these multipotent cells have become of basic interest to many specialties of medicine and may explain variable fat graft behavior. A comparison of whole fat with lipoaspirated fat noted that whole fat contained twice the number of progenitor cells.[50] These results were explained by the fact that ADRCs are primarily located around large vessels, which are mostly left at the donor site during traditional liposuction. In addition, some ADRCs are released into the supernatant portion of the liposuction aspirates and discarded. These important findings offer additional insight into the harvesting and preparation of fat grafts, and potentially support the use of lipoaspirated fat enriched with ADRCs.

Several techniques have been attempted to achieve more consistent long-term outcomes with traditional fat grafting.[26] Many techniques focus on different processing methods before fat injection,[27] and include centrifugation to remove the nonliving components (oil, blood, water, lidocaine),[16] the use of whole fat versus suction-assisted lipectomy, processing fat with nutrients,[51] anabolic hormones, or the use of bioenhancers (eg, insulin, insulin growth factor, type 1 collagen, and so forth).[52] Despite this intense interest, a consensus for producing consistent long-term results has not been reached and no single method of graft preparation is in widespread use.

Enrichment of traditional fat grafts with ADRCs may be the method to stabilize outcomes and produce more predictable results. Over the past decade, many investigators have explored various in vitro and in vivo effects of ADRCs.[26,50,53] The inherent properties of preinjected fat (ie, adipocyte maturity, extracellular scaffold, and the presence of ADRCs) may explain some differences in fat graft behavior.[17,36] The safety and efficacy of ADRC-enriched fat grafting for soft tissue augmentation was reported in the RESTORE-2 trial, where improvements in breast defects occurred using ADRC-enriched fat grafts, with stable results at 12 months.[26] This study also concluded that volume augmentation at 6 months can be considered permanent, with continued improvement in the tissue quality over time, as measured by an increase in skin elasticity and reduction in scar tethering.[26] The emergence of commercially available devices to enrich preinjected fat with autologous ADRCs has introduced a practical way of incorporating stem cells into clinical practice. However, similar to many new technologies, regenerative cell-enriched fat has been received with both promise and skepticism. To decipher the degree of true benefit versus marketing-hype, additional studies need to be done before a scientific consensus can be reached.[26,50,53]

REFERENCES

1. Report on autologous fat transplantation. ASPRS Ad-Hoc Committee on New Procedures, September 30, 1987. Plast Surg Nurs 1987;7:140–1.
2. Coleman SR. Structural fat grafting: more than a permanent filler. Plast Reconstr Surg 2006;118:108S–20S.
3. Coleman WP 3rd. Autologous fat transplantation. Plast Reconstr Surg 1991;88:736.
4. Neuber G. Fettimplantation. Verhandlungen der Deutschen Gesellschaft fur Chirurgie 1893;22:66 [in German].
5. Peer LA, Walker JC Jr, Marzoni FA. Plastic surgery during the years 1949 and 1950. AMA Arch Otolaryngol 1951;54:560–97.
6. Niechajev I, Sevcuk O. Long-term results of fat transplantation: clinical and histologic studies. Plast Reconstr Surg 1994;94:496–506.
7. Horl HW, Feller AM, Biemer E. Technique for liposuction fat reimplantation and long-term volume evaluation by magnetic resonance imaging. Ann Plast Surg 1991;26:248–58.

8. Cervelli V, Palla L, Pascali M, et al. Autologous platelet-rich plasma mixed with purified fat graft in aesthetic plastic surgery. Aesthetic Plast Surg 2009;33:716–21.

9. Hardy TG, Joshi N, Kelly MH. Orbital volume augmentation with autologous micro-fat grafts. Ophthal Plast Reconstr Surg 2007;23:445–9.

10. Illouz YG. The fat cell "graft": a new technique to fill depressions. Plast Reconstr Surg 1986;78:122–3.

11. Phulpin B, Gangloff P, Tran N, et al. Rehabilitation of irradiated head and neck tissues by autologous fat transplantation. Plast Reconstr Surg 2009;123:1187–97.

12. Panettiere P, Accorsi D, Marchetti L, et al. Large-breast reconstruction using fat graft only after prosthetic reconstruction failure. Aesthetic Plast Surg 2011;35(5):703–8.

13. Moseley TA, Zhu M, Hedrick MH. Adipose-derived stem and progenitor cells as fillers in plastic and reconstructive surgery. Plast Reconstr Surg 2006;118:121S–8S.

14. Zuk PA, Zhu M, Mizuno H, et al. Multilineage cells from human adipose tissue: implications for cell-based therapies. Tissue Eng 2001;7:211–28.

15. Zuk PA, Zhu M, Ashjian P, et al. Human adipose tissue is a source of multipotent stem cells. Mol Biol Cell 2002;13:4279–95.

16. Kurita M, Matsumoto D, Shigeura T, et al. Influences of centrifugation on cells and tissues in liposuction aspirates: optimized centrifugation for lipotransfer and cell isolation. Plast Reconstr Surg 2008;121:1033–41 [discussion: 42–3].

17. Matsumoto D, Sato K, Gonda K, et al. Cell-assisted lipotransfer: supportive use of human adipose-derived cells for soft tissue augmentation with lipoinjection. Tissue Eng 2006;12:3375–82.

18. ASAPS/ASPS position statement on stem cells and fat grafting. Aesthet Surg J 2011;31:716–7.

19. Eaves FF 3rd, Haeck PC, Rohrich RJ. ASAPS/ASPS position statement on stem cells and fat grafting. Plast Reconstr Surg 2012;129:285–7.

20. Gir P, Oni G, Brown SA, et al. Human adipose stem cells: current clinical applications. Plast Reconstr Surg 2012;129:1277–90.

21. Brayfield C, Marra K, Rubin JP. Adipose stem cells for soft tissue regeneration. Handchir Mikrochir Plast Chir 2010;42:124–8.

22. Sterodimas A, de Faria J, Nicaretta B, et al. Autologous fat transplantation versus adipose-derived stem cell-enriched lipografts: a study. Aesthet Surg J 2011;31:682–93.

23. Tiryaki T, Findikli N, Tiryaki D. Staged stem cell-enriched tissue (SET) injections for soft tissue augmentation in hostile recipient areas: a preliminary report. Aesthetic Plast Surg 2011;35:965–71.

24. Tremolada C, Palmieri G, Ricordi C. Adipocyte transplantation and stem cells: plastic surgery meets regenerative medicine. Cell Transplant 2010;19:1217–23.

25. Lindroos B, Suuronen R, Miettinen S. The potential of adipose stem cells in regenerative medicine. Stem Cell Rev 2011;7:269–91.

26. Perez-Cano R, Vranckx JJ, Lasso JM, et al. Prospective trial of adipose-derived regenerative cell (ADRC)-enriched fat grafting for partial mastectomy defects: the RESTORE-2 trial. Eur J Surg Oncol 2012;38:382–9.

27. Smith P, Adams WP Jr, Lipschitz AH, et al. Autologous human fat grafting: effect of harvesting and preparation techniques on adipocyte graft survival. Plast Reconstr Surg 2006;117:1836–44.

28. Gonzalez AM, Lobocki C, Kelly CP, et al. An alternative method for harvest and processing fat grafts: an in vitro study of cell viability and survival. Plast Reconstr Surg 2007;120:285–94.

29. Moore JH Jr, Kolaczynski JW, Morales LM, et al. Viability of fat obtained by syringe suction lipectomy: effects of local anesthesia with lidocaine. Aesthetic Plast Surg 1995;19:335–9.

30. Coleman SR. Hand rejuvenation with structural fat grafting. Plast Reconstr Surg 2002;110:1731–44 [discussion: 45–7].

31. Strem BM, Hicok KC, Zhu M, et al. Multipotential differentiation of adipose tissue-derived stem cells. Keio J Med 2005;54:132–41.

32. Kim JH, Jung M, Kim HS, et al. Adipose-derived stem cells as a new therapeutic modality for ageing skin. Exp Dermatol 2011;20:383–7.

33. Wang L, Lu Y, Luo X, et al. Cell-assissted lipotransfer for breast augmentation: a report of 18 patients. Zhonghua Zheng Xing Wai Ke Za Zhi 2012;28:1–6 [in Chinese].

34. Kamakura T, Ito K. Autologous cell-enriched fat grafting for breast augmentation. Aesthetic Plast Surg 2011;35:1022–30.

35. Calabrese C, Orzalesi L, Casella D, et al. Breast reconstruction after nipple/areola-sparing mastectomy using cell-enhanced fat grafting. Ecancermedicalscience 2009;3:116.

36. Yoshimura K, Shigeura T, Matsumoto D, et al. Characterization of freshly isolated and cultured cells derived from the fatty and fluid portions of liposuction aspirates. J Cell Physiol 2006;208:64–76.

37. Yoshimura K, Asano Y, Aoi N, et al. Progenitor-enriched adipose tissue transplantation as rescue for breast implant complications. Breast J 2010;16:169–75.

38. Duncan D, Rubin JP, Golitz L, et al. Refinement of technique in injection lipolysis based on scientific studies and clinical evaluation. Clin Plast Surg 2009;36:195–209, v–vi [discussion: 11–3].

39. Matarasso A, Pfeifer TM. Mesotherapy and injection lipolysis. Clin Plast Surg 2009;36:181–92, v [discussion: 93].

40. Park BS, Jang KA, Sung JH, et al. Adipose-derived stem cells and their secretory factors as a promising therapy for skin aging. Dermatol Surg 2008;34:1323–6.

41. Prantl L, Muehlberg F, Navone NM, et al. Adipose tissue-derived stem cells promote prostate tumor growth. Prostate 2010;70:1709–15.

42. Zhang Y, Daquinag A, Traktuev DO, et al. White adipose tissue cells are recruited by experimental tumors and promote cancer progression in mouse models. Cancer Res 2009;69:5259–66.

43. Muehlberg FL, Song YH, Krohn A, et al. Tissue-resident stem cells promote breast cancer growth and metastasis. Carcinogenesis 2009;30:589–97.

44. Yu JM, Jun ES, Bae YC, et al. Mesenchymal stem cells derived from human adipose tissues favor tumor cell growth in vivo. Stem Cells Dev 2008;17:463–73.

45. Cousin B, Ravet E, Poglio S, et al. Adult stromal cells derived from human adipose tissue provoke pancreatic cancer cell death both in vitro and in vivo. PLoS One 2009;4:e6278.

46. Grisendi G, Bussolari R, Cafarelli L, et al. Adipose-derived mesenchymal stem cells as stable source of tumor necrosis factor-related apoptosis-inducing ligand delivery for cancer therapy. Cancer Res 2010;70:3718–29.

47. Kucerova L, Altanerova V, Matuskova M, et al. Adipose tissue-derived human mesenchymal stem cells mediated prodrug cancer gene therapy. Cancer Res 2007;67:6304–13.

48. Mojallal A, Lequeux C, Shipkov C, et al. Stem cells, mature adipocytes, and extracellular scaffold: what does each contribute to fat graft survival? Aesthetic Plast Surg 2011;35(6):1061–72.

49. Yamada T, Akamatsu H, Hasegawa S, et al. Age-related changes of p75 neurotrophin receptor-positive adipose-derived stem cells. J Dermatol Sci 2010;58:36–42.

50. Yoshimura K, Sato K, Aoi N, et al. Cell-assisted lipotransfer for cosmetic breast augmentation: supportive use of adipose-derived stem/stromal cells. Aesthetic Plast Surg 2008;32:48–55 [discussion: 6–7].

51. Salgarello M, Visconti G, Rusciani A. Breast fat grafting with platelet-rich plasma: a comparative clinical study and current state of the art. Plast Reconstr Surg 2011;127:2176–85.

52. Matsumoto D, Shigeura T, Sato K, et al. Influences of preservation at various temperatures on liposuction aspirates. Plast Reconstr Surg 2007;120:1510–7.

53. Zhu M, Zhou Z, Chen Y, et al. Supplementation of fat grafts with adipose-derived regenerative cells improves long-term graft retention. Ann Plast Surg 2010;64:222–8.

Impact of Advances in Breast Cancer Management on Reconstructive and Aesthetic Breast Surgery

Marek Dobke, MD, PhD

KEYWORDS

- Breast cancer • Breast reconstruction • Prophylactic mastectomy
- Skin sparing and nipple-areola sparing • Stem cells for breast reconstruction

KEY POINTS

- Because plastic surgeons are increasingly involved in prophylactic, ablative and restorative surgeries related to the breast cancer, it is imperative that they can offer all technical variants of these surgeries (e.g., prophylactic mastectomy), matching patient oncological needs with high cosmetic expectations and understand the implications of the technical choice on future risks and surveillance requirements.
- The ability to determine adequate margins after presurgical radiation or neoadjuvant chemotherapy; experience in reconstruction in cases with intraoperative or accelerated partial irradiation; ability to manage breast cancer in patients with previous aesthetic surgery; and the ability to supplement tissue rearrangement repairs with small, well-vascularized flaps or alloplastic materials are characteristic of oncoplastic surgeons who are comfortable with all aspects of breast cancer management and who have mastered advanced techniques.

INTRODUCTION

It is difficult to find an example of a multidisciplinary clinical niche showing more rapid growth and greater diversity than breast cancer care.[1] In the 1980s, indications for breast reconstruction were liberalized as a result of increasing experience with various procedures, including microsurgery; development of implants, including tissue expanders designed for breast reconstruction; recognition of the beneficial psychological effects of breast reconstruction; and, most importantly, because of the clinical evidence that reconstructive procedures did not negatively affect the result of mastectomy (at that time the mainstay of the primary breast cancer treatment). Breast reconstructive procedures seem not to worsen the incidence of local and distant disease-free or overall survival in patients subjected to either mastectomy or different forms of breast conservation surgery (BCS) that were established in the 1990s. However, the natural evolution of breast cancer development risk assessment, the advances in diagnostic and surveillance methods, and the changes in the design of comprehensive breast cancer management necessitate the ongoing evaluation of reconstructive approaches to ensure that they do not hinder cancer detection or treatment. Similar concerns are shared in the context of aesthetic breast procedures. Many advances stem from past controversies; whether or not to reconstruct was itself recently a controversy. Practice

Disclosures: Dr Dobke has no commercial interests and disclosures in connection with the content of this article; however, he is a consultant for Ulthera.
Division of Plastic Surgery, University of California San Diego, 200 West Arbor Drive, San Diego, CA 92103-8890, USA
E-mail address: mdobke@ucsd.edu

plasticsurgery.theclinics.com

guidelines for the management of breast cancer do not include detailed recommendations regarding aesthetic or reconstructive approaches.[2,3] Without knowledge of controversies and recognition of advances in oncological breast care, plastic surgery would not be on par, both conceptually and technically, with quality medicine and surgery.[1,4] This article shows how current diagnostic and therapeutic advances affect plastic surgery and how advances in plastic surgery affect breast care.

IMPACT OF PREVENTIVE, DIAGNOSTIC, AND BREAST MANAGEMENT ADVANCES ON RECONSTRUCTIVE AND AESTHETIC BREAST SURGERY
Prophylactic Mastectomy

One of the most effective options in preventing breast cancer is prophylactic mastectomy (PM). In high-risk patients, PM may be performed as a bilateral procedure; for women undergoing surgical treatment of unilateral breast cancer, there remains much debate about the role of contralateral PM (CPM). Supporters of CPM cite general statistics showing that CPM identifies occult malignancy in approximately 5% of cases and that CPM also decreases the risk of future contralateral breast cancer in more than 90% of cases.[4] A woman is considered to be at high genetic risk for the development of breast cancer if she has a BRCA1 or BRCA2 gene mutation or her family history suggests an autosomal dominant pattern of inheritance.[5] A woman with breast malignancy who presents at a young age or has relatives affected by breast cancer should consider testing for BRCA1 and BRCA2 mutations. Plastic surgeons counseling patient candidates for breast reconstructive or aesthetic surgeries have to be familiar with breast cancer risk assessment and recommend appropriate work-up (genetic testing, imaging).[3,6] Breast cancer reducing strategies, other than PM or CPM, include ovarian ablation, endocrine treatment (eg, tamoxifen), and lifestyle adjustments.[6] It is a difficult decision whether to undergo PM or CPM and, from the technical standpoint, timing of these procedures also matters (discussed later). Skeptics point out that the risk of breast cancer in the contralateral breast is overestimated and that breast cancer prevention strategies other than CPM are underappreciated. However, improvements in outcomes of breast reconstruction (BR) and high patient satisfaction rates from both PM and BR (90% range) boost plastic surgeons' confidence and lower the threshold for PM/BR recommendation as an option.[7,8] Furthermore, in arguing for PM or CPM, it could be claimed that risks and consequences of ovarian ablation and other breast cancer risk–reducing strategies are underestimated.[9]

Because plastic surgeons are increasingly involved in both PM and CPM, it is imperative that they can offer all technical variants of PM to match patient oncological needs and understand the implications of the technical choice for future risks and surveillance requirements. Regarding the simple or skin-sparing type of PM, because all types of mastectomy leave some breast tissue behind, subcutaneous mastectomy (in which nipple-areola complex [NAC] is preserved along with a minuscule layer of supporting breast tissue and terminal ducts segments) is associated with a greater risk of development of breast cancer than total mastectomy. More invasive forms of PM should therefore be recommended to high-risk women; however, strict selection criteria have not been established for the patients with breast cancer who are the best candidates for NAC-sparing mastectomy with an acceptably low risk of NAC tumor involvement.[10] Total mastectomy, which includes the removal of breast tissue, NAC, and the axillary tail, is generally considered the preferred procedure for PM and is often followed by immediate BR.[11,12]

Skin and Nipple-Areola–Sparing Mastectomy

Skin sparing, skin reducing, and NAC sparing are key technical issues in BCS. They are important considerations in either prophylactic or therapeutic setting. Skin-sparing mastectomy is typically defined as the removal of the breast, NAC, previous biopsy incisions, and skin overlying superficial tumors (in therapeutic mastectomy). The cosmetic outcome significantly improves with the preservation of the skin envelope and the inframammary crease in particular.[2,13] Skin-sparing therapeutic mastectomies are predominantly performed in patients with in situ T1 or T2 lesions. Skin-sparing mastectomy and immediate autologous tissue reconstruction is an common method of managing primary malignancies (in particular multifocal lesions) with good aesthetic outcomes.

Could this approach be used for the previously irradiated breast? Observations indicate that skin-sparing mastectomy (SSM) and immediate autologous BR or a combination of flaps and implants give satisfactory cosmetic outcomes and oncological outcomes. Even when SSM and immediate BR are applied for the treatment of recurrent lesions, the rate of further recurrences is acceptably low (approximately 10%, comparable with salvage mastectomy) (**Fig. 1**).[14]

The next step in improving aesthetic outcomes is to preserve the NAC. However, whether the NAC

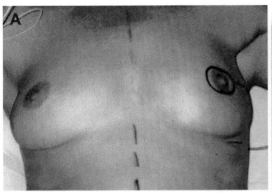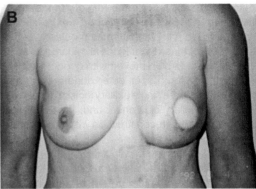

Fig. 1. (*A*) The patient is prepared for SSM and immediate BR in the management of local recurrence after breast-conserving surgery and radiation. (*B*) Latissimus dorsi myocutaneous flap (with small skin paddle to be used for nipple-areola reconstruction in the future) and silicone gel implant were used to reconstruct the left breast.

SSM should be an option is questionable.[10,15,16] In properly selected patients with lesions away from distal ducts, results of NAC sparing in the therapeutic setting would be oncologically acceptable if cancerous or high-risk lesions were histologically contiguous, but this has not been shown.[17,18] The study examining the incidence of malignant areolar and nipple involvement separately concluded that, because the areola is less frequently involved than the nipple with terminal ducts (approximately 10% of nipples harbored cancerous tissue), only the areola should be spared.[19] Subareolar tissue biopsy and extirpation of ducts distant from the nipple may not ensure oncological safety: approximately 6% to 7% of PM specimens harbored occult malignant lesions.[20,21]

It was stated earlier that the next step in improving aesthetic outcomes of BCS, is to preserve the NAC; however, there is no evidence from comparative studies that patient satisfaction from the NAC-sparing mastectomy technique is higher than from NAC reconstruction and that the nipple-areola–sparing option is cosmetically superior to de novo reconstruction, outweighing the oncological risks of nipple preservation, so the effort to spare nipples is a technical advancement.[10] Unavoidable problems such as loss of nipple volume and tone, likely loss of sensitivity, and loss of erectile capability, and healing problems secondary to ischemia (at least 6% in both prophylactic and therapeutic settings) as the result of the nipple-areola–sparing technique, support a bias toward simply offering NAC reconstruction as the primary option for a mastectomy candidate.[10,17,18] In patients with a significant ptosis (eg, a patient who had a history of significant body weight loss after bariatric surgery), a premastectomy surgical delay of NAC has been suggested, even with mastopexy.[17,22]

Other New Technical Issues in Breast Surgery: Oncoplasty

The concept of BCS put new demands on surgeons who had to abandon the concept of 1 size fits all and mastectomy as the universal answer to a breast cancer problem.[1] With the customization of ablative approaches to ensure the best possible cosmetic result and the development of oncoplasty, surgical protocols ensuring adequate mastectomy and the integration of the cancer risk–reducing surgeries into overall breast care became diversified.[2,23] The treatment of breast cancer (except lobular carcinoma in situ) conceptually includes the treatment of local disease with surgery and/or radiation therapy and the treatment of systemic disease with hormonal and cytotoxic chemotherapy. The trend in surgical ablation is toward less radical and disfiguring procedures that do not compromise the treatment of cancer. Configuration of incisions, as long as they provide a negative and adequate margin (at least 2 mm for most primary lesions) and include the lesion biopsy site, should not influence the outcome. Positive margins are more frequently associated with higher stage, positive nodes, lymphovascular invasion, younger age, positive estrogen receptors, and neoadjuvant chemotherapy.[23] Positive margins are managed by local reexcisions or completion of mastectomy.

BR may vary from tissue rearrangements to locoregional flaps or free flaps. Tissue rearrangements and locoregional flaps are conceptually different types of mastopexy and are not new to plastic surgeons. Appropriate technical guides addressing repair guidance for different anatomic requirements are available.[2,13,24] Small, centrally located breast cancers can be removed using Wise-pattern breast reduction incisions with a tumor-directed segmental mastectomy (**Fig. 2**). Lower quadrant tumors can be easily removed via vertical mammoplasty techniques. Both of these techniques allow large tumors in large breasts to be removed with good cosmetic results. In addition, upper outer quadrant tumors can be removed by a single axillary incision for quadrantectomy, axillary clearance, and, if needed for volume restoration, reconstruction with a latissimus dorsi flap.[2,23–25]

In BCS, challenges will lead to technical advances beyond different types of mastopexy. The ability to determine adequate margins, in particular after presurgical radiation or neoadjuvant chemotherapy (resulting in tumor shrinkage); experience in reconstruction in cases with intraoperative or accelerated partial irradiation (both affecting the healing pattern); ability to manage breast cancer in patients with previous breast aesthetic surgery (with and without implants); and ability to supplement tissue rearrangement repairs with small, well-vascularized local flaps (**Fig. 3**) or alloplastic implants will be the trait of oncoplastic surgeons who are comfortable with all aspects of breast cancer management and who have mastered advanced (ie, diverse and customized) techniques.[2,4,17,24,25] Many think that the

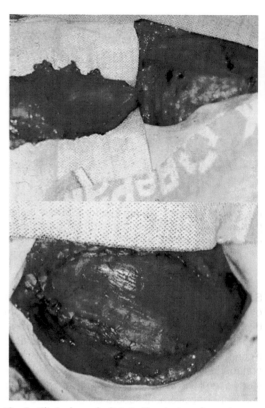

Fig. 3. Clinical needs dictate the choice of supplementary small flaps: the indication for the small split latissimus muscle harvested through the mastectomy wound was the need to provide extra implant coverage with thin and bruised mastectomy skin flaps.

technical challenges of partial BR frequently exceed those of complete mound reconstruction. Specifics of the technical advances of partial BR are presented by Dr M. Hamdi elsewhere in this issue.[26]

BCS, subsequent tissue rearrangement, and delivery of small flaps may result in the site of the original tumor not being located under the scar. In addition, focal tissue necrosis and change in tissue density, especially if implants are used, may cause the surveillance imaging to be difficult.[24,27] Therefore, marking the location of the original lesion site for surveillance or further treatment (eg, radiation) should be a part of state-of-the-art approaches (**Fig. 4**).

Questions and Pitfalls in the Management of the Axilla

The appropriate management of the axilla of patients with T1 and T2 breast cancer treated with breast-conserving therapies and the extent of the axillary dissection in patients with invasive

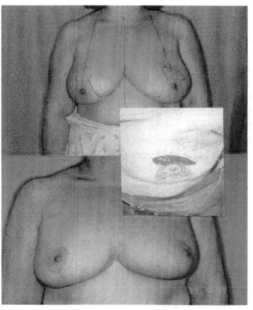

Fig. 2. Simple reconstructive scenario: T1 breast cancer with the lesion cranial to the NAC. Following excision, the defect was repaired using a Wise-pattern, inferior pedicle breast reduction technique. However, a major consideration when choosing the repair is the extent of excision volume and the need to provide breast symmetry.[22] Therefore, the patient underwent breast reduction on the contralateral side.

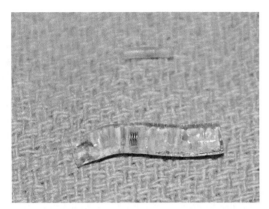

Fig. 4. One of the useful breast biopsy or cancer site markers before and after hydration (HydroMark, Biopsy Sciences, Clearwater, FL). It is visible under ultrasound, mammogram, and magnetic resonance imaging. The marker, which is inserted in nonhydrated form, expands in situ as it becomes hydrated, increasing in length and diameter after it is deployed. As it enlarges it becomes fixed within the site where it is deployed.

cancers has been a topic of controversy for years.[4,28,29] The appropriate extent of axillary dissection, whether axillary dissection alone is sufficient to control the disease, whether axillary irradiation could suffice, and how the morbidity of axillary surgery can effectively be minimized remain unknown and are the subjects of clinical research. Prevention or treatment of upper extremity lymphedema following mastectomy and axillary node dissection is presented by colleagues from Dr C. Becker's group elsewhere in this issue.

Sentinel lymph node biopsy (SNB), in which the first node draining a specific tumor is isolated and removed, is a technique that has become the standard in breast cancer management.[30] Aesthetic surgeons were questioning whether previous breast augmentation and pectoralis major muscle releases would change lymphatic functioning and affect axillary or pectoral area nodes. It seems that SNB can be performed in patients with augmented breasts with low false-negative results regardless of the surgical approach (transaxillary, inframammary, periareolar) and trauma to breast lymphatics.[31,32] Certain reconstructive procedures, such as transfer and passage of the latissimus dorsi myocutaneous flap through the axillary region, affects the ability to follow with periodic axillary physical examinations; lymphoscintigraphy in case of local recurrence; or detection of the rare, but possible, axillary recurrence, and a plastic surgeon has to be aware of potential pitfalls and be able to design breast care so that clinical objectives are met.[28,32]

Prereconstruction, Intraoperative, and Postmastectomy Radiation, Chemotherapy, and BR

The increasing use of radiotherapy after mastectomy, including partial mastectomy, has significant implications for BR. In general, there is a consensus that the combination of radiation and implants is associated with greater than 50% risk of complications in wound healing, capsular contracture, and pain. Scarring from previous surgery being compounded by irradiation (whether preoperative, intraoperative, or postoperative scarring) causes reconstructive procedures to be more difficult and less predictable.[2,14,33] Patients who undergo expander/implant BR after radiotherapy have a higher rate of complications than patients not receiving radiotherapy. More than 20% of patients may require major revision, frequently conversion of BR to that with autologous tissue. However, no significant difference is found in general patient satisfaction with expander/implant between those who did and did not receive radiotherapy.[2,33,34] In contrast, partial breast irradiation or targeted intraoperative radiation with high-dose, focally delivered radiation may lead to the development of fibrosis, scarring that affects the overall outcome of BR without implants (**Fig. 5**).

Autologous fat transfer techniques in delayed BR seem to be promising adjunct modality for patients with tissue expanders or implants and a history of radiation. An improvement of tissue

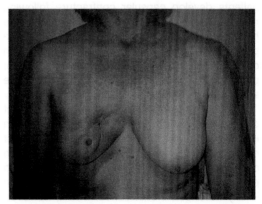

Fig. 5. Lesions in the upper/inner breast quadrant are aesthetically challenging.[22] The patient is shown after superomedial lumpectomy to the right breast, sentinel node biopsy, and radiation. This location is difficult to correct with a laterally based small flap such as the lateral intercostal artery perforator flap. Options: fat grafting, bat-wing full-thickness excision, and rotation of the glandular flap (with contralateral surgery for symmetry); however, the patient has chosen completion mastectomy and reconstruction with a transverse rectus abdominis myocutaneous (TRAM) flap.

quality, with reduction of problems related to scarring and capsular contracture, and improved contour modeling (axillary tail, cleavage, inframammary crease) can be provided.[35]

Expansion of indications for postmastectomy radiotherapy may affect the timing and reconstructive options available, possibly decreasing the use of immediate reconstruction, especially with implants.[36,37] Delayed BR, even with microsurgically transferred free transverse rectus abdominis myocutaneous (TRAM) flaps, was recommended for those undergoing adjuvant radiotherapy because of the increased rate of complications such as fat necrosis, loss of flap volume, fibrosis, and flap contracture.[38] However, for immediate BR, it is not always known whether subsequent radiotherapy will follow.

Given the significant rate of postradiation complications affecting the aesthetic outcomes, saline inflatable, and, in particular, volume-adjustable implants seem to be a more logical implant choice for reconstruction of the breast mound in the initial (perhaps temporary) stage of reconstruction before radiotherapy. Reduction of an implant volume (temporary or permanent, as needed) may be helpful in the management of pain or wound healing problems, whereas temporary overexpansion may be helpful in preventing or managing effects of radiation fibrosis.[39] In previously augmented breasts, radiotherapy has been shown to be as effective as for nonaugmented breast cancer. However, more than 50% of patients develop capsular contracture following radiotherapy and the likelihood of revisions is high.[32] Autologous tissue BR seems to be the preferred immediate breast mound reconstruction option for women with a significant probability of postmastectomy radiotherapy by reconstructive surgeons (Fig. 6).[2,32,38]

Little evidence exists regarding concerns that chemotherapy might affect healing and that both induction and adjuvant chemotherapy may affect results of reconstructive procedures. Induction chemotherapy slightly prolonged the interval to postoperative chemotherapy in patients with locally advanced breast cancer in BR; however, no effect on survival associated with this delay was reported.[40,41] Immediate BR seemed not to delay the start of adjuvant chemotherapy; however, the rate of surgical complications was approximately 15% to 24% compared with 4% to 5% in nonreconstructed patients.[42–44]

Experimental Techniques for BR

Diagnostic and therapeutic advances in breast cancer management used to affect reconstructive approaches. Although there is consensus that surgical reconstructive procedures do not negatively affect results of mastectomy, questions are raised whether new emerging reconstructive modalities such as fat transfer, stem cells, and tissue engineering affect malignancy risks. It seems that, in postmastectomy patients who received radiotherapy, autologous fat grafting, in addition to traditional tissue expander and implant reconstruction, leads to better clinical reconstructive outcomes with the creation of the neosubcutaneous tissue, accompanied by improved skin quality of the reconstructed breast without capsular contracture and without negative impact on oncological outcome. The concept of fat injection to the breast was not accepted until recently. Some propose tissue pretreatment with fat (before delayed reconstruction with implants in irradiated tissue), which seems to reduce the radiation-induced complication rate.[45] Beneficial effects of fat transfer (healing of radiolesions or helping to prevent radiation-related problems) is attributed to the angiogenic capacity of preadipocytes, or stem cells in the fat. Preliminary experimental and clinical studies indicate that autologous fat enriched with adipose tissue–derived stem cells injected to correct limited (postlumpectomy or postradiation) breast defects, or seeded on scaffold structures to form mini-implants, may be useful in BR. Studies are underway to show that fat-derived stem cells taken from a patient with breast cancer behave biologically no differently than those from healthy women.[46,47] Preliminary studies have to led to investigations to address, for example, whether stem cells affect epithelial cell line breast cancer recurrence, how they affect breast stroma, whether patients with BRCA1 and BRCA2 (and other risk-determining gene mutations) respond differently than patients who are BRCA1/2 negative to stem cell engrafting and transdifferentiation, and whether clonal expansion is a prerequisite for malignancy formation.[47]

ADVANCES IN BREAST CANCER TREATMENT: NEW PITFALLS AND CONCERNS
Oncological Follow-Up and Imaging of the Reconstructed Breast

There are no standard practice guidelines for follow-up and imaging of the reconstructed breast.[48] Mammographic surveillance after BCS is recommended. However, difficulties associated with interpretation of mammograms after local surgery, radiotherapy, and adjuvant chemotherapy can be expected.[27,49] Differential diagnosis may be difficult because of residual hematoma, seroma, fat necrosis, skin and fascia

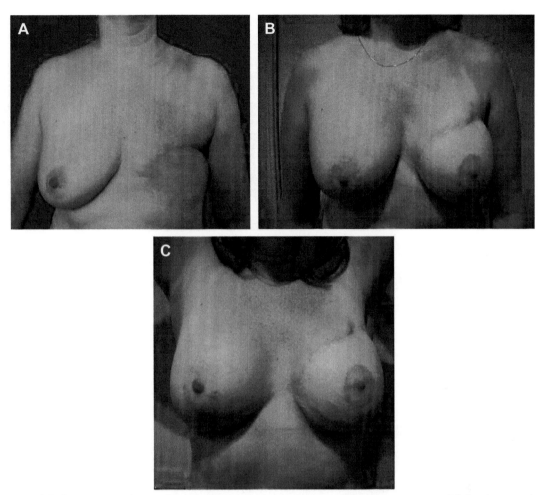

Fig. 6. (*A*) The patient is shown after modified radical mastectomy, radiation treatment, and following completion of chemotherapy. There was no evidence of local recurrence or systemic disease. (*B*) For large volumetric needs, TRAM flap seemed to be the best option. Autologous fat of the TRAM flap seems to increase in bulk as the patient (who was taking tamoxifen) gained some body weight, maintaining satisfactory symmetry between the left reconstructed and the right intact breast. (*C*) Good symmetry of breast mounds on arms abduction.

thickening, increased and nonhomogeneous soft tissue density in the breast, microcalcifications, and implants. Breast tissue rearrangement for reconstructive purposes or increased density secondary to tissue compression caused by breast aesthetic augmentation implants may result in an even higher rate of false-positive and false-negative mammograms. Some institutions have adopted screening mammography after implant or autologous tissue reconstruction, thus enabling the same mammographic look of the skin, chest wall, and remaining breast tissue as for a women who has not had a mastectomy, whereas others prefer magnetic resonance imaging (MRI) even for screening purposes in these situations.[27,50] A reported case of local recurrence involving flap tissue reaffirms the notion of a need for diligent

Box 1
Case 1. A 23-year-old nulliparous woman who tested positive for BRCA2

Her mother and grandmother had prophylactic mastectomies 20 years ago because of family history. A 32-year-old maternal aunt succumbed to breast cancer. A 28-year-old maternal cousin was recently diagnosed with breast cancer. There was a high odds ratio and relative risk for breast cancer.[3] Options: careful observation (understanding that the reliability of mammograms may be poor in a young patient with glandular, dense breasts), oophorectomy (systemic consequences unknown at such young age), tamoxifen (long-term benefit and systemic consequences unknown), bilateral prophylactic mastectomy (which was ultimately her choice; **Fig. 7**).

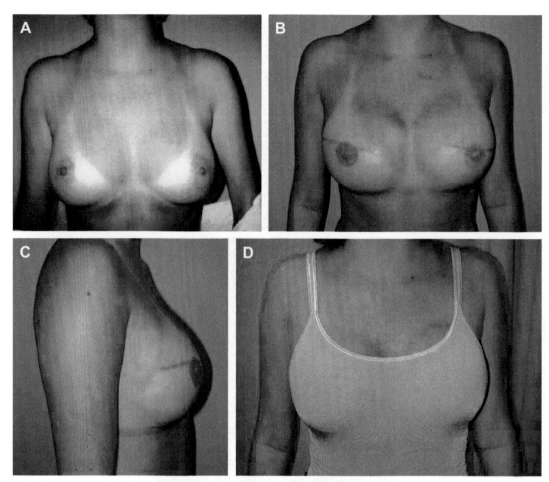

Fig. 7. (*A*) The patient before prophylactic bilateral mastectomy that included the NAC. (*B*) Status post immediate BR using tissue expanders followed by permanent implants and subsequent nipple-areola reconstruction (frontal view). (*C*) Same patient after reconstruction (lateral view). (*D*) Good symmetry in athletic outfit with attractive décolleté.

oncological follow-up and evaluation even of the tissue delivered to the breast area.[51]

For difficult radiated reconstruction contrast-enhanced MRI or positron emission tomography scanning enables differentiation of recurrent tumors from scars or fat necrosis.[27,52] In a study comparing the sensitivity and specificity of clinical examination, screening ultrasound, and screening MRI in detecting local recurrence in patients who underwent mastectomy for invasive breast cancer, the sensitivity and specificity for clinical examination were poor (70% and 35.2% respectively) but could be significantly improved by the use of ultrasound (90% and 88.2% respectively) or MRI (100% and 100% respectively). Considering that ultrasound is an inexpensive and easily repeatable procedure, and because most recurrences occur in the quadrant of the original tumor, directed, focused, frequent ultrasound follow-up examination may be warranted.[52]

Box 2

Case 2. A 45-year-old woman with multiple, metachronous left breast T1N0 invasive lobular cancer lesions

Treated several times with lumpectomy and radiation. Developed another lesion of the left breast and declined the recommendation and offer of prophylactic mastectomy on the right side. A few years later she developed lobular carcinoma of the right breast and underwent mastectomy. Breast reconstruction was performed using latissimus dorsi as opposed to earlier TRAM myocutaneous unit, resulting in an unfavorable outcome. Although the patient was well informed about her options, her decisions were oncologically and cosmetically suboptimal.[8] This patient exemplifies the need for early identification of those who are at high risk of developing breast cancer, as well as the importance of patient education (**Fig. 8**).

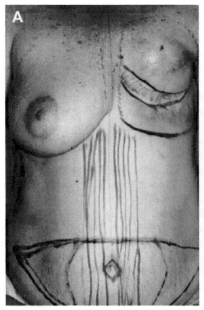
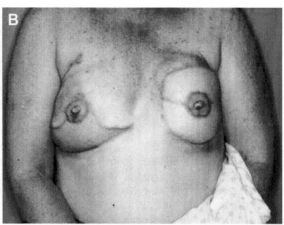

Fig. 8. (*A*) Status post multiple breast-conserving surgeries and repeated radiation for lobular carcinoma lesions of the left breast. The patient developed another lesion, was admitted for completion mastectomy, and had reconstruction using a pedicled TRAM flap. (*B*) Five years later, the same patient developed lobular carcinoma of the right breast, which was treated by mastectomy and latissimus dorsi myocutaneous flap and implant reconstruction. Use of the TRAM unit on the left side necessitated a different type of reconstruction on the right side with an overall suboptimal cosmetic result.

The plastic surgeon who performs BR must become skilled in and attentive to the follow-up examination of the patient who has breast cancer. Anything suspicious or worrisome must be further examined. An aesthetic surgeon has to be committed to the same standards despite implant augmentation of breasts not increasing the risk of breast cancer or worsening prognosis if breast cancer does develop, and self-examination and clinical breast examination being as effective as in the nonaugmented breast.[3,32] In contrast, the surgical oncologist must not assume that new areas of thickening, fullness, mass, pain, skin change, and so forth are just caused by the BR; these findings should be treated with the same level of cancer suspicion as the same findings in the nonreconstructed breast.

ILLUSTRATIVE CASES

The plethora of problems and concerns that have to be addressed by plastic surgeons practicing breast surgery, either aesthetic or reconstructive, has to be addressed with long-term patient wellness in mind. Understanding of the breast cancer biology, risk stratification, and changing principles of surgical and nonsurgical management of breast cancer is essential to ensure the oncological safety

of patients subjected to breast care by plastic surgeons. This article presents cases that show the impact of patient education; the impact of the multispecialty breast team on management decisions, both satisfactory and less satisfactory; and the role of plastic surgery doctoring and surgical techniques in resolving breast cancer problems (**Boxes 1** and **2**).

Box 3
Key technical advances in plastic surgery for breast cancer

- Adaptation of existing mammoplasty techniques for oncoplasty purposes and development of techniques to serve quadrant per quadrant reconstruction needs

- Development of new locoregional flaps such as the lateral intercostal perforator flap

- Development of small perforator free flaps

- Development of techniques for transfer of fat and fat enriched with adipose tissue–derived stem cells for correction of breast defects

- Microlymphatic surgery for the treatment of upper extremity lymphedema

- Use of acellular dermal matrices

SUMMARY

The focus on individualization and customization of approaches, as well as an evidence-based approach, has become the technical standard of aesthetic and reconstructive breast surgery. The merits of surgical techniques are interlaced with breast cancer risk stratification, diagnostic and surveillance issues, and selection and sequencing of the best treatment modalities. The key technical considerations and skills acquisition to ensure the necessary versatility in a modern breast plastic surgeon are listed in **Box 3**.

REFERENCES

1. Zannis VJ. Presidential address: 2010. The American Society of Breast Surgeons. There is no "boring" in breast surgery. Ann Surg Oncol 2010; 17(3):S197–201.

2. Rosson GD, Magarakis M, Shridharani SM, et al. A review of the surgical management of breast cancer: plastic reconstructive techniques and timing implications. Ann Surg Oncol 2010;17(7):1890–900.

3. Sharabi SE, Bullocks JM, Dempsey PJ, et al. The need for breast cancer screening in women undergoing elective breast surgery: and assessment of risk and risk factors for breast cancer in young women. Aesthet Surg J 2010;30(6):821–31.

4. Boughey JC, Mittendorf EA, Solin LJ, et al. Controversies in breast surgery. Ann Surg Oncol 2010; 17(3):S230–2.

5. Mielnicki LM, Asch HL, Asch BB. Genes, chromatin, and breast cancer: an epigenetic tale. J Mammary Gland Biol Neoplasia 2001;6(2):169–82.

6. Schragg D. Life expectancy gains from cancer prevention strategies for women with breast cancer and BRCA1 or BRCA2 mutations. JAMA 2000; 283(5):617–24.

7. Frost M, Hoskin TL, Hartman LC, et al. Contralateral prophylactic mastectomy: long term consistency of satisfaction and adverse effects and the significance of informed decision-making, quality of life, and personal traits. Ann Surg Oncol 2011;18(11):3110–6.

8. Lee CN, Belkora J, Chang Y, et al. Are patients making high-quality decisions about breast reconstruction after mastectomy. Plast Reconstr Surg 2011;127(1):18–26.

9. Arrington A, Tuttle T. Author reply: contralateral prophylactic mastectomy overtreatment: expectations from personal genomics for tailored breast cancer surgery. Ann Surg Oncol 2010;17(3):940.

10. Wagner JL, Fearmonti R, Hunt KK, et al. Prospective evaluation of the nipple-areola complex sparing mastectomy for risk reduction and for early-stage breast cancer. Ann Surg Oncol 2012; 19(4):1137–44.

11. Meijers-Heliboer H, Van Geel B, Van Putten WL. Breast cancer after prophylactic mastectomy in women with a BRCA 1 or BRCA 2 mutation. N Engl J Med 2001;345(3):159–64.

12. Simmons RM, Osborne MP. Prophylactic mastectomy. Breast J 1997;6(3):372–9.

13. Nair A, Jaleel S, Abbott N, et al. Skin-reducing mastectomy with immediate implant reconstruction as an indispensable tool in the provision of oncoplastic breast services. Ann Surg Oncol 2010; 17(9):2480–5.

14. Linford AJ, Meretoja TJ, von Smitten KA, et al. Skin-sparing mastectomy and immediate breast reconstruction in the management of locally recurrent breast cancer. Ann Surg Oncol 2010;17(6):1669–74.

15. Babiera G, Simmons R. Nipple-areola complex sparing mastectomy: feasibility, patient selection, and technique. Ann Surg Oncol 2010;17(3):S245–8.

16. Laronga C, Robb GL, Singletary SE. Feasibility of skin-sparing mastectomy with preservation of the nipple-areola complex. Breast Diseases 1998;9: 125–7.

17. Jensen JA, Orrigner JS, Giuliano AE. Nipple-sparing mastectomy in 99 patients with a mean follow-up of 5 years. Ann Surg Oncol 2011;18(6):1665–70.

18. Spear SL, Willey SC, Feldman ED, et al. Nipple-sparing mastectomy for prophylactic and therapeutic indications. Plast Reconstr Surg 2011; 128(5):1005–14.

19. Simmons RM, Brennan M, Christos P. Analysis of nipple/areolar involvement with mastectomy: can the areola be preserved? Ann Surg Oncol 2001; 9(2):165–8.

20. Filho P, Capko D, Barry JM, et al. Nipple-sparing mastectomy for breast cancer and risk-reducing surgery: the Memorial Sloan-Kettering Cancer Center experience. Ann Surg Oncol 2011;18(11):3117–22.

21. Reynolds C, Davidson JA, Lindor NM, et al. Prophylactic and therapeutic mastectomy in BRCA mutation carriers: can the nipple be preserved? Ann Surg Oncol 2011;18(11):3102–9.

22. Spear SL, Rottman SJ, Seiboth LA, et al. Breast reconstruction using a staged nipple-sparing mastectomy following mastopexy or reduction. Plast Reconstr Surg 2012;129(3):572–81.

23. Bong J, Parker J, Clapper R, et al. Clinical series of oncoplastic mastopexy to optimize cosmesis of large-volume resections for breast carcinoma. Ann Surg Oncol 2010;17(12):3247–51.

24. Clough KB, Kaufman GJ, Nos C, et al. Improving breast cancer surgery: a classification and quadrant per quadrant atlas for oncoplastic surgery. Ann Surg Oncol 2010;17(5):1375–91.

25. Shrotria S. Single axillary incision for quadrantectomy, axillary clearance and immediate reconstruction with latissimus dorsi. Br J Plast Surg 2001; 54(2):128–31.

26. Hamdi M, van Landuyt K, Blondeel P, et al. Autologous breast augmentation with the lateral intercostal artery perforator flap in massive weight loss patients. J Plast Reconstr Aesthet Surg 2009;62(1):65–70.

27. Mendelson E. Radiation changes in the breast. Semin Roentgenol 1993;28(4):344–61.

28. Perez CA. Current perspectives in the management of the axilla in patients with stage T1 or T2 breast cancer treated with breast conserving therapy. Breast Diseases 2001;11(4):370–4.

29. Sondak VK. How do we know when a lymph node dissection is adequate? Ann Surg Oncol 2011;18(9):2419–21.

30. Giuliano A. Sentinel lymphadenectomy in breast cancer. J Clin Oncol 1997;15(6):2345–50.

31. Roxo AC, Aboudib JH, DeCastro CC, et al. Evaluation of the effects of transaxillary breast augmentation on sentinel lymph node integrity. Aesthet Surg J 2011;31(4):392–400.

32. Tang SS, Gui GP. A review of the oncologic and surgical management of breast cancer in the augmented breast: diagnostic, surgical and surveillance challenges. Ann Surg Oncol 2011;18(8):2173–81.

33. Hirsch EM, Seth AK, Dumanian GA, et al. Outcomes of tissue expander/implant breast reconstruction in the setting of prereconstruction radiation. Plast Reconstr Surg 2012;129(2):354–61.

34. Kruegger EA, Wilkins EG, Strawderman M. Complications and patient satisfaction following expander/implant breast reconstruction with and without radiotherapy. Int J Radiat Oncol Biol Phys 2001;49(3):713–21.

35. Serra-Renom J, Munoz-Olmo J, Serra-Mestre J. Fat grafting in postmastectomy breast reconstruction with expanders and prostheses in patients who have received radiotherapy: formation of new subcutaneous tissue. Plast Reconstr Surg 2010;125(1):12–8.

36. Disa JJ, Cordeiro PG, Heerdt AH. Skin-sparing mastectomy and immediate autologous tissue reconstruction after whole-breast irradiation. Plast Reconstr Surg 2003;111(1):118–24.

37. Morrow M, Scott SK, Menck HR. Factors influencing the use of breast reconstruction postmastectomy. A National Cancer Database Study. J Am Coll Surg 2001;192(1):1–8.

38. Tran NV, Chang DW, Gupta A. Comparison of immediate and delayed free TRAM flap breast reconstruction in patients receiving postmastectomy radiation therapy. Plast Reconstr Surg 2001;108(1):78–82.

39. Spear SL, Onyewu C. Staged breast reconstruction with saline-filled implants in irradiated breast: recent trends and therapeutic implications. Plast Reconstr Surg 2000;105(3):930–42.

40. Broadwater JR, Edwards MJ, Kugler C. Mastectomy following preoperative chemotherapy. Ann Surg 1991;213(2):126–9.

41. Recht A. Timing of chemotherapy and radiotherapy after breast-conserving surgery. Breast Diseases 1997;8(1):91–3.

42. Allweis TM, Boisvert ME, Otero SE. Immediate breast reconstruction after mastectomy for breast cancer does not prolong the time to starting adjuvant chemotherapy. Am J Surg 2002;183(3):218–21.

43. Mortenson MM, Schneider PD, Khatri VP, et al. Immediate breast reconstruction after mastectomy increases wound complications: however, initiation of adjuvant chemotherapy is not delayed. Arch Surg 2004;139(9):988–91.

44. Zhong T, Hofer SO, McCready DR, et al. A comparison of surgical complications between immediate breast reconstruction and mastectomy: the impact on delivery of chemotherapy-an analysis of 391 procedures. Ann Surg Oncol 2012;19(2):560–6.

45. Salgarello M, Visconti G, Barone-Adesi L. Fat grafting and breast reconstruction with implant: another option for irradiated breast cancer patients. Plast Reconstr Surg 2012;129(2):317–29.

46. Kitamura K. Stem cell augmented reconstruction: a new hope for reconstruction after breast conservation therapy. Breast Cancer Res Treat 2007;106(Suppl 1) [abstract 4071].

47. Pearl RA, Leedham SJ, Pacifico MD. The safety of autologous fat transfer in breast cancer: lessons from stem cell biology. J Plast Reconstr Aesthet Surg 2012;65(3):283–8.

48. National Comprehensive Cancer Network: update: NCCN practice guidelines for the treatment of breast cancer. Oncology 1999;13(5A):187–212.

49. Ashkanani F, Sarkar T, Needham G. What is achieved by mammographic surveillance after breast conservation for breast cancer? Am J Surg 2001;182(3):207–10.

50. Leibman AJ, Styblo TM, Bostwick J. Mammography of the postreconstruction breast. Plast Reconstr Surg 1997;99(3):698–704.

51. Mund DF, Wolfson P, Gorczyca DP. Mammographically detected recurrent nonpalpable carcinoma developing in a transverse rectus abdominis myocutaneous flap: a case report. Cancer 1994;74(10):2804–7.

52. Yilmaz M, Esen G, Ayarcan YI. The role of US and MR imaging in detecting local chest tumor recurrence after mastectomy. Diagn Interv Radiol 2007;13(1):13–8.

Advances in Autologous Breast Reconstruction with Pedicled Perforator Flaps

Moustapha Hamdi, MD, PhD[a],*,
Mohamed Zulfikar Rasheed, MBBS, MRCSEd, MMed(Surgery)[a,b]

KEYWORDS

- Perforator flap • Pedicled perforator flap • Breast conservation therapy • Partial mastectomy
- Autologous breast augmentation • Fat grafting • Tissue scaffold • Tissue matrix

KEY POINTS

- Breast conservation therapy (BCT) is an accepted treatment of selected breast cancers.
- Certain post-BCT defects require volume replacement; pedicled perforator flaps (PPFs) are ideal for the reconstruction of these defects.
- Other applications for PPFs in breast surgery include salvage of partial necrosis of breast flaps, chest wall coverage, total breast reconstruction, and autologous breast augmentation.
- PPFs may function as vascularized tissue scaffolds that support subsequent fat grafting.
- The main advantage of PPFs is minimal donor site morbidity from functional muscle preservation.
- Preoperative perforator mapping with Doppler ultrasound or multidetector CT (MDCT)/MRI is important step for deciding which perforator to use and reduces operative time and complication rate.

OVERVIEW

The advent of perforator flaps in the past 2 decades has expanded the horizons of reconstructive surgery. Harvesting a flap without sacrificing the underlying muscle and its functional motor nerves characterizes this technique, which aims to reduce donor site morbidity to an absolute minimum. PPFs are a more recent development and have been widely used for breast reconstruction.

BCT is the surgical excision of a breast cancer with a tumor-free margin while preserving the remainder of the uninvolved breast. Adjuvant breast irradiation is mandatory. This treatment modality has become the first choice for patients with early breast cancers because it has proved oncologically sound with survival rates similar to that of total mastectomy while providing associated aesthetic and psychological benefits.[1,2] Patient selection, however, is important. A relative contraindication is a woman with a large tumor in a small breast; in these patients, the aesthetic outcome of BCT is poor.[3,4] To overcome this, oncoplastic techniques that resect the tumor along breast reduction patterns or redistribute the remaining parenchyma via breast rearrangement may be used, along with reduction or mastopexy of the contralateral breast for symmetry.[5–10] There is a limit, however, to how much volume displacement techniques are able to achieve in

Funding sources: Nil.
Conflict of interest: Nil.
[a] Department of Plastic and Reconstructive Surgery, Brussels University Hospital, Free University of Brussels, UZ Brussel, Laarbeeklaan 101, Brussels B-1090, Belgium; [b] Department of Plastic, Reconstructive and Aesthetic Surgery, Singapore General Hospital, Outram Road, Singapore 169608, Singapore
* Corresponding author.
E-mail address: moustapha.hamdi@uzbrussel.be

Clin Plastic Surg 39 (2012) 477–490
http://dx.doi.org/10.1016/j.cps.2012.07.016
0094-1298/12/$ – see front matter © 2012 Elsevier Inc. All rights reserved.

masking the volume discrepancy and contour abnormality from tumor resection. Patients with larger tumor-to-breast ratios were not considered suitable candidates for this procedure and were treated with total mastectomy with or without reconstruction. Volume replacement techniques import tissues, mainly from the regions surrounding the breast. The latissimus dorsi (LD) flap is a prime example of a musculocutaneous flap that has been used for partial breast reconstruction.[11,12] The sacrifice of a substantial muscle, however, results in significant donor site morbidity, in particular, seroma formation and detrimental effects on shoulder function.

PPFs are a recent development in the field of breast reconstruction.[13–15] Their main role is in the reconstruction of partial mastectomy defects with minimal donor site morbidity by preservation of the underlying muscles. They allow breast surgeons to resect a tumor with as much margins as oncologically necessary without fear of a poor cosmetic result.[16,17] Moreover, these flaps act as a vascularized tissue scaffold that support the survival of free fat grafts. This is especially important given that adjuvant breast irradiation is mandatory in BCT, and fat transfer may be used to reverse the late sequelae of radiation and function as filler to correct residual volume and contour abnormalities.

Based on the authors' successful experience with PPFs and fat grafting in partial breast reconstruction, the indications of PPFs could be expanded to include total breast reconstruction. In this novel concept, the PPF functions as a vascularized tissue scaffold for subsequent sessions of fat grafting, to achieve a larger desired volume and contour in the reconstructed breast. This article reviews the concept of PPFs and their current use in breast surgery.

PEDICLED PERFORATOR FLAPS IN BREAST SURGERY

The PPFs that are useful for breast reconstruction may be classified according to the source vessel the perforator arises from, namely the thoracodorsal artery, the intercostal artery, the branch to the serratus anterior, and the superior epigastric artery (SEA) **(Table 1)**.[15–20]

A variable segment of the LD muscle may need to be included due to anatomic variations that become apparent only intraoperatively. In these cases, the thoracodorsal artery perforator (TDAP) flap is converted to a muscle-sparing TDAP (MS-TDAP). The flap is harvested based on the status of the TDAPs,[16,18] as indicated in the following algorithm.

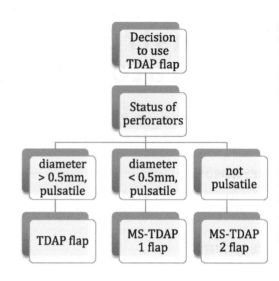

The MS-TDAP type I flap is elevated when the perforator is small but pulsatile, because there is a risk of avulsion of the perforator. It is also recommended when a surgeon anticipates excessive tension on the flap in reaching a distal (medial quadrant) defect. A segment of the LD muscle measuring 4 cm long and 2 cm wide posterior to the perforator is included. This serves to protect the posterior wall of the perforator from excessive traction placed on the pedicle.

When there are multiple perforators but are of small caliber, or when the perforators are nonpulsatile, then the MS-TDAP type II flap is harvested. A larger segment of muscle (up to 5 cm width) at the anterior border of the LD is included with the flap. This serves to capture the maximum number of perforators from the vertical branch of the thoracodorsal artery, which are located within the anterior 5 cm of the LD muscle between 8 cm and 13 cm caudal to the axillary crease. An MS-TDAP type II flap may also be used when a segment of the LD muscle is needed, such as when more bulk is required or to cover an implant. A similar technique can be used by surgeons with limited experience in perforator flaps during their initial cases of TDAP flaps. Isolating the perforator with the anterior cuff of the LD muscle enables breast surgeons to achieve a satisfactory reconstruction expediently and safely, with limited donor site morbidity, even in difficult cases.[16,18]

INDICATIONS AND CONTRAINDICATIONS

There are few contraindications to PPFs for breast surgery. Adequate expertise in perforator flap harvest is requisite, and surgeons may choose to familiarize themselves with other perforator flaps, such as the deep inferior epigastric perforator flap or the superior gluteal artery perforator flap,

Table 1
Pedicled perforator flaps and muscle-sparing modifications in breast surgery

Flap	Source Vessel	Location of Perforator	Muscle Component	Reach	Notes
TDAP flap	Thoracodorsal artery (vertical branch)	Within 5 cm posterior to the anterior border of the LD, 8–13 cm caudal to the axillary crease	—	All quadrants	—
MS-TDAP type I flap	—	—	4 cm × 2 cm of LD posterior to perforator	—	—
MS-TDAP type II flap	—	—	5 cm width of LD from its anterior border	—	—
LICAP flap	Intercostal artery, costal segment, anterior to the LD	Mean distance of 3.5 cm from the anterior border of the LD in the 4th–8th ICS	—	Lateral quadrant	Preserves TDAP/MS-TDAP/LD flaps for future use
SAAP flap	Serratus anterior branch (vascular connection to intercostal artery)	Same as LICAP flap	—	Retroareolar, 6–9 cm pedicle length	Vascular connection is present in only 21% of cases
AICAP flap	Intercostal artery, muscular/rectus segment	Rectus muscle/sheath	—	Inferomedial quadrant	—
SEAP flap	SEA	Rectus muscle/sheath, between costal margin and the first tendinous intersection	—	Inferomedial quadrant	—

Abbreviations: ICS, intercostal space; SAAP flap, serratus anterior artery perforator flap.

which have larger and more numerous perforators and are more forgiving.

Damage to the thoracodorsal artery pedicle due to previous axillary or thoracic surgery is an absolute contraindication to raising a TDAP flap, as it is for a traditional LD flap. A lateral intercostal artery perforator (LICAP) flap, however, may still be harvested for lateral breast defects. Previous surgery to the axilla, lateral thoracotomy, or radiotherapy may also damage the perforator complexes.

Current indications for PPFs in breast surgery are summarized in (**Box 1**).

Immediate Partial Breast Reconstruction

PPFs replace volume by recruiting well-vascularized tissues from around the breast. They therefore expand the indications of breast conservation surgery to include women with larger tumor-to-breast volume ratios than was previously possible while maximizing aesthetic outcome. The

> **Box 1**
> Indications for pedicled perforator flaps in the breast
>
> - Immediate partial breast reconstruction
> - Delayed partial breast reconstruction
> - Thoracic coverage after radical excision
> - Salvage procedure after significant partial necrosis of flap in breast reconstruction
> - Postmastectomy breast reconstruction with or without an implant
> - Autologous breast augmentation

major indications of the PPFs are defects that are larger than 30% of the breast or in cases where the tumor resection results in unacceptable aesthetic result (**Fig. 1**). Another relative indication is in women who, despite having adequate tissue for

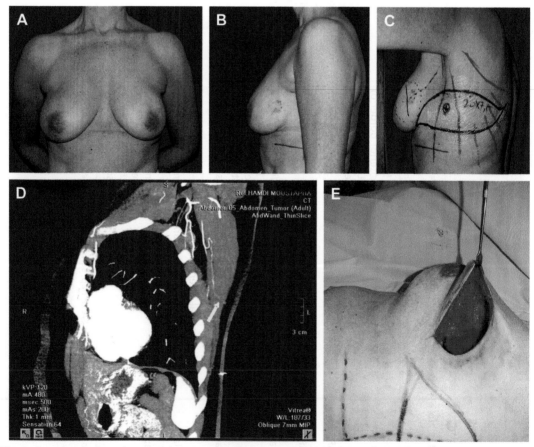

Fig. 1. A patient undergoing partial mastectomy for a 3-cm ductal carcinoma located in the superolateral quadrant of the left breast. Reconstruction was performed with a completely de-epithelialized TDAP flap. (*A, B*) Preoperative views. (*C*) Flap design. (*D*) The dominant perforator (*arrow*) was localized preoperatively using MDCT. (*E*) Tumor resection with wide margins and skin (specimen weight 195 g).

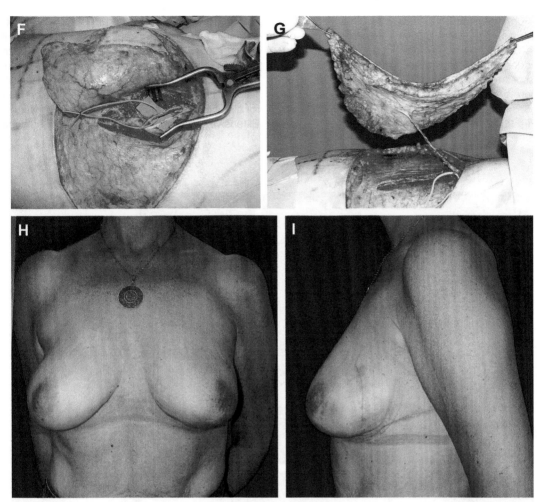

Fig. 1. (*F*) The LD muscle is split and the perforator dissected proximally to the main pedicle. (*G*) TDAP flap based on a single perforator. (*H, I*) Outcome of reconstruction after irradiation.

breast rearrangement (volume displacement) surgery, prefer to maintain their original breast volume without reducing the contralateral breast.

The choice of flap depends on the location of the tissue defect, the available donor sites, and the volume and type of tissue to be replaced.[16,17] From an anatomic standpoint, the breast is divided into quadrants relative to a horizontal and a vertical line passing through the nipple. This is also a useful description when planning reconstruction. The LICAP flap is primarily indicated for lateral defects because of its short pedicle.[15,16,19,21] The TDAP flap with its longer pedicle is usually able to cover all quadrants. Medial quadrants may be reconstructed with the anterior intercostal artery perforator (AICAP) or SEA perforator (SEAP) flaps, which are harvested from the upper abdominal areas.[15,19,20] The following algorithm shows flap choice as related to breast quadrants.

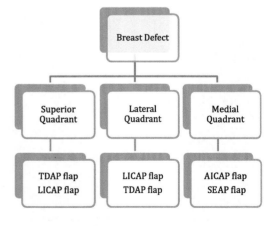

Delayed Partial Breast Reconstruction

Delayed partial breast reconstruction should be considered when post-BCT deformities occur. Several classification systems have been developed to characterize delayed breast deformities and their suggested reconstructive options.[3,10,17] Most of these deformities can be treated with serial fat injections. However, when moderate to severe radiation sequelae are associated with major deformity involving 2 or more breast quadrants or are larger than 20% of the initial breast size, then PPFs are indicated (**Fig. 2**).

Due to previous surgery and irradiation, the postoperative complication rate after delayed partial breast reconstruction is higher than in immediate partial breast reconstruction. Therefore, careful handling of irradiated breast tissue is essential. The scar tissue should be excised and submitted for histopathologic analysis to rule out malignancy. Extensive undermining of the breast should be

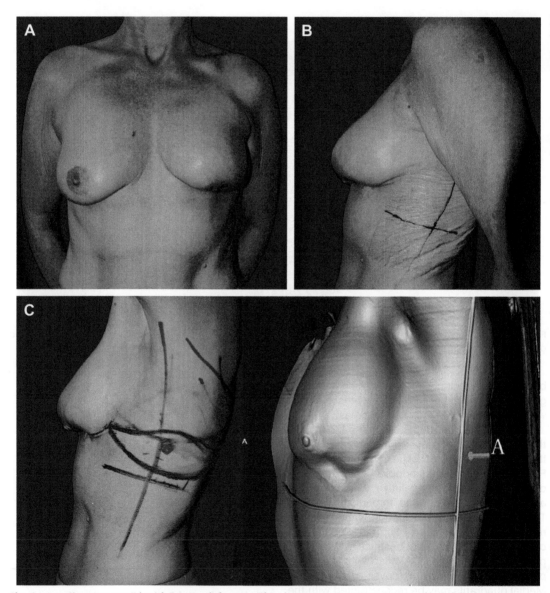

Fig. 2. A patient presented with severe deformity after breast conservation surgery for left breast cancer. An attempt to lengthen the inferior pole with Z-plasty was performed by another surgeon without success. The breast was extremely scarred and fibrotic at the lower pole with atrophic overlying skin. A TDAP flap was used to provide adequate tissue after scar excision and release. Fat injection with contralateral breast remodeling was performed 3 months later. (*A, B*) Preoperative views. (*C*) Design of the TDAP flap incorporating the thoracodorsal perforator (*marked*) localized preoperatively by MDCT.

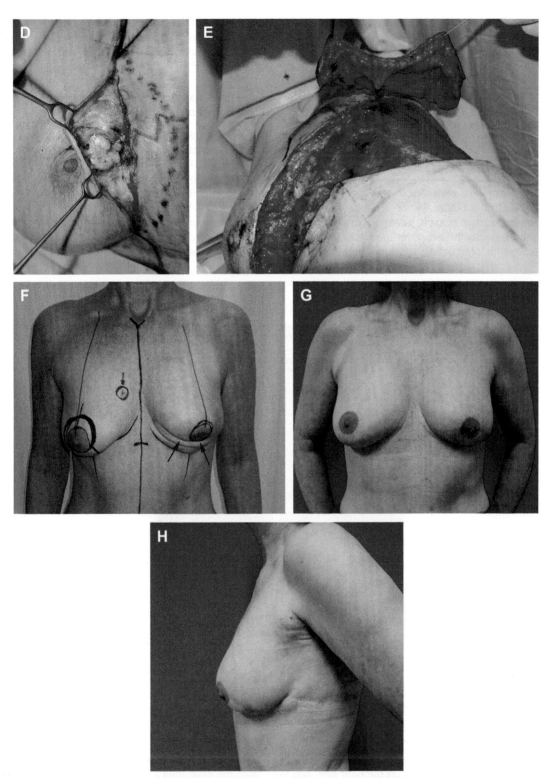

Fig. 2. (*D*) Scar tissue with a cartilage-like nodule from multiple surgeries and irradiation. (*E*) The defect postscar excision and the TDAP flap. (*F*) The patient at 3-months post-TDAP flap reconstruction (*arrows*) planned for fat injection and contralateral breast remodeling. (*G, H*) Outcome of the reconstruction. Areola tattoo was also performed.

avoided to preserve vascularity, but releasing all scar tissue is vital for a good aesthetic outcome. The resultant defect is always significantly larger after scar release; this should be anticpated and a larger flap designed. In the majority of cases, contralateral breast remodeling is necessary to achieve breast symmetry. Further surgical corrections with or without fat grafting might be needed if the initial deformity was severe.[10,17]

Thoracic/Axillary Wall Reconstruction

PPFs are well suited for resurfacing defects around the shoulder.[15,22,23] Defects related to cancer excision, trauma, infection, or burns have been treated with skin coverage based on thoracodorsal or intercostal perforators (**Fig. 3**). Based

on the free-style perforator flap concept, 1 or more perforators may be identified adjacent to the defect and a flap designed and elevated accordingly.[23]

Salvage Procedure after Partial Necrosis of Flap in Breast Reconstruction

Salvage procedure after partial necrosis of flap in breast reconstruction is an ultimate indication for PPFs (**Fig. 4**). Raising a skin flap without sacrificing the LD muscle is ideal for patients who suffer from major partial flap or fat necrosis. In the majority of cases, the PPF can be harvested without sacrificing the thoracodorsal pedicle; the LICAP and AICAP flap cover the necrosed areas at the lateral and medial extremities of the breast flap,

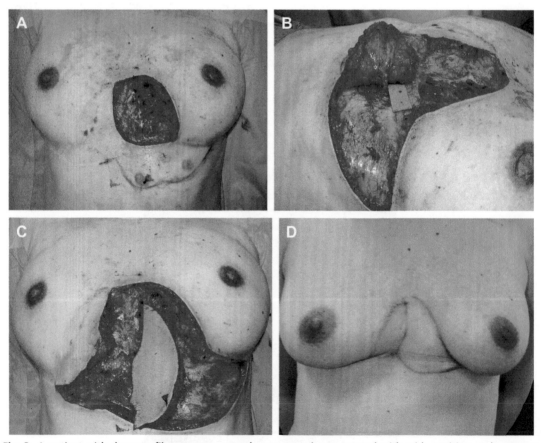

Fig. 3. A patient with dermato-fibrosarcoma over the presternal area treated with wide excision and coverage with an AICAP flap harvested on the right side. Two years later, she developed a local recurrence extending to the medial quadrant of the left breast. (*A*) Wide resection was done and an AICAP flap was designed over the upper left abdomen. Perforators were localized preoperatively using a handheld Doppler. (*B*) The anterior intercostal perforator was dissected within the left rectus abdominis muscle. (*C*) The flap was completely islanded and rotated 90° anticlockwise to cover the defect. The donor site was primarily closed with abdominal advancement. (*D*) The final result with complete wound healing.

respectively. The TDAP flap, however, is preferred when the necrosis involves more than 40% of the breast.

Postmastectomy Reconstruction with or without Implant

The combination of an expander or implant with the LD musculocutaneous flap is well accepted as a safe and reliable method for postmastectomy reconstruction. The versatile LD flap has undergone a resurgence in popularity because many new applications are being described. Replacing the classical LD musculocutaneous flap by a TDAP flap looks appealing for postmastectomy reconstruction because it spares one of the largest muscles in the body. The TDAP, however, provides less volume than the classical LD musculocutaneous flap, and placing an expander or implant under a TDAP flap may be needed but could lead to perforator compression and consequently flap failure. The authors presented strategies of combining the TDAP flap with an implant to achieve a safe technique of breast reconstruction with minimal donor site morbidity.[24]

To enhance the level of safety and durability of the technique, total breast reconstruction using PPFs without implants is the next step. Avoiding alloplastic materials is ideal because it results in fewer short-term and long-term complications with fewer revision procedures. When the axillary/back fat fold is sufficiently thick, total breast reconstruction solely with a pedicled TDAP flap is feasible, especially when the required breast size is small to medium. In the majority of cases, however, pedicled flaps alone do not have sufficient volume to allow for total breast reconstruction. Total breast reconstruction using a combination of pedicled LD musculocutaneous flap and abdominal advancement flap followed by serial sessions of fat grafting was previously described by Sinna and colleagues.[25] With the resurgence of fat grafting during the last decade, using the PPF as a vascularized tissue scaffold for subsequent fat grafting is a good alternative to free perforator flaps for total autologous breast reconstruction while reducing donor site morbidity to the minimum.

Autologous Breast Augmentation

PPFs can be used for breast augmentation in situations, such as breast asymmetry, bilateral breast augmentation without the use of implants, and as a combined augmentation-mastopexy procedure in massive weight loss patients.[26] In most massive weight loss patients, the breast deformity is accompanied by lateral skin redundancy, or side

rolls, in the lateral thoracic area. The excess axillary extension of the breast can be used to autoaugment patients with insufficient breast volume using a variety of surgical techniques. The authors described the use of the lateral redundant dermoglandular tissue based on LICAPs.[19,26] The technique evolved from an initial experience with LICAP flaps for partial breast reconstruction within a clinical algorithm based on the location of the defect and the availability of these perforators. As the skin redundancy extends further posteriorly, the flap can be based on perforators from the thoracodorsal artery. The TDAP flap is thus another valuable tool that redistributes redundant tissue from the back to reshape the breast via the autoaugmentation principle.

TECHNIQUES
Surgical Anatomy

The surgical anatomy of the TDAP flap and the intercostal artery perforator flaps were described in the authors' previous publications. The thoracodorsal artery is the main pedicle of the LD muscle and divides into the descending and transverse branches. The descending branch is the preferred choice for the flap as the perforators take on a more direct and perpendicular intramuscular course, making dissection easier.[18] The musculocutaneous perforators are located within an area 5 cm posterior to the anterior border of the LD at a level 8 cm to 13 cm caudal to the axillary crease.[18,27] In 55% of patients, a septocutaneous perforator arises from the thoracodorsal artery and runs anterior to the border of the LD muscle, obviating intramuscular dissection.[27] To include this perforator, the skin paddle of the flap should, therefore, extend beyond the anterior border of the LD muscle.

The lateral intercostal artery perforators are located in the 4th to 8th intercostal spaces at a mean distance of 3.5 cm anterior to the anterior border of the LD muscle.[19] Flap dissection is, therefore, possible without needing to sacrifice the thoracodorsal vessels or LD muscle. These perforators arise from the costal segment of the intercostal artery, which run in the subcostal groove between the internal and innermost intercostal muscles. The perforators pierce the internal and external intercostal muscles, pass obliquely under a slip of the origin of the serratus anterior muscle, and run medially posteriorly superficial to the LD muscle, usually accompanied by a sensory cutaneous nerve.

A vascular connection between the intercostal perforators and the serratus anterior branch is found in 21% of cases.[19] When present, this

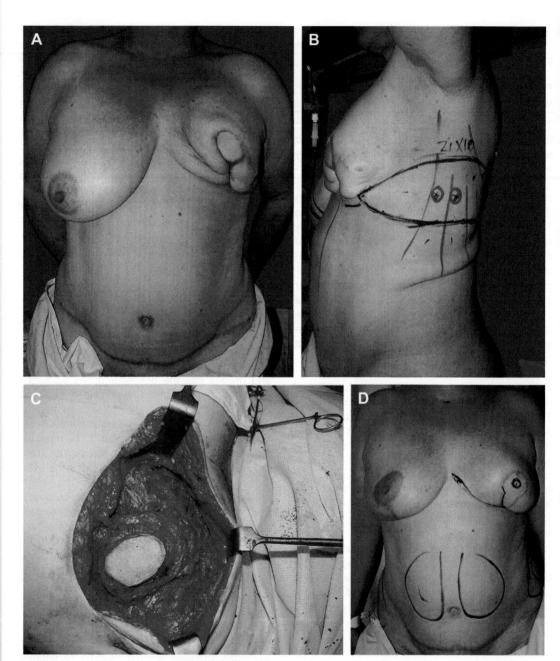

Fig. 4. A 58-year-old patient who underwent skin sparing mastectomy and primary deep inferior epigastric perforator flap breast reconstruction developed major partial flap and fat necrosis. Corrective surgery was planned in 2 stages: débridement and TDAP flap reconstruction in the first stage, followed by fat injection and contralateral breast remodeling in the second stage. (A) Preoperative photograph showing major flap volume loss after multiple revisions of venous microanastomoses. (B) Design of TDAP flap with perforators localized preoperatively with Doppler ultrasound. (C) Débridement resulted in more than 80% loss from the initial flap volume. (D) Three months postreconstruction with TDAP flap. The flap was de-epithelialized under the native breast skin leaving a skin paddle for the nipple areolar complex. In the second stage, 300 cm³ of fat was injected with reduction of the contralateral breast.

enables the harvest of the serratus anterior perforator flap, which has the benefits of a long pedicle that can reach medial breast defects while preserving the thoracodorsal vessels.[19]

Anterior intercostal perforators originate from the muscular or rectus segments of the intercostal artery and are the basis of the AICAP flaps.[13,15]

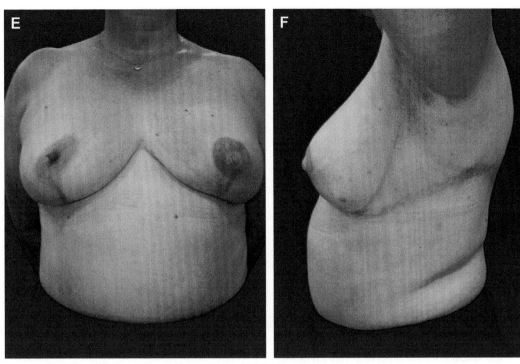

Fig. 4. (*E*) The result at 6 months postoperatively. (*F*) The donor site.

The SEA is the inferior continuation of the internal mammary artery and enters the rectus abdominis muscle on its deep surface, approximately 7 cm below the costal margin.[20] Several perforators arise from the branches of the SEA, between the costal margin to the first tendinous intersection. The perforators pierce the rectus muscle or the sheath beside the lateral border of the muscle.[20]

Preoperative Perforator Mapping

It is essential to locate the perforators preoperatively. Careful perforator mapping is a decisive step for the choice of perforator in PPFs and reduces the operative time and complication rate significantly. The potential perforators are identified using a unidirectional Doppler (8 Hz) whereupon the flap is designed to incorporate the chosen perforator.[28] For the TDAP and LICAP flaps, Doppler examination is performed with patients in a lateral decubitus position with 90° of shoulder abduction and 90° of elbow flexion. This replicates the position at surgery and stretches the skin, placing the perforators in a perpendicular orientation for accurate Doppler localization. The mapping of an intercostal or superior epigastric perforator is done on the patient in supine position. In difficult cases, a duplex examination is performed.[28] More recently, the MDCT and MRI

examinations have been introduced for the preoperative localization of various perforators.[28–30]

Flap Design

TDAP/LICAP/serratus anterior artery perforator flap

The borders of the LD muscle are marked with the patient standing with both hands pressed on the hips. Doppler examination is performed as described previously. The flap is designed like the classic LD myocutaneous flap but to include any possible septocutaneous perforators from the thoracodorsal artery or lateral intercostal artery perforators, the anterior aspect of the flap should always overlie the anterior border of the LD, reaching the lateral border of the inframammary fold.[16–19] The flap measures 20 cm × 8 cm on average, with the width determined by the size of the defect and the ability for primary closure of the donor site.

AICAP/SEAP flap

The skin paddle is marked over the upper abdomen and incorporates the identified perforator.[20] The flap is usually designed over the midline and extends laterally under the inframammary fold. The flap width is determined by pinch test and varies between 4 cm and 8 cm. The donor site is closed primarily but refixation of the inframammary fold may be necessary in the case of high-tension closure. The flap can be completely islanded or designed as a rotation flap.

Surgical Technique

The surgical technique of the TDAP flap has been widely described in the authors' previous reports and is discussed in general terms[10,13–19]:

- The patient is positioned depending on the location of breast defect and/or the clinical indication. Most of PPFs are harvested in lateral decubitus with 90° of shoulder abduction and 90° of elbow flexion.
- The skin is first incised at the anteroinferior border of the flap; this allows identification of the anterior border of the LD muscle and the possibility of repositioning the anterior border of the flap if necessary. Skin and subcutaneous tissue are incised down to the level of the muscle fascia, bevelling outwards to include more fat.
- Suprafascial flap elevation under loupe magnification proceeds cranially above the LD fascia until the preoperatively identified perforators are encountered.
- A posterior approach is generally used when a TDAP flap is planned; however, an anterior approach is used for LICAP flap. By approaching the perforator in this manner, surgeons still have other options available in the case of unfavorable perforator anatomy.
- Once a suitable perforator has been identified, the LD muscle is split around the perforator in the direction of the muscle fibers, maintaining their longitudinal integrity.
- The perforator is dissected from the surrounding muscle fibers, where they tend to lie in a fibrofatty layer. Wide exposure is essential to perforator dissection within the muscle. The dissection should be performed close to the pedicle, ligating muscular branches with surgical clips or bipolar cautery. Nerve branches to the LD muscle should be freed from the pedicle with atraumatic dissection technique. The main thoracodorsal pedicle is dissected free until the required pedicle length is obtained. The branch to the serratus may be divided if it impedes reach.
- When dissection of the perforator is complete, the flap is detached from the serratus fascia and from the LD muscle and intercostal perforators that may be encountered in front of the anterior border of the LD muscle.

- The flap is now based totally on the TDAP. A subcutaneous tunnel between the LD and the breast that is wide enough to accommodate the flap is developed. The flap is passed through the split LD into the tunnel and transposed into the defect with its anterior border becoming the medial or inferior part of the reconstruction. Extreme care should be taken in order not to damage the perforator during the passage of the flap.
- The donor site is closed in layers over a drain and the patient turned supine for shaping and inset.
- The pliable flap lends itself to being easily folded as required to fill the defect and may be partially or completely de-epithelialized depending on the need for a skin paddle.

When a LICAP flap is planned, the flap is designed with its anterior aspect overlying this perforator extending posteriorly along the axis of the rib. A similar approach to that of the TDAP flap is used.

- The serratus anterior muscle surrounding the perforator is split along the direction of the muscle fibers.
- The perforator is dissected close to the vessel, ligating any side branches with clips or bipolar cautery. The course of the perforator is traced through the serratus anterior, external intercostal, and internal intercostal muscles to its origin from the intercostal artery in the subcostal groove. This allows sufficient pedicle length to rotate the flap 180° for inset without torsion of the pedicle.
- If a longer pedicle is required, the intercostal artery may be dissected anteriorly subperiosteally within the subcostal groove. This maneuver, however, carries a potential risk of pneumothorax and is usually unnecessary.

CLINICAL OUTCOME OF PEDICLED PERFORATOR FLAPS

It is difficult to predict the long-term outcome of partial breast reconstruction with PPFs due to the indefinite impact of irradiation on the final outcome. Nevertheless, the authors' experience has shown a stable result in the long term. Moreover, the majority of the authors' PPFs were used in partial breast reconstruction without contralateral breast remodeling. Breast asymmetry, therefore, might be expected due to the different aging processes between the 2 breasts. The nonirradiated side may become more ptotic with time compared with the irradiated side. Alternatively, the irradiated side may show signs of total breast atrophy. When the breast asymmetry becomes obvious, fat grafting alone or with contralateral breast remodeling is indicated.

The use of fat grafting, alone or most commonly in combination with other reconstructive options for the treatment of breast defects after tumor resection, is gaining popularity. In contrast to what was believed in the past, fat grafting of the breast is now accepted as a safe, reliable method for treating volume and contour abnormalities of the breast.[31]

COMPLICATIONS AND CONCERNS WITH PEDICLED PERFORATOR FLAPS

The main benefit of PPFs over traditional myocutaneous flaps in partial breast reconstruction is the reduction in donor site morbidity associated with functional muscle preservation.[32] Only a few seroma formations have been observed, which can be managed conservatively. Wound dehiscence at the donor site may occur when the wound is closed under tension but this is an infrequent event and is managed with local treatment. Displeasing scars, flap contractures, and volume loss are other sequelae that may require secondary surgical correction. Flap reconstruction of a partial breast defect may give a plugged-in appearance; this seems to improve slightly after radiation therapy. Finally, some patients who undergo partial breast reconstruction with a TDAP flap report an initial decrease in forward arm elevation and passive abduction, which recovers over time.

SUMMARY

BCT has a proved track record for treating breast cancer while preserving uninvolved breast tissue. PPFs are available to address many of the post-BCT defects while limiting donor site morbidity and preserving good aesthetic outcome. The introduction of these flaps showed clearly that sacrificing the LD muscle is not needed and flaps can be based solely on a single perforator. Using the free style-perforator flap concept, many challenging defects can be now be covered by adjacent PPFs. Moreover, these flaps can also function as a vascularized tissue matrix for subsequent fat grafting. Based on this novel concept, total reconstruction of moderate-sized breasts can be achieved. The surgical techniques of elevating PPFs have been established. Preoperative perforator mapping with Doppler ultrasound remains a challenge; advances in CT and MRI

imaging technology promise to simplify this task and increase precision and reliability.

REFERENCES

1. Veronesi U, Cascinelli N, Mariani L, et al. Twenty-year follow-up of a randomized study comparing breast-conserving surgery with radical mastectomy for early breast cancer. N Engl J Med 2002; 347(16):1227–32.
2. Dillon MF, Hill AD, Quinn CM, et al. A pathologic assessment of adequate margin status in breast-conserving therapy. Ann Surg Oncol 2006; 13(3):333–9.
3. Clough KB, Kroll SS, Audretsch W. An approach to the repair of partial mastectomy defects. Plast Reconstr Surg 1999;104(2):409–20.
4. Slavin SA, Love SM, Sadowsky NL. Reconstruction of the radiated partial mastectomy defect with autogenous tissues. Plast Reconstr Surg 1992; 90(5):854–65.
5. Audretsh WP. Fundamentals of oncoplastic surgery. In: Losken A, Hamdi M, editors. Partial breast reconstruction: techniques in oncoplastic surgery. St Louis (MO): Q.M.P.Inc; 2009. p. 3–26.
6. Anderson BO, Masetti R, Silverstein MJ. Oncoplastic approaches to partial mastectomy: an overview of volume-displacement techniques. Lancet Oncol 2005;6(3):145–57.
7. Kronowitz SJ, Kuerer HM, Buchholz TA, et al. A management algorithm and practical oncoplastic surgical techniques for repairing partial mastectomy defects. Plast Reconstr Surg 2008;122(6):1631–47.
8. Kronowitz SJ. Immediate versus delayed reconstruction. Clin Plast Surg 2007;34(1):39–50.
9. Song HM, Styblo TM, Carlson GW, et al. The use of oncoplastic reduction techniques to reconstruct partial mastectomy defects in women with ductal carcinoma in situ. Breast J 2010;16(2):141–6.
10. Hamdi M, Wolfli J, Van Landuyt K. Partial mastectomy reconstruction. Clin Plast Surg 2007;34(1):51–62.
11. Gendy RK, Able JA, Rainsbury RM. Impact of skin-sparing mastectomy with immediate reconstruction and breast-sparing reconstruction with miniflaps on the outcomes of oncoplastic breast surgery. Br J Surg 2003;90(4):433–9.
12. Dixon JM, Venizelos B, Chan P. Latissimus dorsi mini-flap: a technique for extending breast conservation. Breast 2002;11(1):58–65.
13. Hamdi M, Van Landuyt K, Monstrey S, et al. Pedicled perforator flaps in breast reconstruction: a new concept. Br J Plast Surg 2004;57(6):531–9.
14. Levine JL, Soueid NE, Allen RJ. Algorithm for autologous breast reconstruction for partial mastectomy defects. Plast Reconstr Surg 2005;116(3):762–7.

15. Hamdi M, Van Landuyt K, de Frene B, et al. The versatility of the inter-costal artery perforator (ICAP) flaps. J Plast Reconstr Aesthet Surg 2006;59(6):644–52.

16. Hamdi M. Pedicled perforator flap reconstruction. In: Losken A, Hamdi M, editors. Partial breast reconstruction: techniques in oncoplastic surgery. St Louis (MO): Q.M.P.Inc; 2009. p. 387.

17. Losken A, Hamdi M. Partial breast reconstruction: current perspectives. Plast Reconstr Surg 2009; 124(3):722–36.

18. Hamdi M, Van Landuyt K, Hijjawi JB, et al. Surgical technique in pedicled thoracodorsal artery perforator flaps: a clinical experience with 99 patients. Plast Reconstr Surg 2008;121(5):1632–41.

19. Hamdi M, Spano A, Van Landuyt K, et al. The lateral intercostal artery perforators: anatomical study and clinical application in breast surgery. Plast Reconstr Surg 2008;121(2):389–96.

20. Hamdi M, Van Landuyt K, Ulens S, et al. Clinical applications of the superior epigastric artery perforator (SEAP) flap: anatomical studies and preoperative perforator mapping with multidetector CT. J Plast Reconstr Aesthet Surg 2009;62(9):1127–34.

21. Veber M, Ho Quoc C, Fakiha M, et al. Lateral Intercostal Artery Perforator (LICAP) flap for lateral breast defect reconstruction. Ann Chir Plast Esthet 2011;56(6):568–73.

22. Ortiz CL, Mendoza MM, Sempere LN, et al. Versatility of the pedicled thoracodorsal artery perforator (TDAP) flap in soft tissue reconstruction. Ann Plast Surg 2007;58(3):315–20.

23. Stillaert FB, Casaer B, Roche N, et al. The inframammary extending lateral intercostal artery perforator flap for reconstruction of axillary contractures: a case report. J Plast Reconstr Aesthet Surg 2008; 61(12):e7–11.

24. Hamdi M, Salgarello M, Barone-Adesi L, et al. Use of the thoracodorsal artery perforator (TDAP) flap with implant in breast reconstruction. Ann Plast Surg 2008;61(2):143–6.

25. Sinna R, Delay E, Garson S, et al. Breast fat grafting (lipomodelling) after extended latissimus dorsi flap breast reconstruction: a preliminary report of 200 consecutive cases. J Plast Reconstr Aesthet Surg 2010;63(11):1769–77.

26. Hamdi M, Van Landuyt K, Blondeel P, et al. Autologous breast augmentation with the lateral intercostal artery perforator flap in massive weight loss patients. J Plast Reconstr Aesthet Surg 2009;62:65–70.

27. Heitmann C, Guerra A, Metzinger SW, et al. The thoracodorsal artery perforator flap: anatomic basis and clinical application. Ann Plast Surg 2003;51(1):23–9.

28. Hamdi M, Van Landuyt K, Van Hedent E, et al. Advances in autogenous breast reconstruction: the role of preoperative perforator mapping. Ann Plast Surg 2007;58(1):18–26.

29. Masia J, Clavero JA, Larrañaga JR, et al. Multidetector-row computed tomography in the planning of abdominal perforator flaps. J Plast Reconstr Aesthet Surg 2006;59(6):594–9.

30. Masia J, Navarro C, Clavero JA, et al. Noncontrast magnetic resonance imaging for preoperative perforator mapping. Clin Plast Surg 2011;38(2):253–61.

31. Petit JY, Lohsiriwat V, Clough KB, et al. The oncologic outcome and immediate surgical complications of lipofilling in breast cancer patients: a multicenter study—Milan-Paris-Lyon experience of 646 lipofilling procedures. Plast Reconstr Surg 2011;128(2): 341–6.

32. Hamdi M, Decorte T, Demuynck M, et al. Shoulder function after harvesting a thoracodorsal artery perforator flap. Plast Reconstr Surg 2008;122(4):1111–7.

Microsurgical Advances in Extremity Salvage

Milomir Ninkovic, MD, PhD[a],*, Sebastian Voigt, MD[a],
Ulf Dornseifer, MD[a], Sarah Lorenz, MD[a],
Marina Ninkovic, MD[b]

KEYWORDS

- Complex extremity injury • Free flap • Timing of reconstruction • Microsurgical extremity salvage

KEY POINTS

- Isolated complex extremity injury requires immediate specialized attention via an interdisciplinary approach.
- Key steps in surgical management include radical tissue debridement, adequate fracture stabilization, and reconstruction of viable structures—if necessary, by use of autologous blood vessels or nerve grafts.
- A key step in surgical management and one of the most powerful tools for infection control is an early and radical debridement of devitalized, and potentially contaminated, tissue.
- Although still considered essential components in reconstructive surgery, local flaps and skin grafting are often associated with an increased rate of wound complications and compromises concerning results, enabling new techniques of free tissue transfer, functional composite free flaps, and preexpanded and chimeric flaps to become better options in extremity salvage surgery.

INTRODUCTION

During the past 40 years, evolution in reconstructive microsurgery has substantially influenced limb salvage surgery. Despite continuous improvement in trauma management leading to a significant reduction in primary limb amputations, complex injuries involving extremities remain a particular challenge for reconstructive surgeons. In the past, limb salvage procedures were often impended by local tissue status; modern methods of microsurgical free tissue transfer now allow an early, "custom-fit" wound management, aimed to optimally meet the individual functional and esthetic requirements of the affected trauma region.

State-of-the-art reconstructive microsurgery has opened a wide range of possibilities in limb salvage surgery allowing immediate fracture and soft tissue repair with only minimal compromise in functional outcome. Key steps in surgical management include radical tissue debridement, adequate fracture stabilization, and reconstruction of viable structures (if necessary, by use of autologous blood vessels or nerve grafts). Subsequently, tissue defects should be covered by sufficient well-vascularized tissue, optimally matched to meet the individual tissue requirements at the recipient site.[1] The authors outline the impact of recent microsurgical advances on extremity salvage and reconstruction.

Disclosures: The following authors have identified no professional or financial affiliation for themselves or their spouse/partner: Milomir Ninkovic, MD, PhD; Sebastian Voigt, MD; Sarah Lorenz, MD; Marina Ninkovic, MD; and Ulf Dornseifer, MD.
[a] Department of Plastic, Reconstructive, Hand and Burn Surgery, Klinikum Bogenhausen, Städtisches Klinikum München GmbH, Munich, Germany; [b] Unit of Physical Medicine and Rehabilitation, Center of Operative Medicine, Innsbruck Medical University, Anichstrasse 35, Innsbruck A-6020, Austria
* Corresponding author. Department of Plastic, Reconstructive Hand and Burn Surgery, Klinikum Bogenhausen, Städtisches Klinikum München GmbH, Englschalkinger Straße 77, Munich 81825, Germany.
E-mail address: milomir.ninkovic@klinikum-muenchen.de

Clin Plastic Surg 39 (2012) 491–505
http://dx.doi.org/10.1016/j.cps.2012.08.003

INITIAL PREOPERATIVE ASSESSMENT

Initial stabilization and diagnosis should be performed via a multidisciplinary approach according to the established Advanced trauma life support protocol.[2] For extremity trauma, immediate attention primarily targets hemorrhage control. Once the patient is stabilized, a focused clinical evaluation is performed. Assessment of injured extremities must consider trauma mechanisms, wound dimensions, and all functional components (soft tissue, nerves, vessels, and bones). These components must be examined individually and in combination.

Radiographic imaging should also be focused on the trauma zone including directly adjacent joints. In case of potential vascular involvement, Doppler sonography or angiography is essential for evaluation and planning of surgical treatment, especially because vascular damage can potentially exclude the use of local flaps.

INDICATIONS FOR RECONSTRUCTION VERSUS AMPUTATION

Indications for limb salvage procedures versus primary amputation must be evaluated individually for each patient, considering not only local trauma site but also patient age, presence of other concomitant injuries, patient comorbidities, patient socioeconomic status, and patient motivation. Despite major advancements in reconstructive microsurgery, severe lower extremity trauma (Gustilo III-B-IIIC) is still associated with amputation rates of up to 40%.[3,4] In general, indications for microsurgical free flap reconstruction include the following[5]:

- Trauma-induced injures with substantial bone and muscle defects
- Osteomyelitis
- Deep burns
- Tumor excisions
- Vascular disease

The most commonly used classification system for lower extremity trauma has been the Gustilo classification, introduced in 1976 and subsequently modified in 1984 (**Table 1**). This classification analyzes not only wound dimensions and the presence or absence of neurovascular injury but also wound contamination and trauma energy impact.[6]

Numerous algorithms have been established, designed to estimate the viability of damaged tissue and to assist in determining whether amputation is necessary or whether limb salvage of traumatized extremities is recommended and promising. These include the Mangled Extremity

Table 1 Gustilo classification	
Gustilo Classification	Definition
Type I	Wound <1 cm, minimal contamination, low-energy and simple fracture
Type II	Laceration >1 cm; moderate soft tissue damage with adequate bone coverage
Type IIIA	Extensive soft tissue damage, massive contamination but adequate bone coverage
Type IIIB	Extensive soft tissue damage with periosteal stripping and bone exposure, flap coverage is usually required
Type IIIC	Arterial injury associated and requiring repair

Severity Score, the Limb Salvage Index, the Predictive Salvage Index, and the Hannover Fracture Scale.[7-11] Besides providing an analysis of local tissue status, these scores also specifically consider arterial and venous vascular injury as a prognostic factor and warm ischemia and shock time. A prospective evaluation of 556 consecutive patients from 2001 on showed that, because of high specificity, low scores reliably predicted limb salvage potential. In contrast, because of low sensitivity, trauma evaluation scores did not reliably identify patients possibly requiring an amputation.[12] Current data suggest that these scores can be useful tools in the decision-making process (when used cautiously). They should not be used as the principal means for reaching difficult decisions.[13] From an economic point of view, unless amputation is inevitable, surgeons should always consider limb salvage, which will yields lower costs and higher utility compared with amputation.[14]

Special attention must be paid to complete traumatic limb amputation. If the patient's life is at stake, the principle of "life before limb" will obviously be the primary objective. In this case, immediate replantation remains fairly uncommon.[15] Indications for primary amputation may include advanced patient age, severe crush injuries with complete transsection of essential anatomic structures, prolonged warm ischemia time, or presence of potentially life-threatening concomitant injuries. In the case of traumatic amputation, warm ischemia can be tolerated up to 8 hours and cooling may extend the time-frame for replantation to 24 hours.[16,17] A study published in 2005 demonstrated that plantar sensation is no longer a limiting prognostic factor when evaluating possible limb salvage, because it showed comparable functional outcomes in plantar sensation between patients initially lacking and patients with permanently preserved plantar sensitivity.[18]

Thus, a surgeon must perform realistic risk-benefit stratification to determine whether amputation is justified. When considering salvage procedures, expectations must be tempered by a realistic assessment of potential outcome, because protracted attempts for limb salvage may have a negative impact on the patient's social, physiologic and psychological subsistence.[19] In some cases, limb amputation may even be the preferable strategy because it may reduce the duration of hospitalization and rehabilitation. Several studies even suggest that patients with primary amputation show equally good functional outcomes as those who underwent limb reconstruction.[20] The lower extremity assessment project demonstrated reconstruction results in 2-year outcomes equivalent to those of amputation.[20]

In conclusion, individual patient assessment remains the key step in determining whether limb salvage or primary amputation is indicated. Through a careful risk-benefit assessment, surgeons should try to optimally meet outcome expectations while keeping morbidity at the lowest possible level.

TIMING

Since Marco Godina introduced the concept of the "emergency" free tissue transfer in the 1980s, surgical treatment of severe tissue trauma has experienced a substantial change.[21] Early, fastidious trauma zone debridement followed by immediate restoration of affected longitudinal structures and early defect coverage by transferring adequately vascularized tissue has proved to reduce the incidence of osteomyelitis and fracture nonunion. In his study from 1986, Godina showed that delayed microsurgical reconstruction following trauma (between 72 hours and 90 days) was associated with the highest risk of infection and flap loss. Thus, he proposed the concept of "early" microsurgical reconstruction within 72 hours after trauma. Despite the proved advantage, the optimal timing for free tissue wound coverage remains controversial. Several consecutive studies analyzing the correlation between time until reconstruction and complication rate or functional outcome proved to be consistent with Godina's initial results, showing that early microsurgical reconstruction significantly reduced

bone union time, number of surgical procedures, and infection rate.[22–25] In contrast, a study from 2008 showed no potential disadvantage associated with delayed lower extremity reconstruction.[26] Byrd and colleagues[22] demonstrated the importance of early soft tissue coverage after removing all devitalized tissue, thereby preventing bacterial colonization. Complex and contaminated wounds should be converted into surgically clean wounds to allow primary closure.[24]

There remains a wide and misleading variety of terms used for defining windows during which posttraumatic free flap wound closure is recommended. To reliably compare reconstructive results between individual institutions, a standardized terminology for the timing of free flap coverage is essential. Thus, Ninkovic and colleagues implemented a simple and versatile terminology, analogous to the established nomenclature defining the phases of normal wound healing.[27]

According to this terminology, flap closure timing is subdivided into 3 categories:

1. "Primary free flap closure" (12–24 hours)
2. "Delayed primary free flap closure" (2–7 days)
3. "Secondary free flap closure" (>7 days)

Primary flap cover for crucial closure prevents further tissue damage caused by desiccation and facilitates vascular ingrowth from the new surrounding soft tissue. Well-vascularized muscle free flaps provide healthy tissue, thereby allowing a radical debridement of the trauma zone. Because the primary goal in the treatment of complex extremity injury is a quick and functionally optimal recovery, the treatment of choice is the primarily free flap cover within the first 24 hours after injury. This minimizes morbidity, tissue infection rate, requirement for secondary surgical procedures, rehabilitation time, and total duration of hospital stay.[28]

Primary free flap closure with primary reconstruction is defined as a combination of definite functional reconstruction of longitudinal structures (bone, vessels, nerves, and tendons using grafts if it is necessary) combined with free or pedicled flap coverage following surgical debridement as a single-step procedure within a period of 24 hours (**Figs. 1** and **2**).

Delayed primary reconstruction is defined by free flap defect closure within 2 to 7 days after the trauma. Again, definite reconstruction of longitudinal structures can be performed within this time frame or later according to the wound condition and type of injury. It is important to consider that by delaying timing of definite defect closure, surgical options for reconstruction of longitudinal structures are significantly reduced without

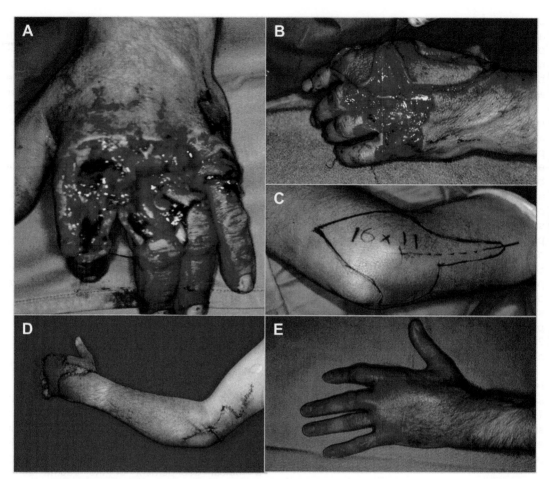

Fig. 1. (*A*) Complex hand injury with severe soft tissue defect, MCP joint destruction, and extensor tendon defect following motor-saw accident post primary reconstruction of all injured. (*B*) Structures as joint capsule and extensor tendon by using tendon graft. (*C*) Planning of extended lateral arm flap for primary soft tissue coverage. (*D*) Two weeks after surgery at the time of discharging. (*E*) One-year follow-up.

possibilities to replace the missing structure (eg, bone, tendon, nerve) with graft because of a higher rate of infection. However, this coverage allows the possibility of starting immediate physical medicine and, soon, definitive secondary reconstruction (**Figs. 3** and **4**).

Secondary free flap closure signifies closure with a free flap later than 1 week after the trauma. In general, reconstruction of soft tissue and temporary bone stabilization may be achieved. However, definite reconstruction of longitudinal structures and bone defects is performed later (**Figs. 5** and **6**).

SURGICAL TECHNIQUE
Radical Debridement

A key step in surgical management and one of the most powerful tools for infection control is an early and radical debridement of devitalized, and potentially contaminated, tissue. Debridement should be performed like resection of malignancy, which means through healthy tissue and always under tourniquet control. It minimizes blood loss during debridement and alleviates evaluation of traumatized tissue. Tendons and essential neurovascular structures should be debrided and preserved, provided they are intact. In case of damage or complete transsection, essential structures should be primarily repaired either through direct coaptation or via interposition of vessels, tendon, nerve, or bone grafts.[29,30]

Fracture Stabilization

For skeletal stabilization, external fixation is the initial method of choice. In case of minimal soft tissue destruction and wound contamination, primary internal fixation can be performed.

Since the imposition of microsurgery in the 1960s, the traditional concept of the "reconstructive

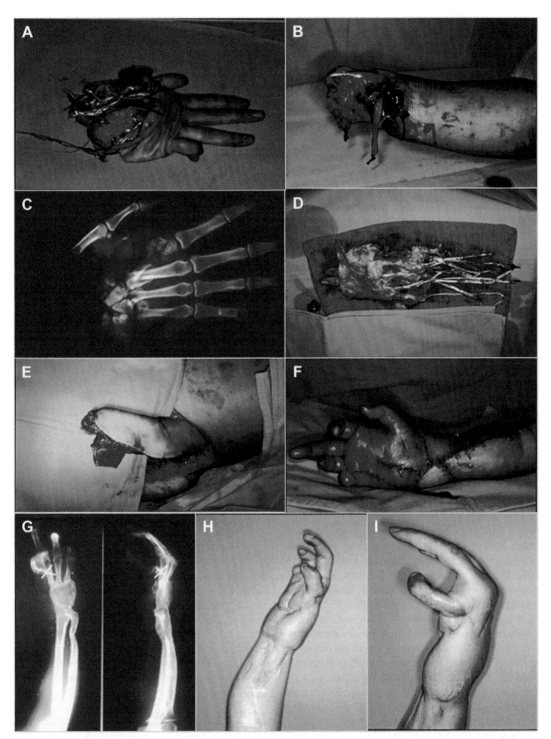

Fig. 2. Primary free flap closure with delayed thumb reconstruction: avulsed right-hand amputation following contact with helicopter blade. (*A–D*) Surgical steps included radical debridement, replantation performing bone stabilization, vessels, tendons, nerve repair, and soft tissue reconstruction using a composite groin flap including vascularized iliac crest bone graft for carpal-metacarpal bone defect. (*E, F*) Two years after delayed thumb reconstruction by pollicization with index finger following primary surgery. (*G–I*) Note primary bone healing after composite groin flap.

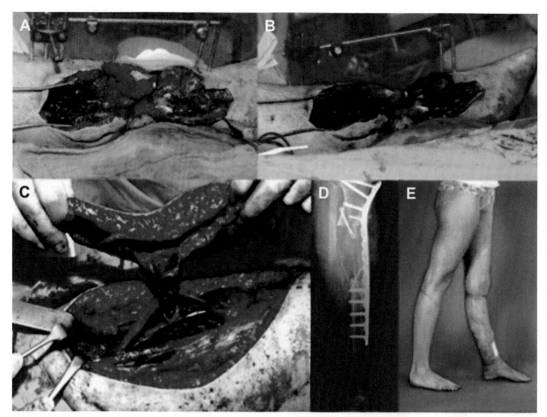

Fig. 3. Delayed free flap closure with secondary bone reconstruction: 2 Days after extensive trauma to the left sided lower extremity following motor vehicle accident. (*A*) Initial surgical management consisted of radical surgical debridement, temporary fracture stabilization and soft tissue coverage using a anterior lateral thigh flow-though free flap for lower extremity revascularisation. (*B, C*) Definite bone stabilization was performed in a second procedure using a vascularized iliac crest bone graft anastomosed to the descending branch of the circumflex femoral artery. (*D*) 2 Year follow up (*E*).

ladder" has undergone a rapid and substantial evolution. In the past, the primary objective was a simple wound closure using local flaps and skin grafts. Modern microsurgery allows reconstruction of complex bone and soft tissue defects with excellent esthetic and functional outcomes.[31,32] Thus, the reconstructive ladder has undergone "surgical acceleration" toward becoming the "reconstructive elevator."[33,34] Although local flaps and skin grafting are still considered essential components in reconstructive surgery, they are often associated with an increased rate of wound complications and compromises concerning results.[35] Consequently, the importance of local flaps is increasingly receding into the background. Today, local and pedicled flaps are still recommended for small to medium-sized defects, which cannot sufficiently be treated by direct closure or skin grafts.[36] In case of complex extremity trauma, local flaps are often damaged and therefore unusable. Further compromise of a severely injured extremity by sacrificing local tissue should be avoided.

Therefore, free tissue transfer provides the most appropriate repair for severely injured extremities.[37]

Modern techniques range from supermicrosurgical free tissue transfer, functional composite free flaps, and preexpanded and chimeric flaps to innervated functional myocutaneous flaps.[38,39] Today, through constant improvement in surgical technique and understanding of perforator anatomy, microsurgical free tissue transfer is considered a routine technique that opens almost endless possibilities in extremity salvage surgery.[1,40–42]

Reconstruction of Soft Tissue

In general, there are 3 principal indications for free flap coverage of traumatized lower extremities: soft tissue defects in the distal third, extensive soft tissue defects at any level, and "salvage free flaps" in case of nonreplantable amputation.[28] Because of the huge variety of flaps available for reconstruction, flap selection must aim to optimally meet the specific functional and esthetic requirements of

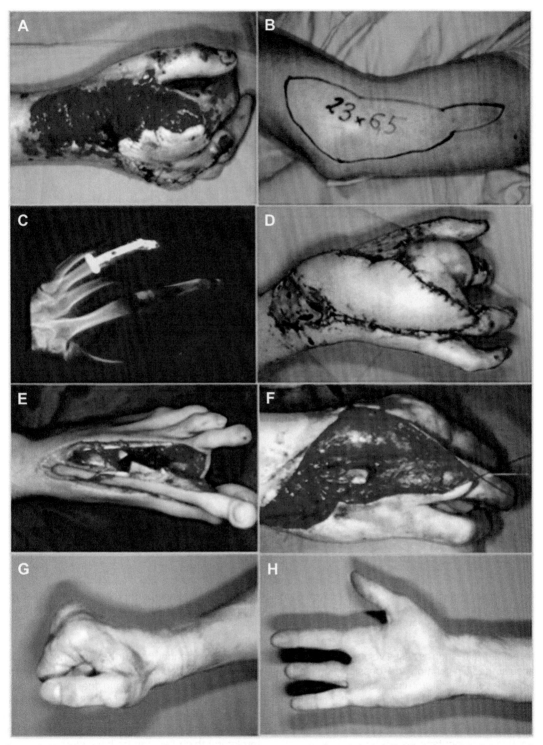

Fig. 4. (*A*) Delayed primary free flap closure with late reconstruction: 6 days following traumatic injury to the right hand after motor vehicle accident. (*B–D*) Free flap coverage using extended lateral arm flap and joint stabilization. (*E–F*) Delayed free vascularized metacarpophalangeal joint reconstruction using vascularized metatarsophalangeal joint of second toe 2 months after injury. (*G, H*) Functional result after 1 year.

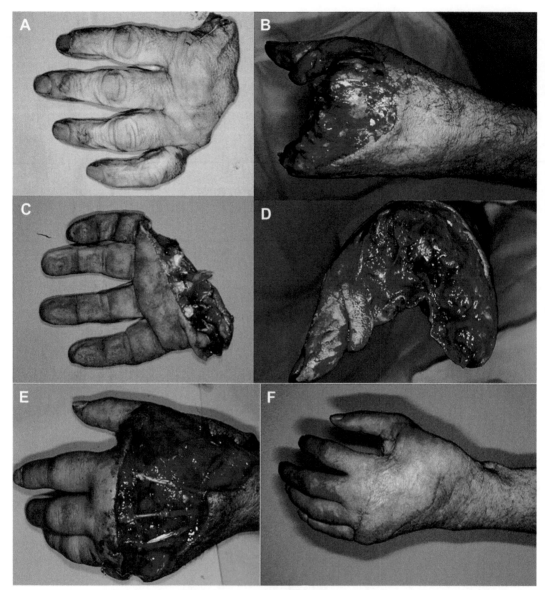

Fig. 5. Finger replantation and secondary free flap closure: traumatic amputation. (*A–D*) Replantation and temporary skin graft coverage. (*E*) One month following removal of split skin graft and definite soft tissue coverage with extended lateral arm free flap (*F*).

the recipient site such as tissue volume and surface, vascular pedicle length, and possible functional exigencies. In general, free flaps consist of a composition of different tissues (bone, muscle, adipose, fascia, and skin); consequently, they are referred to as "composite free flaps." Examples include (functional) myocutaneous, fasciocutaneous, or osteo(myo)cutaneous flaps. All flaps have unique characteristics in terms of functionality, durability, vascular supply, and blood flow. For instance, myo(cutaneous) flaps have a blood supply that is 3 times that of fasciocutaneous flaps. This improved perfusion has great influence on bone healing and

infection resistance.[28,43] Furthermore, muscle flaps provide large wound coverage and they can be separated longitudinally along the muscle fibers, allowing optimal coverage of defects with complex surface topography and obliteration of dead space.[1,22,35,44,45] Fasciocutaneous flaps like the anterolateral thigh flap can be harvested as sensate flaps, allowing various combinations of tissue components. They additionally show excellent surface texture, allowing perfect tissue contouring with superb esthetic results.[46–48] Their lack of bulk makes them especially applicable in areas requiring minimal-thickness soft tissue transfer for defect

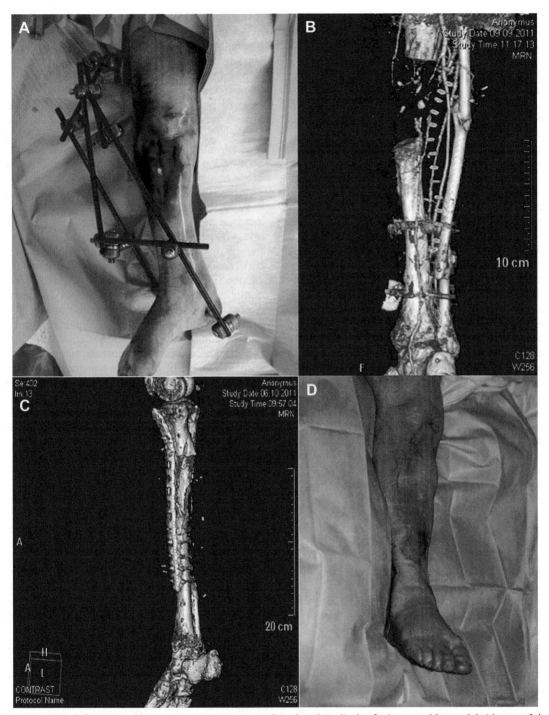

Fig. 6. Tibial defect caused by posttraumatic osteomyelitis. (*A, B*) Radical soft tissue and bone debridement followed by soft tissue reconstruction with anterolateral thigh flow-through free flap as a first stage procedure, followed by bone reconstruction using vascularized iliac crest bone graft anastomosed to descending branch of anterolateral thigh flap combined with a pedicled fibula flap 3 weeks later as a second stage procedure (*C, D*).

coverage.[49–51] Also, several studies could demonstrate the positive impact of fasciocutaneous flaps on chronic osteomyelitic wounds.[49–52] Therefore, there is an upcoming trend toward using

cutaneous flaps in reconstructive surgery. A study from 2005 analyzed the versatility of free fasciocutaneous flaps as an alternative to free muscle flaps for the reconstruction of traumatic open tibial fractures.

There was no statistical difference in terms of flap survival, rate of postoperative infections, chronic osteomyelitis, and stress fractures. Although free muscle transfer is still recommended for extensive 3-dimensional defects with a large dead space, fasciocutaneous flaps proved to be a reliable and effective alternative for covering traumatic open tibial fractures.[53] Deepithelialization of fasciocutaneous flaps even allows obliteration of dead space in extensive defects, thus representing a feasible alternative to muscle flaps.[54–57]

Special attention must be paid to the reconstruction of the highly sensitive weight-bearing area of the foot. Here, choice of flap remains controversial and is mainly determined by localization and extent of the foot defect.[58–61] For restoration of weight-bearing areas, the use of free muscle flaps combined with split-thickness skin grafts is recommended. In non–weight bearing areas, fasciocutaneous flaps should be preferred.[62] Because of its size, the latissimus dorsi free flap proved to be ideally suited for covering extensively damaged soft tissue. Used as a "cross leg free flap," it even allows simultaneous coverage of both feet in a single-step procedure.[63] A study from 1998 demonstrated lower rates of ulcerations with the use of free muscle flaps compared with faciocutaneous flaps. The glabrous skin surface of the foot sole and palm has very distinctive characteristics; it is thick and dense in structure and histologically shows a high concentration of sweat pores and nerve endings. A unique structure of adipose tissue stabilized by multidirectional fibrous septae ensures its capacity to withstand pressure and shearing force.[58] Current clinical evidence shows no significant necessity for special sensory reconstruction, although it improves quality of life and reduces time for rehabilitation.[64,65]

Although a variety of free flaps are commonly preferred for specific indications in extremity reconstruction, a fixed assignment of flaps for certain defects or flap standardization is not recommended. A key principle must be individual flap selection depending on individual recipient site requirements. Preoperative planning must consider patient age, anatomic and physiologic preconditions, dimensions, volume and composition of tissue required, pedicle length and diameter, possible need for motoric or sensory innervation, and donor site morbidity.

Supermicrosurgery, or "perforator-to-perforator surgery," represents a modern technique of free tissue transfer in which the diameter of anastomosis does not exceed 0.8 mm.[66] Donor site tissue is harvested in a superficial approach, leaving the underlying fascia intact and thereby, presumably, reducing donor site morbidity. Consequently, this dissection results in pedicles of limited length and caliber. Additionally, this technique uses small-caliber perforators as recipient site vessels, leaving major vessels unaffected. Subsequently, because of minimal pedicle length, in most cases, one cannot respect the basic principle of performing anastomosis outside of the trauma zone.[67] A study from 2009 analyzed the versatility of supermicrosurgery for extremity reconstruction in 42 consecutive patients. Results showed the technique to be feasible and efficient in the hands of an experienced surgeon.[68,69] The proposed benefits are described as a reduction in flap harvest time and donor site morbidity, an increase in the number of available perforators, and a decrease in swelling as a result of minimal muscle manipulation.[70,71] In extremity reconstruction, however, these advantages must be critically weighed against the increased risk of anastomosis complications and flap failure caused by direct exposure to the trauma zone. If anastomotic failure occurs, surgical options for anastomosis repair and revision are usually limited because of minimal vessel dimensions. Consequently, patient safety and prevention of any potential surgery-related complications are of highest priority. Optimal outcome must not be compromised by a sophistication of operating techniques, and individual indication for a supermicrosurgical approach must be well justified.

RECONSTRUCTION OF BONE

The main objectives of fracture management are stabilization, length maintenance, preservation of function, and early rehabilitation. In the past, extensive skeletal defects (ie, segmental bone loss) were primarily managed by interposition of nonvascularized autografts and allografts in combination with external/internal fixation or by the Ilizarov bone-lengthening technique. Because of narrow blood supply, these methods showed high rates of infection, nonunion, and early fracture.[72] Ultimately, these methods were limited to segmental defects of less than 6 cm in length. Reconstructive microsurgery has opened new possibilities in skeletal reconstruction. Vascularized bone transplants provide excellent structural support while at the same time reducing rates of infection and bone nonunion.[73] Furthermore, microvascular bone transfer reduces infection rate while at the same time increasing the stability of bone union and functional outcome. Timing of bone reconstruction is mainly determined by local wound contamination and/or infection, because inflammation is associated with a higher rate of delayed bone healing, pseudarthrosis, and vascular thrombosis.[74] In the case of heavily contaminated wounds, a staged bone reconstruction might be recommended.[73–76] The strategy consists of radical debridement and soft tissue coverage in a first step followed by delayed bone reconstruction (**Fig. 6**).

Potential donor sites suited for vascularized bone graft harvest include fibula, iliac crest, scapula, and radius.[77] The vascularized fibula and iliac crest flaps are primarily used in (lower) extremity bone reconstruction because they exhibit a reliable anatomy, provide a stabile bone matrix, and can optionally be harvested as osteo(myo)cutaneous flaps. Because of excellent periosteal perfusion, fibula flaps can be inserted as double-barreled grafts, thus further improving functional stability.[77–79] Additionally, with appropriate dissection, donor site morbidity remains negligible.

The Ilizarov technique is based on the principle of inducing bone regeneration through callus distraction. It has proved to be a useful technique in cases of (infected) tibial nonunion and for small to moderate bone skeletal defects.[80] Especially in chronically infected and severely traumatized extremities, a combination of the distraction osteogenesis with free tissue transfer has proved to be a powerful technique for limb salvage surgery.[81] In case of an extensive trauma zone, even a combination of osteosynthesis, free osteocutaneous iliac crest flap, and pedicled fibula flap proved to be well realizable.

FUNCTIONAL MUSCLE TRANSFER

Besides adequate bone stabilization and soft tissue coverage, restoration of impaired physiologic function is one of the key objectives in extremity salvage. Microsurgical tissue transfer has opened a wide variety of possibilities for reestablishing function of impaired extremities. If local repair or tendon transfer and/or nerve grafting is not practicable because of localized trauma, free functional muscle transplantation will be the treatment of choice. Several previous studies proved the applicability of this concept.[82–88] Basic functions of skeletal muscles include posture maintenance, joint stabilization, and active movement. Several different muscles are available for functional muscle transfer, each of which has distinctive features in terms of size, shape, and type of tactile strength. There are 2 main types of muscles, which differ regarding their mechanism of contraction: parallel (strap) and pennate muscles. In parallel muscles, fascicles are arranged in line with the

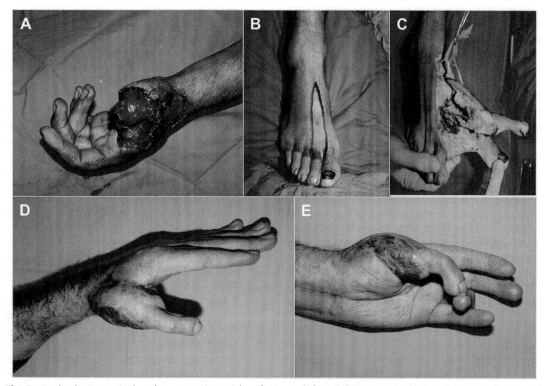

Fig. 7. Avulsed traumatic thumb amputation with soft tissue defect. (*A*) Primary reconstruction using free vascularized second toe. (*B*) Donor site planning. Toe elevation. (*C*) Functional result 6 months following surgery (*D, E*).

axis of the muscle. During contraction, these muscles shorten and increase in diameter. These muscles show adequate tactile strength but extensive range of motion. Examples include the biceps brachii, gracilis, and Sartorius muscles. In pennate muscles, fascicles attach in an oblique angle (pennation angle) to its tendon. When these muscles contract, the pennation angle increases. Examples include the biceps femoris, soleus, and gastrocnemius. Compared with parallel muscles, pennate muscles show potentially higher tactile strength but less range of motion.[89]

In functional muscle transfer, the surgical goal is to supply sufficient resting tension while at the same time providing an optimal range of motion. Therefore, muscle selection must target to optimally meet these functional requirements. If necessary, functional muscle flaps can be transplanted as composite free flaps including bone and soft tissue.[90] Commonly used muscles include the gracilis, rectus femoris, latissimus dorsi, and Tensor Fascia Lata flap.[91–96] The main functional goal for free muscle transfer in lower extremity reconstruction is restoration of active hip, knee, and ankle dorsiflexion/extension. Gracilis, rectus femoris, and latissimus muscle transfers have successfully been used in the restoration of impaired function.[90,93–95] Ninkovic and colleagues[96] showed a new technique in drop foot reconstruction using neuromusculotendinous transfer of the gastrocnemius muscle, hereby achieving voluntary normal walking pattern.

In upper extremity salvage, the gracilis and pectoralis muscles are considered the main muscles used for reanimation of elbow and long finger flexion/extension.[97,98] Usually, functional restoration after trauma or severe nerve injury consists of a complex combination of tendon transfer, nerve transplantation, and functional muscle transfer.[99]

A study from 2011 demonstrated that even a selective coaptation of individual gracilis nerve branches to specific branches of the anterior interosseous nerve is possible, thereby successfully establishing independent thumb and finger flexion. In reconstructive hand surgery, another highly sophisticated and well-established technique is free toe-to-hand transfer, which aims to restore length, stability, optical appearance, and especially pinch-and-grasp function of traumatized hands. Single or multiple toe transplantations can effectively help the patient to regain acceptable function and appearance, even after traumatic multiple digit amputations.[100–103] In case of nonrestorable finger amputation, primary toe-to-hand transfer has proved to be a valid reconstructive option (**Fig. 7**).

SUMMARY

During the past decades, reconstructive microsurgery has strongly influenced the management of complex extremity trauma. According to the current authors' experience, isolated complex extremity injury requires immediate specialized attention via an interdisciplinary approach. Whenever possible, all efforts must focus on primary surgical reconstruction and soft tissue coverage at the earliest point of time. Any delay in treatment may lead to a higher rate of complications, prolonged hospital stay, an increase in invalidity, and higher costs of treatment.

In conclusion, the main goal of reconstructive microsurgery must be an optimal functional and esthetic reconstruction, meeting the individual trauma site requirements with minimal donor site morbidity.

REFERENCES

1. Heller L, Levin LS. Lower extremity microsurgical reconstruction. Plast Reconstr Surg 2001;108(4): 1029–41 [quiz: 1042].
2. Kortbeek JB, Al Turki SA, Ali J, et al. Advanced trauma life support, 8th edition, the evidence for change. J Trauma 2008;64(6):1638–50.
3. O'Sullivan ST, O'Sullivan M, Pasha N, et al. Is it possible to predict limb viability in complex Gustilo IIIB and IIIC tibial fractures? a comparison of two predictive indices. Injury 1997;28(9–10):639–42.
4. Puno RM, Grossfeld SL, Henry SL, et al. Functional outcome of patients with salvageable limbs with grades III-B and III-C open fractures of the tibia. Microsurgery 1996;17(3):167–73.
5. Ninkovic M, Hussl H, Hefel L, et al. Timing of management of severe injuries of the upper extremity by free flap-plasty. Handchir Mikrochir Plast Chir 1995;27(6):297–306 [in German].
6. Gustilo RB, Anderson JT. Prevention of infection in the treatment of one thousand and twenty-five open fractures of long bones: retrospective and prospective analyses. J Bone Joint Surg Am 1976;58(4):453–8.
7. Helfet DL, Howey T, Sanders R, et al. Limb salvage versus amputation. Preliminary results of the mangled extremity severity score. Clin Orthop Relat Res 1990;256:80–6.
8. Kumar MK, Badole C, Patond K. Salvage versus amputation: utility of mangled extremity severity score in severely injured lower limbs. Indian J Orthop 2007;41(3):183–7.
9. Russell WL, Sailors DM, Whittle TB, et al. Limb salvage versus traumatic amputation. A decision based on a seven-part predictive index. Ann Surg 1991;213(5):473–80 [discussion: 480–1].

10. Howe HR Jr, Poole GV Jr, Hansen KJ, et al. Salvage of lower extremities following combined orthopedic and vascular trauma. A predictive salvage index. Am Surg 1987;53(4):205–8.

11. Seekamp A, Kontopp H, Tscherne H. Hannover fracture scale '98—reevaluation and new prospects for an established score system. Unfallchirurg 2001;104(7):601–10 [in German].

12. Bosse MJ, MacKenzie EJ, Kellam JF, et al. A prospective evaluation of the clinical utility of the lower-extremity injury-severity scores. J Bone Joint Surg Am 2001;83(1):3–14.

13. Durrant CA, Mackey SP. Orthoplastic classification systems: the good, the bad, and the ungainly. Ann Plast Surg 2011;66(1):9–12.

14. Chung KC, Saddawi-Konefka D, Haase SC, et al. A cost-utility analysis of amputation versus salvage for Gustilo type IIIB and IIIC open tibial fractures. Plast Reconstr Surg 2009;124(6):1965–73.

15. Reddy V, Stevenson TR. MOC-PS(SM) CME article: lower extremity reconstruction. Plast Reconstr Surg 2008;121(Suppl 4):1–7.

16. Chen ZW, Zeng BF. Replantation of the lower extremity. Clin Plast Surg 1983;10(1):103–13.

17. Gustilo RB, Merkow RL, Templeman D. The management of open fractures. J Bone Joint Surg Am 1990;72(2):299–304.

18. Bosse MJ, McCarthy ML, Jones AL, et al. The insensate foot following severe lower extremity trauma: an indication for amputation? J Bone Joint Surg Am 2005;87(12):2601–8.

19. Lange RH. Limb reconstruction versus amputation decision making in massive lower extremity trauma. Clin Orthop Relat Res 1989;243:92–9.

20. Bosse MJ, MacKenzie EJ, Kellam JF, et al. An analysis of outcomes of reconstruction or amputation after leg-threatening injuries. N Engl J Med 2002; 347(24):1924–31.

21. Godina M. Early microsurgical reconstruction of complex trauma of the extremities. Plast Reconstr Surg 1986;78(3):285–92.

22. Byrd HS, Cierny G 3rd, Tebbetts JB. The management of open tibial fractures with associated soft-tissue loss: external pin fixation with early flap coverage. Plast Reconstr Surg 1981;68(1):73–82.

23. Herter F, Ninkovic M, Ninkovic M. Rational flap selection and timing for coverage of complex upper extremity trauma. J Plast Reconstr Aesthet Surg 2007;60(7):760–8.

24. Lister G, Scheker L. Emergency free flaps to the upper extremity. J Hand Surg Am 1988;13(1):22–8.

25. Sundine M, Scheker LR. A comparison of immediate and staged reconstruction of the dorsum of the hand. J Hand Surg Br 1996;21(2):216–21.

26. Karanas YL, Nigriny J, Chang J. The timing of microsurgical reconstruction in lower extremity trauma. Microsurgery 2008;28(8):632–4.

27. Ninkovic M, Mooney EK, Ninkovic M, et al. A new classification for the standardization of nomenclature in free flap wound closure. Plast Reconstr Surg 1999;103(3):903–14 [discussion: 915–7].

28. Ninkovic M, Schoeller T, Benedetto KP, et al. Emergency free flap cover in complex injuries of the lower extremities. Scand J Plast Reconstr Surg Hand Surg 1996;30(1):37–47.

29. Ninkovic M, Schoeller T, Wechselberger G, et al. Primary flap closure in complex limb injuries. J Reconstr Microsurg 1997;13(8):575–83.

30. Ninkovic M, Schoeller T, Wechselberger G, et al. Infection prophylaxis in complex limb trauma through immediate definitive reconstruction via a free tissue transfer. Chirurg 1997;68(11):1163–9 [in German].

31. Turner AJ, Parkhouse N. Revisiting the reconstructive ladder. Plast Reconstr Surg 2006; 118(1):267–8.

32. Lineaweaver WC. Microsurgery and the reconstructive ladder. Microsurgery 2005;25(3):185–6.

33. Knobloch K, Vogt PM. The reconstructive sequence in the 21st century. A reconstructive clockwork. Chirurg 2010;81(5):441–6 [in German].

34. Dunn R, Watson S. Why climb a ladder when you can take the elevator? Plast Reconstr Surg 2001; 107(1):283.

35. Pollak AN, McCarthy ML, Burgess AR. Short-term wound complications after application of flaps for coverage of traumatic soft-tissue defects about the tibia. The Lower Extremity Assessment Project (LEAP) study group. J Bone Joint Surg Am 2000; 82(12):1681–91.

36. Engel H, Lin CH, Wei FC. Role of microsurgery in lower extremity reconstruction. Plast Reconstr Surg 2011;127(Suppl 1):228S–38S.

37. Ninkovic M, Deetjen H, Ohler K, et al. Emergency free tissue transfer for severe upper extremity injuries. J Hand Surg Br 1995;20(1):53–8.

38. Hallock GG. Preexpansion of free flap donor sites used in reconstruction after burn injury. J Burn Care Rehabil 1995;16(6):646–53.

39. Takushima A, Harii K, Asato H. Expanded latissimus dorsi free flap for the treatment of extensive post-burn neck contracture. J Reconstr Microsurg 2002;18(5):373–7.

40. Lange RH, Bach AW, Hansen ST Jr, et al. Open tibial fractures with associated vascular injuries: prognosis for limb salvage. J Trauma 1985;25(3):203–8.

41. Gustilo RB, Mendoza RM, Williams DN. Problems in the management of type III (severe) open fractures: a new classification of type III open fractures. J Trauma 1984;24(8):742–6.

42. Janis JE, Kwon RK, Attinger CE. The new reconstructive ladder: modifications to the traditional model. Plast Reconstr Surg 2011;127(Suppl 1): 205S–12S.

43. Richards RR, Orsini EC, Mahoney JL, et al. The influence of muscle flap coverage on the repair of devascularized tibial cortex: an experimental investigation in the dog. Plast Reconstr Surg 1987;79(6):946–58.

44. Guzman-Stein G, Fix RJ, Vasconez LO. Muscle flap coverage for the lower extremity. Clin Plast Surg 1991;18(3):545–52.

45. Mathes SJ, Alpert BS, Chang N. Use of the muscle flap in chronic osteomyelitis: experimental and clinical correlation. Plast Reconstr Surg 1982;69(5):815–29.

46. Wei FC, Jain V, Celik N, et al. Have we found an ideal soft-tissue flap? an experience with 672 anterolateral thigh flaps. Plast Reconstr Surg 2002;109(7):2219–26 [discussion: 2227–30].

47. Lin CH, Wei FC, Lin YT, et al. Lateral circumflex femoral artery system: warehouse for functional composite free-tissue reconstruction of the lower leg. J Trauma 2006;60(5):1032–6.

48. Engel H, Gazyakan E, Cheng MH, et al. Customized reconstruction with the free anterolateral thigh perforator flap. Microsurgery 2008;28(7):489–94.

49. Wyble EJ, Yakuboff KP, Clark RG, et al. Use of free fasciocutaneous and muscle flaps for reconstruction of the foot. Ann Plast Surg 1990;24(2):101–8.

50. Chen D, Jupiter JB, Lipton HA, et al. The parascapular flap for treatment of lower extremity disorders. Plast Reconstr Surg 1989;84(1):108–16.

51. Colen LB, Pessa JE, Potparic Z, et al. Reconstruction of the extremity with the dorsal thoracic fascia free flap. Plast Reconstr Surg 1998;101(3):738–44.

52. Weinzweig N, Davies BW. Foot and ankle reconstruction using the radial forearm flap: a review of 25 cases. Plast Reconstr Surg 1998;102(6):1999–2005.

53. Yazar S, Lin CH, Lin YT, et al. Outcome comparison between free muscle and free fasciocutaneous flaps for reconstruction of distal third and ankle traumatic open tibial fractures. Plast Reconstr Surg 2006;117(7):2468–75 [discussion: 2476–7].

54. Lee JC, St-Hilaire H, Christy MR, et al. Anterolateral thigh flap for trauma reconstruction. Ann Plast Surg 2010;64(2):164–8.

55. Ali RS, Bluebond-Langner R, Rodriguez ED, et al. The versatility of the anterolateral thigh flap. Plast Reconstr Surg 2009;124(Suppl 6):e395–407.

56. Rodriguez ED, Bluebond-Langner R, Copeland C, et al. Functional outcomes of posttraumatic lower limb salvage: a pilot study of anterolateral thigh perforator flaps versus muscle flaps. J Trauma 2009;66(5):1311–4.

57. Hong JP, Shin HW, Kim JJ, et al. The use of anterolateral thigh perforator flaps in chronic osteomyelitis of the lower extremity. Plast Reconstr Surg 2005;115(1):142–7.

58. Noever G, Bruser P, Kohler L. Reconstruction of heel and sole defects by free flaps. Plast Reconstr Surg 1986;78(3):345–52.

59. Rautio J, Kekoni J, Hamalainen H, et al. Mechanical sensibility in free and island flaps of the foot. J Reconstr Microsurg 1989;5(2):119–25.

60. Potparic Z, Rajacic N. Long-term results of weight-bearing foot reconstruction with non-innervated and reinnervated free flaps. Br J Plast Surg 1997;50(3):176–81.

61. Hollenbeck ST, Woo S, Komatsu I, et al. Longitudinal outcomes and application of the subunit principle to 165 foot and ankle free tissue transfers. Plast Reconstr Surg 2010;125(3):924–34.

62. Rainer C, Schwabegger AH, Bauer T, et al. Free flap reconstruction of the foot. Ann Plast Surg 1999;42(6):595–606 [discussion: 606–7].

63. Ninkovic MM, Schwabegger AH, Hausler JW, et al. Limb salvage after fulminant septicemia using a free latissimus dorsi cross-leg flap. J Reconstr Microsurg 2000;16(8):603–7.

64. Ducic I, Hung V, Dellon AL. Innervated free flaps for foot reconstruction: a review. J Reconstr Microsurg 2006;22(6):433–42.

65. Kuran I, Turgut G, Bas L, et al. Comparison between sensitive and nonsensitive free flaps in reconstruction of the heel and plantar area. Plast Reconstr Surg 2000;105(2):574–80.

66. Koshima I, Yamamoto T, Narushima M, et al. Perforator flaps and supermicrosurgery. Clin Plast Surg 2010;37(4):683–9, vii–iii.

67. Rainer C, Meirer R, Gardetto A, et al. Perforator-pedicled skin island flap for coverage of microvascular anastomoses in myocutaneous flaps in the lower extremity. Plast Reconstr Surg 2003;112(5):1362–7.

68. Hong JP, Koshima I. Using perforators as recipient vessels (supermicrosurgery) for free flap reconstruction of the knee region. Ann Plast Surg 2010;64(3):291–3.

69. Hong JP. The use of supermicrosurgery in lower extremity reconstruction: the next step in evolution. Plast Reconstr Surg 2009;123(1):230–5.

70. Acland RD. Refinements in lower extremity free flap surgery. Clin Plast Surg 1990;17(4):733–44.

71. Muramatsu K, Shigetomi M, Ihara K, et al. Vascular complication in free tissue transfer to the leg. Microsurgery 2001;21(8):362–5.

72. Chen CM, Disa JJ, Lee HY, et al. Reconstruction of extremity long bone defects after sarcoma resection with vascularized fibula flaps: a 10-year review. Plast Reconstr Surg 2007;119(3):915–24 [discussion: 925–6].

73. Cavadas PC, Landin L, Ibanez J, et al. Reconstruction of major traumatic segmental bone defects of the tibia with vascularized bone transfers. Plast Reconstr Surg 2010;125(1):215–23.

74. Pelissier P, Pistre V, Casoli V, et al. Reconstruction of short lower leg stumps with the osteomusculocutaneous latissimus dorsi-rib flap. Plast Reconstr Surg 2002;109(3):1013–7.

75. Masquelet AC, Fitoussi F, Begue T, et al. Reconstruction of the long bones by the induced membrane and spongy autograft. Ann Chir Plast Esthet 2000;45(3):346–53 [in French].

76. Lopez-Casero R, De Pedro JA, Rodriguez E, et al. Distal vascular pedicle-hemisoleus to tibial length ratio as a main predictive index in preoperative flap planning. Surg Radiol Anat 1995; 17(2):113–9, 115–7.

77. Hierner R, Wood MB. Comparison of vascularised iliac crest and vascularised fibula transfer for reconstruction of segmental and partial bone defects in long bones of the lower extremity. Microsurgery 1995;16(12):818–26.

78. Donski PK, Buchler U, Ganz R. Combined osteocutaneous microvascular flap procedure for extensive bone and soft tissue defects in the tibia. Ann Plast Surg 1986;16(5):386–98.

79. Lin CH, Wei FC, Chen HC, et al. Outcome comparison in traumatic lower-extremity reconstruction by using various composite vascularized bone transplantation. Plast Reconstr Surg 1999;104(4):984–92.

80. Wani N, Baba A, Kangoo K, et al. Role of early Ilizarov ring fixator in the definitive management of type II, IIIA and IIIB open tibial shaft fractures. Int Orthop 2011;35(6):915–23.

81. Chim H, Sontich JK, Kaufman BR. Free tissue transfer with distraction osteogenesis is effective for limb salvage of the infected traumatized lower extremity. Plast Reconstr Surg 2011;127(6):2364–72.

82. O'Brien BM, Morrison WA, MacLeod AM, et al. Free microneurovascular muscle transfer in limbs to provide motor power. Ann Plast Surg 1982;9(5): 381–91.

83. Manktelow RT, Zuker RM, McKee NH. Functioning free muscle transplantation. J Hand Surg Am 1984;9A(1):32–9.

84. Manktelow RT. Free muscle transplantation for facial paralysis. Clin Plast Surg 1984;11(1):215–20.

85. Manktelow RT, McKee NH, Vettese T. An anatomical study of the pectoralis major muscle as related to functioning free muscle transplantation. Plast Reconstr Surg 1980;65(5):610–5.

86. Manktelow RT, McKee NH. Free muscle transplantation to provide active finger flexion. J Hand Surg Am 1978;3(5):416–26.

87. Doi K, Kuwata N, Kawakami F, et al. Limb-sparing surgery with reinnervated free-muscle transfer following radical excision of soft-tissue sarcoma in the extremity. Plast Reconstr Surg 1999;104(6): 1679–87.

88. Grotting JC, Buncke HJ, Lineaweaver WC, et al. Functional restoration in the upper extremity using free muscle transplantation. Ann Chir Main Memb Super 1990;9(2):98–106.

89. Martini F. Fundamentals of anatomy and physiology. 5th edition. Upper Saddle River (NJ): Prentice Hall; 2001.

90. Lin CH, Lin YT, Yeh JT, et al. Free functioning muscle transfer for lower extremity posttraumatic composite structure and functional defect. Plast Reconstr Surg 2007;119(7):2118–26.

91. Wechselberger G, Pichler M, Pulzl P, et al. Free functional rectus femoris muscle transfer for restoration of extension of the foot after lower leg compartment syndrome. Microsurgery 2004;24(6):437–41.

92. Willcox TM, Smith AA, Beauchamp C, et al. Functional free latissimus dorsi muscle flap to the proximal lower extremity. Clin Orthop Relat Res 2003; 410:285–8.

93. Hallock GG. Restoration of quadriceps femoris function with a dynamic microsurgical free latissimus dorsi muscle transfer. Ann Plast Surg 2004; 52(1):89–92.

94. Ihara K, Shigetomi M, Kawai S, et al. Functioning muscle transplantation after wide excision of sarcomas in the extremity. Clin Orthop Relat Res 1999;358:140–8.

95. Kobayashi S, Sekiguchi J, Sakai Y, et al. Functioning free muscle transplantation to the lower leg. J Reconstr Microsurg 1995;11(5):319–25.

96. Ninkovc M, Sucur D, Starovic B, et al. A new approach to persistent traumatic peroneal nerve palsy. Br J Plast Surg 1994;47(3):185–9.

97. Bahm J, Ocampo-Pavez C. Free functional gracilis muscle transfer in children with severe sequelae from obstetric brachial plexus palsy. J Brachial Plex Peripher Nerve Inj 2008;3:23.

98. Hierner R, Berger A. Pectoralis major muscle transfer for reconstruction of elbow flexion in posttraumatic brachial plexus lesions. Oper Orthop Traumatol 2009;21(2):126–40 [in German].

99. Berger A, Hierner R. Free functional gracilis muscle transplantation for reconstruction of active elbow flexion in posttraumatic brachial plexus lesions. Oper Orthop Traumatol 2009;21(2):141–56 [in German].

100. Lister GD, Kalisman M, Tsai TM. Reconstruction of the hand with free microneurovascular toe-to-hand transfer: experience with 54 toe transfers. Plast Reconstr Surg 1983;71(3):372–86.

101. Morrison WA, O'Brien BM, MacLeod AM. Thumb reconstruction with a free neurovascular wrap-around flap from the big toe. J Hand Surg Am 1980;5(6):575–83.

102. Tsai TM, Aziz W. Toe-to-thumb transfer: a new technique. Plast Reconstr Surg 1991;88(1):149–53.

103. Wei FC, Chen HC, Chuang CC, et al. Microsurgical thumb reconstruction with toe transfer: selection of various techniques. Plast Reconstr Surg 1994; 93(2):345–51 [discussion: 352–7].

The Latissimus Dorsi Detrusor Myoplasty for Functional Treatment of Bladder Acontractility

Milomir Ninkovic, MD, PhD[a,*], Arnulf Stenzl, MD, PhD[b],
Georgios Gakis, MD[b], Marina Ninkovic[c],
Sebastian Voigt, MD[a], Ulf Dornseifer, MD[a]

KEYWORDS

• Motor neuron disease • Urinary bladder • Neurogenic • Latissimus dorsi • Detrusor myoplasty

KEY POINTS

- The main goal of the latissimus dorsi detrusor myoplasty is to get patients with bladder acontractility independent from lifelong self-catheterization with its related disadvantages.
- The free neurovascular latissimus dorsi muscle (LDM) is particularly appropriate for the detrusor myoplasty because it provides a suitable neurovascular pedicle, muscle size and configuration of muscle fibers.
- The coaptation of the thoracodorsal nerve to a branch of the intercostal nerve results in a synergistic function of the transferred latissimus muscle and the muscles of the abdominal wall
  - The success of the latissimus dorsi detrusor myoplasty (LDDM) is dependent on an excellent cooperation between both surgical disciplines—urology and plastic surgery.

INTRODUCTION

Poor detrusor contractility and related impaired bladder emptying is a debilitating and irreversible disorder presenting a major medical and social problem. It is estimated that several thousand patients with this disease in the United States depend on *clean intermittent catheterization* several times a day.[1] The underlying pathology of bladder acontractility may be damage to the detrusor muscle itself, its autonomic nerve supply, or the spinal micturition center. Possible causes include congenial anomalies (eg, myelomeningocele and myelodysplasia), acquired infections, inflammatory or autoimmune diseases, chronic overdistension due to subvesical outlet obstruction, and central or peripheral nerve injuries secondary to trauma or degenerative diseases. The hypoflexic or areflexic bladder characteristically results in urinary retention and overflow incontinence associated with urinary tract infections, stone formation, and vesicoureteral reflux.

Disclosures: The authors listed below have identified no professional or financial affiliation for themselves or their spouse/partner: Milomir Ninkovic, MD, PhD; Arnulf Stenzl, MD, PhD; Georgios Gakis, MD; Marina Ninkovic, MD; and Ulf Dornseifer, MD.

[a] Department of Plastic, Reconstructive, Hand and Burn Surgery, Klinikum Bogenhausen, Städtisches Klinikum München GmbH, Englschalkinger Straße 77, Munich 81825, Germany; [b] Department of Urology, Eberhard-Karls University, Hoppe-Seyler-Straße 3, Tuebingen 72076, Germany; [c] Unit of Physical Medicine and Rehabilitation, Center of Operative Medicine, Innsbruck Medical University, Anichstraße 35, Innsbruck 6020, Austria
* Corresponding author. Department of Plastic, Reconstructive Hand and Burn Surgery, Klinikum Bogenhausen, Städtisches Klinikum München GmbH, Englschalkinger Straße 77, Munich 81825, Germany.
E-mail address: milomir.ninkovic@klinikum-muenchen.de

If left untreated, this condition inevitably leads to impairment of the upper and lower urinary tract.

The main goals in treating patients with neurogenic bladder dysfunction are

- Preservation of upper urinary tract integrity
- Insurance of adequate continence
- Minimization of stone formation and urinary infection

All these therapeutic goals aim to improve patient quality of life and prolong life expectancy.

Catheterization

Until now, the gold standard treatment has been lifelong clean intermittent catheterization that has reduced renal-related mortality in the past 4 decades but is also associated with serious adverse effects[2–4]:

- Urinary tract infections; prevalence varies widely in literature (from 12 to 88%).[2]
- Epididymitis
- Epididymo-orchitis
- Urethral trauma and stricture
- Bladder injury
- Urolithiasis
- Deteriorating renal function

In addition, the socioeconomic and psychological burdens of lifelong intermittent catheterization must be considered.[2,5,6]

All these disadvantages associated with this procedure emphasize the importance of effective alternative treatment options for the acontractile bladder.

Sacral Neuromodulation

One approach to restore bladder contraction is the so-called sacral neuromodulation that enables a voluntary bladder emptying by electrical stimulation[7,8] but requires an intact spinal cord, micturition center, and spinal roots.[9] If these conditions are not fulfilled, voluntary micturition can be achieved only by a functional muscle transfer.

Functional Muscle Transfer

The free neurovascular LDM is particularly appropriate for this procedure because it provides a suitable neurovascular pedicle, muscle size, and configuration of muscle fibers that could be initially proved in an experimental model.[10,11] In this procedure, the LDM is partially wrapped around the acontractile bladder with its thoracodorsal nerve coaptated to the lowest branch of the intercostal nerve. After the reinnervation of the LDM,

a contraction of the rectus abdominis muscle results in a simultaneous contraction of the transferred latissimus, which leads to an voluntary emptying of the bladder. As the contraction of both muscles then increases the intravesicular pressure, the nerve coaptation enables a synergistic function of both muscles. In 1998, successful clinical applicability of the LDDM for the treatment of bladder acontractility was reported for the first time.[12]

PREOPERATIVE CONSIDERATIONS AND ASSESSMENTS

Candidates for LDDM are patients with bladder acontractility that is not ascribed to an upper motor neuron lesion (ie, multiple sclerosis, apoplectic stroke, or spinal trauma above the 12th thoracic vertebra) (**Box 1**). Main causes of acontractility that indicate the procedure are spinal trauma below Th12, tethered cord syndrome, lumbar hernia of nuclei pulposi, megacystis/bladder outlet obstruction, sacral myelomeningocele, and idiopathic and chronic retention after hysterectomy. Considering the complex procedure, life expectancy should be more than 10 years. There should be no improvement of the bladder dysfunction for at least 1 year. Suitable patients should handle clean intermittent catheterization with safety for at least 1 year and be able to continue performing this catheterization in case of LDDM failure. There should be no signs of infravesical obstruction at urethrocystoscopy.[13]

Routine preoperative evaluation includes

- Video-urodynamics
- Diagnostic urethrocystoscopy
- Excretory urography

Box 1
Indications for the latissimus dorsi detrusor myoplasty

- Bladder acontractility without upper motor neuron lesion
- No indication for neuromodulation
- Life expectancy greater than 10 years
- No improvement of bladder dysfunction longer than 1 year
- Patient should handle clean intermittent catheterization greater than 1 year
- No infravesical obstruction
- Intact 12th intercostal motor nerve

In addition, electromyography of the lower portion of the rectus abdominis muscle should be performed to confirm an intact 12th intercostal motor nerve for the neural coaptation. In patients with idiopathic cause of the disease, a neurophysiologic assessment of the sacral district, including MRI or CT, is recommended to exclude an upper motor neuron lesion. Preoperative targeted diagnostics are also essential to identify those patients who are eligible for a detrusor myoplasty and those who can also benefit from sacral neuromodulation. Urodynamics are essential to evaluate suspected acontractility. In cases of equivocal urodynamic findings, sacral neuromodulation should be applied to rule out the presence of bladder hypocontractility rather than acontractility. Direct electrostimulation of the sacral nerves may then help identify those patients with hypocontractility who might be candidates for implantation of a permanent device for sacral neuromodulation.[13]

OPERATIVE TECHNIQUE

Patients are placed in a supine position with the respective shoulder elevated and the arm overhead to enable synchronous work at the nondominant LDM and the bladder by 2 surgical teams (urologic and plastic surgery). An axillary zigzag-shaped incision offers direct access to the anterior border of the LDM and a clear dissection of the thoracodorsal neurovascular bundle as proximal as possible. It is mandatory to document the resting muscle tension before separating the muscle at its origin and attachment. Accordingly, 2 marking sutures at defined distances are placed on the muscle and every effort is made to re-extend the muscle to its original length during its fixation in the pelvis. The LDM is then completely elevated except for the neurovascular bundle, which is not transected until the recipient vessels have been prepared for microanastomosis (**Fig. 1**). Donor site closure is terminally performed using several interrupted absorbable sutures between the skin flap and the thoracic wall to reduce the large wound cavity and with it the risk of postoperative seroma formation.

A Pfannenstiel incision is usually made to prepare the bladder, which is freed down to the trigone. In cases of a small capacity bladder, an autoaugmentation can be performed by excision or incision of the diseased detrusor. Subsequently, the inner surfaces of both ischial bones and insertions of the sacrospinal ligaments are identified. In male patients, after preparation of Denonvilliers fascia, a polyglactin mesh is placed at the posterior bladder wall and secured with single sutures at the pubic arc, whereas in women, the uterus takes over the function of a counter bearing for the LDM. The sutures for the fixation of the LDM in the pelvis are all fixed in advance at the fascial and ligamentous structures. **Fig. 2** shows fixation of LDM around the urinary bladder and **Fig. 3** shows reconstructed bladder.

After identifying the deep inferior epigastric vessels, the thoracodorsal vessels and nerve are divided, the LDM is transferred to the recipient side, and microsurcial vascular anastomosis is performed immediately to keep the ischemia time as short as possible (not more than 30 minutes). The anastomosis should be performed with the LDM upside down as the flap is accordingly positioned in the pelvis.

Subsequently the flap is attached to the fascial and ligamentous structures in the pelvis. A slightly spiral configuration of the LDM is performed taking the original muscle resting tension into consideration. The appropriate muscle resting tension is restored by stretching the muscle to recreate the original length between the markers.

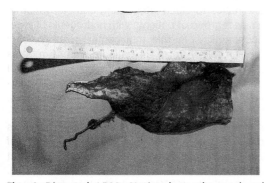

Fig. 1. Dissected LDM. Notice long thoracodorsal nerve and tendon part of the LDM.

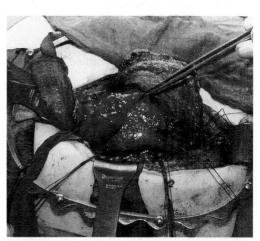

Fig. 2. Fixation of the LDM around the urinary bladder.

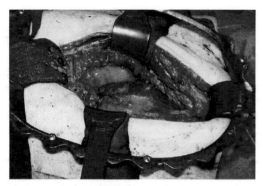

Fig. 3. Reconstructed bladder—LDDM.

Finally, the thoracodorsal nerve is microsurgically coaptated to the lowest branches of the intercostal nerves originally innervating parts of the rectus abdominis muscle. Careful dissection is crucial to identify the donor nerve segment directly supplying motor innervation to the muscle, routinely using nerve stimulation. Nerve selection and repair are the most critical parts of this procedure. Meticulous nerve coaptation is essential for reinnervation. The nerve repair should be placed as close as possible to the neuromuscular junction to provide a minimal distance for nerve regeneration and to avoid a long period of muscle denervation.

Pearls for LDDM bladder reconstruction:

- A generous zigzag-shaped incision in the axilla enables the essential long dissection of the neurovascular thoracodorsal pedicle

- The neurovascular thorcodorsal pedicle has to be dissected as long as possible to attain enough length for a stressless nerve coaptation

- The resting muscle tension has to be documented before separating the LDM and the transferred muscle must be re-extend in the pelvis according to these marks

- Motor branches of the intercostal nerves should be additionally identified by electro-stimulation

---

Pitfalls in LDDM bladder reconstruction

- The diameter of the thoracodorsal vein and the recipient vein (deep inferior epigastric vein) may strongly differ, which can impede the venous anastomosis

- Inadequate selection of the recipient nerve and nerve coaptation (eg, under tension) can compromise the whole reconstruction

---

POSTOPERATIVE CARE

The bladder has to be initially drained with an indwelling transurethral catheter and subsequently with clean intermittent catheterization for a total of 12 weeks. Afterward, the patients are instructed to void under physiotherapeutic guidance by voluntarily contracting the lower abdominal muscles and to perform timed voiding if there was lack of sensation. Postvoid residual urine volumes have to be measured by self-catheterization, and catheterization intervals are gradually increased accordingly. Muscle flap vascularization has to be confirmed by Doppler ultrasonography regularly during the first postoperative days and in 3-month intervals in the first year. In addition, the first video-urodynamic evaluations have to be performed at 6 months postoperatively and yearly thereafter.[12–14]

RESULTS

The experimental study has already shown that the pressure obtained by a stimulated LDM, wrapped around a bladder-like reservoir, was more than sufficient to evacuate this reservoir. Additionally, it has been demonstrated that microneurovascular free transfer of the LDM to the bladder resulted in a reinnervated, functional muscle in the canine model.[10,11]

The first clinical results described the successful microneurovascular free transfer of the latissimus muscle to functionally restore a deficient detrusor muscle.[12] In a first larger clinical series, 14 of 20 patients were able to void spontaneously within 4 months postoperatively, with postvoid residual volumes of less than 100 mL. Voluntary voiding was restored by bladder neck incision in 4 of the 20 patients and only 2 patients (10%) still required self-catheterization. None of the patients had morphologic and functional changes of the upper tract or de novo incontinence postoperative.[14]

Current long-term results underline these first findings and confirm that the LDDM is an effective alternative to clean intermittent catheterization in a select group of patients with neurogenic bladder acontractility. In this multicenter investigation[13] median follow-up of 24 patients was 46 months (range 8–89). Of the 24 patients, 17 (71%) gained complete spontaneous voiding with a mean postvoid residual urine volume of 25 mL (range 0–100). In 3 patients (13%), the frequency of clean intermittent catheterization was reduced to 2 to 4 times daily with a mean postvoid residual urine volume of 200 mL (range 150–250). Recurrent urinary tract infections ceased in 21 of 23 patients (91%). Four patients (17%) required clean intermittent catheterization with the same frequency as before the procedure. No chronic pain at the donor site or vesicoureteral reflux was observed in any patient of this series. The procedure was associated with 6 major complications, which did not require ICU management:

1. Deep vein thrombosis
2. Pulmonary embolism
3. Pelvic abscess requiring temporary drainage
4. Compartment syndrome of the nonoperated shoulder
5. Wound healing disorder
6. Persistent seroma of the operated shoulder requiring surgical intervention

All patients who experienced a major complication recovered completely. No free flap failure was encountered intraoperatively or postoperatively. In this series, the mean operating time was 536 ± 22 minutes and the median length of hospital stay was 13 days (range 7–32).[13]

DISCUSSION

Aside from the LDM, only the rectus abdominis is discussed as a potential appropriate muscle for functional transfer to restore voluntary voiding.

Based on the principles of cardiomyoplasty, the option to envelop the bladder with a pedicled, innervated, unilateral rectus abdominis muscle has been first described in 1994.[15] The use of the rectus abdominis seems attractive because this surgical procedure is, in comparison to the LDD, much less complex. In addition, the rectus abdominis has no risk of failed reinnervation. The existing data indicate, however, that the initial enthusiasm concerning the use of the functional rectus abdominis muscle for detrusor myoplasty must be curbed. Micturition pattern and voiding volume did not alter between rats with spinal cord injury and rectus abdominis detrusor myoplasty and those without detrusor myoplasty. Clinical results concerning the rectus abdominis were limited to only 1 case, in which the patient was able to void by contracting the transferred rectus abdominis muscle.[16] Muscle innervation is mandatory for functional reconstruction and it is doubtful whether this can routinely be achieved with the rectus abdominis muscle, because the segmental nerve supply varies considerably. Perhaps this relevant uncertainty has led to the later experimental attempts to optimize the rectus abdominis detrusor myoplasty by electrical stimulation.[17,18] To stimulate the transferred innervated rectus abdominis muscle in a dog model, 2 bipolar myocardial pacing lead electrodes have been inserted near the entry of the intercostal nerves. This modification, however, has not led to promising results. The chronically stimulated myoplasty did not maintain efficient bladder emptying.[17]

In contrast, the clinical results of the LDDM[12–14,19] demonstrate that this procedure is reliable to restore voluntary voiding for a select group of patients with neurogenic bladder acontractility. This success is due, among other things, to the proper selection of the donor muscle. The LDM has a sufficient cross-section and mass for exerting force and a suitable fiber length for excursion. The anatomic arrangement of the muscle fibers within a strap muscle configuration, as opposed to that of a pennate configuration, provides a muscle, such as the LDM, with a greater range of excursion. In addition, the reliable neurovascular anatomy and its large surface make the LDM, in comparison to other donor muscles, predestined for this application. Advocates of the rectus abdominis myoplasty have discussed that use of the LDM would create a large thoracic wall defect, pointing out that paraplegic patients rely on their upper extremities and torso strength for mobility.[17] Morbidity of the LDM donor site, however, is well analyzed in large series studies and considered low.[20,21] Muscle flaps of the lower extremity, which are more favorable for paraplegic patients, do not meet the requirements. Additionally, the morbidity associated with the harvest of the latissimus flap is in no proportion to the benefit of the regained ability of voluntary micturition.

The LDDM is a curative treatment option for patients (discussed previously) who would otherwise require lifelong clean intermittent catheterization with its related disadvantages. Elimination of the need for self-catheterization leads to growing self-confidence among patients and facilitates managing their usual daily and occupational activities.

The success of LDDM is dependent, however, on excellent cooperation between both surgical disciplines—urology and plastic surgery. Due to the complexity of this procedure, this technique should stay in referral centers to maximize the outcome for patients.

REFERENCES

1. Madjar S, Appell RA. Impaired detrusor contractility: anything new? Curr Urol Rep 2002;3(5):373–7.
2. Vaidyanathan S, Krishnan KR, Soni BM, et al. Unusual complications of intermittent self-catheterisation in spinal cord injury patients. Spinal Cord 1996;34(12):745–7.
3. Koleilat N, Sidi AA, Gonzalez R. Urethral false passage as a complication of intermittent catheterization. J Urol 1989;142(5):1216–7.

4. Di Benedetto P. Clean intermittent self-catheterization in neuro-urology. Eur J Phys Rehabil Med 2011;47(4): 651–9.

5. Wyndaele JJ. Complications of intermittent catheterization: their prevention and treatment. Spinal Cord 2002;40(10):536–41.

6. Kuhn W, Rist M, Zaech GA. Intermittent urethral self-catheterisation: long term results (bacteriological evolution, continence, acceptance, complications). Paraplegia 1991;29(4):222–32.

7. Tanagho EA, Schmidt RA. Electrical stimulation in the clinical management of the neurogenic bladder. J Urol 1988;140(6):1331–9.

8. Brindley GS, Rushton DN. Long-term follow-up of patients with sacral anterior root stimulator implants. Paraplegia 1990;28(8):469–75.

9. Stohrer M, Blok B, Castro-Diaz D, et al. EAU guidelines on neurogenic lower urinary tract dysfunction. Eur Urol 2009;56(1):81–8.

10. Ninkovic M, Stenzl A, Hess M, et al. Functional urinary bladder wall substitute using a free innervated latissimus dorsi muscle flap. Plast Reconstr Surg 1997;100(2):402–11 [discussion: 412–4].

11. Stenzl A, Ninkovic M, Willeit J, et al. Free neurovascular transfer of latissimus dorsi muscle to the bladder. I. Experimental studies. J Urol 1997; 157(3):1103–8.

12. Stenzl A, Ninkovic M, Kolle D, et al. Restoration of voluntary emptying of the bladder by transplantation of innervated free skeletal muscle. Lancet 1998; 351(9114):1483–5.

13. Gakis G, Ninkovic M, van Koeveringe GA, et al. Functional detrusor myoplasty for bladder acontractility: long-term results. J Urol 2011;185(2):593–9.

14. Ninkovic M, Stenzl A, Schwabegger A, et al. Free neurovascular transfer of latisstmus dorsi muscle for the treatment of bladder acontractility: II. Clinical results. J Urol 2003;169(4):1379–83.

15. Chancellor MB, Rivas DA, Acosta R, et al. Detrusor-myoplasty, innervated rectus muscle transposition study, and functional effect on the spinal cord injury rat model. Neurourol Urodyn 1994;13(5):547–57.

16. Chancellor MB, Rivas DA, Salzman SK. Detrusor-myoplasty to restore micturition. Lancet 1994;343(8898):669.

17. Van Savage JG, Perez-Abadia G, Palanca LG, et al. Comparison of the experience with acute and chronic electrically stimulated detrusor myoplasty. Neurourol Urodyn 2002;21(5):516–21.

18. Van Savage JG, Perez-Abadia GP, Palanca LG, et al. Electrically stimulated detrusor myoplasty. J Urol 2000;164(3 Pt 2):969–72.

19. Stenzl A, Ninkovic M. Restoring voluntary urinary voiding using a latissimus dorsi muscle free flap for bladder reconstruction. Microsurgery 2001;21(6):235–40.

20. Garusi C, Lohsiriwat V, Brenelli F, et al. The value of latissimus dorsi flap with implant reconstruction for total mastectomy after conservative breast cancer surgery recurrence. Breast 2011;20(2):141–4.

21. Delay E, Gounot N, Bouillot A, et al. Autologous latissimus breast reconstruction: a 3-year clinical experience with 100 patients. Plast Reconstr Surg 1998; 102(5):1461–78.

Competency Versus Performance in Plastic Surgery
Navigating Through New Technologies and Medical Devices

Salim C. Saba, MD[a],*, Salvatore J. Pacella, MD, MBA[b],
Stephen H. Miller, MD, MPH[c], Marek K. Dobke, MD, PhD[a,d]

KEYWORDS

- Plastic surgery • Novel technology • Surgeon competence

KEY POINTS

- Plastic surgeons' cooperation with industry has played a pivotal role in the development of many of the new technologies that characterize reconstructive and aesthetic procedures.
- While many of these technologies represent non-invasive ancillary devices, their uses are characterized by variable levels of complexity.
- Underappreciation of the subtle nuances of seemingly simple devices by inadequately trained practitioners could lead to diminished patient safety and optimal clinical outcomes. Even though industry plays a big role in educating practitioners on the use of the latest medical devices, it does not fully satisfy conditions of competent use.
- Plastic surgery professional associations and individuals with expert level knowledge in specific devices, must take ownership of educating its members and setting competency benchmarks.

OVERVIEW

Invasive and noninvasive plastic surgical procedures have undergone exponential growth over the last 30 years, due in part to an expansion of extensive basic and clinical research. During the 1960s and 1970s, introduction of contemporary microsurgical techniques by plastic surgeons ushered in a vast catalog of skin and muscle flaps that, to this day, are used for the most challenging reconstructive cases. In the 1980s, innovation of refined aesthetic surgery techniques yielded continuing advances in facial aesthetic surgery and body contouring,

thereby complementing advances in reconstructive surgery. It was during this decade that plastic surgeons took on the moniker of being plastic and reconstructive surgeons. In the 1990s, the introduction of surgical products, devices, and noninvasive technologies further advanced the plastic and reconstructive surgeon's toolkit, at times supplanting them all together. Examples include botulinum toxin injections or soft tissue fillers to reduce the appearance of facial rhytids, minimally invasive office-based procedures, and a variety of laser-assisted skin and other tissue treatments. In this

Disclosures: Dr Pacella is on the speaker's bureau for Lifecell Corporation; Dr Dobke is a consultant for Ulthera, Incorporated.

[a] Department of Surgery, Division of Plastic and Reconstructive Surgery, University of California at San Diego, MS 8890, 200 West Arbor Drive, San Diego, CA 92103, USA; [b] Plastic & Reconstructive Surgery, Scripps Clinic & Green Hospital, 10666 North Torrey Pines Rd, La Jolla, CA 92037, USA; [c] Department of Surgery, University of California at San Diego, 200 West Arbor Drive, San Diego, CA 92103, USA; [d] Division of Plastic and Reconstructive Surgery, University of California at San Diego, San Diego, CA, USA
* Corresponding author.
E-mail address: mdobke@ucsd.edu

Clin Plastic Surg 39 (2012) 513–520
http://dx.doi.org/10.1016/j.cps.2012.07.018

article, the authors address the adoption of these technologies as well as strategies that plastic surgeons may adopt for mastery of these techniques. Mention of specific technologies in this article is done for demonstrative purposes to illustrate how practitioners of plastic surgery gain competence in their safe and effective use.

NEW METHODS IN PLASTIC SURGERY: INTERPLAY OF TECHNOLOGY AND TECHNIQUE

The practice of plastic surgery combines knowledge of basic and clinical science in addition to development of technical skill. The acquisition of technical and manual skill, however, is closely associated with the use of surgical technology. Learning to use a surgical instrument and applying it appropriately to human tissue is defined as technique. Advances in surgical methods in plastic surgery combine new techniques, new applications of existing techniques, and new medical devices (**Table 1**). The 1 paramount requirement for successful application of any and all of these 3 modalities is the plastic surgeon's closest mentor: detailed knowledge of surgical anatomy and physiology.

Data elucidated from evidence-based research and clinical trials as well as structured technical cases form the building blocks for the clinician to safely extrapolate indications for the use of new or existing technologies to treat existing surgical challenges or address aesthetic concerns. The first reported use of botulinum toxin was in 1980 for the treatment of strabismus and blepharospasm.[1] Since then, indications, (albeit some off-label) have grown to include treatment of glabellar frown lines, facial and cervical dystonias, and as of October 2010,

migraine headaches as described by multiple authors.[2,3] Successful application of botulin toxin for nonsurgical management of migraines helped advance surgeons' understanding of muscle function alteration and its impact on adjacent nerve structures, and a permanent solution to migraine headaches using transection of the corrugator supercilii muscles, a technique described as part of the classical browlift procedure, was proposed and effectively applied.[4]

Techniques in microsurgery first developed in 1921 with the indication to surgically repair a labyrinthine fistula of the middle ear. Vascular surgeon Jules Jaconson is credited for the first true microvascular anastomosis, coupling 1.4 mm vessels in 1960. In 1963, this application was extended for replantation of a partially amputated digit, and, in 1966, transfer of a second toe for thumb reconstruction was performed by Dong-yue Yang and Yu-dong Gu in Shanghai, China. Since then, microsurgical techniques have been applied toward peripheral nerve reconstruction by extension of cable grafts, and in microlymphatic surgery in the treatment of chronic lymphedema. With the advent of face transplantation over the last 5 years, this technique has evolved exponentially to something that may have never been conceptualized had it not been for earlier advancements.[5,6] The history of microsurgery and teaching of microsurgery at different levels (beginner, intermediate, and advanced) exemplifies the importance of appropriately targeted continuing education and maintenance of skills.

While plastic surgeons have pioneered many of the technologies through laboratory-based research, cooperation with industry has also played a major role. This is perfectly exemplified by the modern era of breast augmentation. After observing

Table 1
Examples of advancements in plastic surgery methods

New Techniques	• Tissue engineering using molded polymer or organic tissue scaffolds • Robotic surgery
New Indications of Existing Techniques	• Botulinum toxin (Allergan, Inccorporated, Irvine, California) injection for Raynaud disease and migraine headaches • Endoscopic and surgical decompression for migraine headaches • Biomaterial use in tissue reconstruction or healing: Gore BioA (W. L. Gore & Associates, Incorporated, Flagstaff, Arizona), Acell (Acell, Incorporated, Columbia, Maryland), Graftjacket (Wright Medical Technology, Incorporated, Arlington, Tennessee) • Microsurgery for face transplantation and microlymphatic reconstruction
New Medical Devices	• Breast enhancement: style 410 form-stable Natrelle implants (Allergan, Incorporated), Brava (Brava LLC, Miami, Florida), • Energy-based facial rejuvenation systems: Ulthera (Ulthera, Incorporated, Mesa, Arizona), Thermage (Solta, Incorporated, Hayward, California)

disastrous results with injection of paraffin for breast reconstruction during the early part of the 20 century, plastic surgeons Thomas Cronin and Frank Gerow developed the first silicone breast prosthesis in conjunction with the Dow Corning Corporation, which subsequently led to the first augmentation mammoplasty in 1962. Silicone implants have undergone numerous modifications since then to increase the viscosity of silicone polymer and to house it within a more durable shell. These developments have led to enhancements in breast shape with minimization of comorbidities and such problems as silicone gel extravasation, gross implant rupture, or formation of capsular contracture. Newer examples of applications of silicone implant technology include sixth generation form-stable implants, development of advanced texturing techniques for implant adherence, and combined use of implants with acellular dermal matrix products to optimize implant pocket and inframammary fold position in breast reconstruction.

Plastic surgery has evolved through the innovation of its practitioners. A great part of this innovation has come as a result of plastic surgeons responsibly embarking on off-label use of US Food and Drug Administration (FDA)-approved products (note that the use of products not approved by the FDA is illegal unless they are done in the setting of an approved clinical study or during life-threatening emergencies where the product is already under clinical investigation). This legal practice has been the driving force behind extending the indications for

Botulinum toxin for use on facial rhytids other than the glabellar region (which in and of itself was FDA-approved in 2002)

Closed capsulotomy for capsular contracture

Breast implant overfilling and endoscopic breast augmentation

The leukotriene inhibitor Singulair has been used to prevent capsular contracture or hypertrophic scarring, and human growth hormone has been used for its antiaging effects. Nonetheless, off-label use has to be tempered with a thorough knowledge of reported clinical and scientific precedents in the literature. Additionally, the practitioner has to educate the patient, through informed consent, before embarking on off-label uses of approved products. This not only strengthens the bond between physician and patient, but also serves to legally protect the surgeon from intent-to-harm clauses if litigation should ensue.[7] Current examples of creative, sometimes off-label application of biomaterials are discussed elsewhere in this issue by Kim and Evans et al.

As surgical technology continues to grow, so does the responsibility of plastic surgeons at every level from medical student to independent practitioner, to achieve proficiency in various techniques using new technology. Given the dynamic nature of plastic surgery as a field, continuing medical education (CME) and maintenance of competency have become vital to sustainability in an increasingly regulated and competitive health care arena. In the next section, the authors discuss how knowledge and skill levels are acquired at different levels of training (**Table 2**) and how independent practitioners maintain high performance and patient safety standards.

ACQUISITION OF SKILLS IN PLASTIC SURGERY: STUDENT AND RESIDENT EDUCATION

Beginning with medical school, a plastic surgeon's education evolves constantly to accommodate an individual student level of surgical skill. Medical students generally have no prior experience when

Table 2
Learning new technology and technique at different levels of training

	Baseline Surgical Knowledge	Surgical Skills	Learning of New Techniques and Technology
Student	Very little	Very little	Part of general curriculum
Resident in training	Basic surgery	Basic and ACGME- defined requirements (see **Box 1**)	• Done within context of clinical or service load • Dependent on supervising faculty practice patterns
Practitioner	Advanced surgery	Advanced and versatile	• Transfer of skills from other practitioners and champions of industry[a]

[a] The term, champion of industry, defines a physician with special training or expertise in a particular technological development or medical device who, with or without the manufacturer's support, is heavily involved in educating and training potential and future users of the device.

initially rotating through a plastic surgery clerkship. Thus the main emphasis of learning is on associating clinical observations with knowledge gained from the preclinical years. Time spent in a plastic surgery rotation for a typical medical student is 1 month. Such an abbreviated exposure affords little time to learn the clinical science of plastic surgery, and even less time to learn basic surgical skills such as suturing. Regarding more complex plastic surgery issues, at best one can teach the concepts of flaps and defect management, rather than the technical details of those flaps. In recent years, a greater emphasis has been placed on the use of various simulator technologies including those to teach basic clinical tasks. These have been used to teach isolated procedures such as venipuncture, intubation, and suturing.[8] Simulators have also been used to teach more complex clinical functions in the setting of a multidisciplinary team approach. New-generation of computer-based simulation devices uses acquired computed tomography (CT) scan data to simulate 3-dimensional imagery and more importantly, to offer haptic force feedback in a 3-dimensional field.[9] Despite advancement in student teaching methods, new technologies as part of the finer details of the specialty are only learned through passive exposure in the hospital wards, while in-office technology is rarely encountered.[10]

On commencement of training, a typical plastic surgery resident has already completed a surgical clerkship, a plastic surgery rotation, followed then by an additional month of plastic surgery subinternship. Possessing only a basic surgical skill set on which to build, residents spend a great deal of time learning fundamental procedures that define the specialty. Learning new technologies, which is often dictated by attending-specific practice patterns, is not defined as part of the American College of Graduate Medical Education (ACGME) guidelines that dictate training level-specific proficiency in key procedures (**Box 1**).[11] Thus, resident education is mainly concerned with transfer of well-established skills and techniques by experienced practitioners.

Resident exposure to new technologies can be sporadic and generally takes place in a protected physician environment. Examples of such protected environments include operating room and outpatient clinic settings with faculty as teachers or proctors. Ironically, while the physicians often counsel patients on many in-office nonsurgical laser and injectable technologies, middle-level practitioners such as physician assistants or nurses are the ones formally in-serviced, and ultimately perform the actual procedures. In contrast, residents frequently spend a greater deal of time

---

Box 1
Partial representation of ACGME-defined competency benchmarks for plastic surgery residency training programs

Patient care-directed areas of clinical experience
- Skin graft
- Z-plasty flap
- Local flap reconstruction of soft tissue defects
- Flexor and extensor tendon repair
- Excision of skin malignancy
- Repair of mandible fractures
- Placement of tissue expanders and implants for breast reconstruction
- Breast reduction and augmentation
- Autologous flaps for breast reconstruction
- Flap reconstruction of pressure sores
- Microtia
- Cleft lip and palate repair
- Facelift
- Rhinoplasty
- Blepharoplasty
- Otoplasty

Data from ACGME competencies. In: ACGME Program Requirements for Graduate Medical Education in Plastic Surgery. Section IV.5.A:10–11.

---

learning the theory behind these technologies with fewer patient hours logged in training. Although simulators are being used to a greater extent in surgical training, most are concerned with developing cognitive and technical skills of long-standing surgical procedures. Examples of these simulators include; Smile Train Cleft Lip and Palate Viewer (BioDigital, New York City), SurgSim Trainers (SimQuest LLC, Silver Spring, Maryland), and patient-specific anatomic reconstruction programs. These simulators range from anatomic illustrations to CT- and magnetic resonance imaging (MRI)-guided soft tissue animations coupled with simulator devices with haptic feedback.[12] Such devices assist the surgical trainee in tasks that range from something as simple as endoscopic manipulations, to more complex tasks that incorporate a set of maneuvers centered around a specific procedure.

Plastic surgery residency programs face numerous contemporary challenges concerning limitations on resident work hours, optimization of consistency in training experience, and teaching of new technologies and innovations. From the resident standpoint, increasing service obligations must be balanced with the opportunity for meaningful educational opportunities.[13] To address this, the ACGME has been restructuring its 6-domain clinical competency system introduced in 1999, into the Next Accreditation System (NAS). Phased implementation of the NAS, which begins in July of 2013, is meant to accelerate ACGME program accreditation based on educational outcomes of residents and to reduce the burden of the process-based approach that is enforced on all residency programs uniformly. In effect, the NAS is more pliable than the old system, as it relaxes restrictions on programs that have consistently met resident educational goals. In return for good performance, programs are given additional freedom to innovate their curricula by teaching their residents new competencies and, in turn, technologies that are not strictly defined by the ACGME.[14] This will optimize the training of plastic surgery residents and reward an effort to transition into independent practice seamlessly without the added obstacle of navigating through the vast maze of mastering surgical technology and medical devices.

SKILL TRAINING BEYOND RESIDENCY: CREDENTIALING AND COMPETENCE

The importance of acquiring and maintaining skills in new technological devices is greatly amplified at the level of the independent practitioner. While students and residents train under close faculty supervision, independent practitioners face only indirect monitoring locally at the hospital level, from state medical boards, or national specialty organizations such as the American Board of Medical Specialties (ABMS), of which the American Board of Plastic Surgery (ABPS) is a branch. By administration of the maintenance of certification (MOC) program, the ABPS ensures that all practicing plastic surgeons meet minimal procedure-centered criteria for safe practice. However, as an ever-increasing portion of plastic surgery procedures is reliant on the use of medical devices and technologies, MOC does not, and likely is unable to provide clear, detailed, and adequate credentialing and competency guidelines for the use of each new technology and device.

MOC poorly elucidates the finer complexities of medical devices that distinguish the novice user from the expert practitioner. Thus, practitioner perception of level of difficulty for the safe and successful use of medical devices is often inaccurate. Intuitive as it may be, the notion of mastery of medical devices through a trial-and-error approach is suboptimal. Industry-driven CME

activities on the use of medical devices, while attempting to be comprehensive, often present an incongruous picture of the level of successful mastery to the inexperienced user. KCI (Kinetic Concepts, Incorporated, San Antonio, Texas) provides extensive courses on the use of a negative pressure wound therapy device that can be taught to a medical student or nursing assistant in a few sessions. Likewise, independent performance of minimally invasive procedures in many laparoscopic training programs is contingent upon demonstration of competency in the easy-to-use energy-based harmonic scalpel (Ethicon endo surgery, Incorporated, Cincinnati, Ohio) that is easily taught to, and routinely operated by, junior-level surgical residents.

In contrast, Ultherapy (Ulthera, Inc, Mesa, Arizona), an example of a non-nvasive modality, relying on ultrasound waves to induce connective tissue-controlled damage and, therefore tightening below the skin surface, is often operated by middle-level practitioners. While not necessarily inappropriate, the safe and effective use of this technology assumes a familiarity with human anatomy as represented by an ultrasonographic image. The educational challenge with such a technology is to teach individuals who may have an inconsistent level of surgical training or even an inadequate level of understanding of human anatomy. As a result, occasional underappreciation of the difficulties of the use of this seemingly simple technology leads to diminished success in achieving the desired clinical outcomes. Education involves, among other things, setting up on-site training courses, ranging from 1 to 3 days, to offer expert-level support to physicians and staff members of cosmetic-based practices. Underappreciation of certain technical nuances, such as inaccurately gauging the depth of delivery or even misapplication of the ultrasound gel, may occasionally lead to undesirable side effects or results that fall short of the patient's and practitioner's expectations. Therefore, credentialing for this deceptively complex energy-based skin tightening modality is entrusted, in Ulthera's case, to champions of industry. These experienced educators are proficient, not only in application of ultrasound treatment and Ulthera technology, but also in identifying learners who have adequately mastered the use of this technology to a level ensuring its safe and successful use, as well as those who would require additional training.

The overall lack of organized credentialing and education in the use of medical devices and technologies would perhaps explain the diversity in methods of learning by independent practitioners (**Table 3**). What is striking is the intimate level of involvement of industry in CME activities. In fact,

Table 3
Independent practitioner expanded list of methods of learning new techniques and technology

Techniques	Examples
Lecture-based learning	• Regional and national professional meetings • University-organized grand rounds activities • Industry-sponsored events
Procedure demonstrations	• University or industry-sponsored cadaver laboratories • Point-of-care learning under the tutelage of industry representatives and sponsored champions of industry • Direct preceptorship of experts in the operating room • Remote preceptorship of experts via telemedicine technology
Simulation training	Industry-sponsored university simulation centers that include animal and cadaver laboratories and robotic training

by 2008, overall hours spent by physicians on industry-funded CME activities was greater than that spent by those sponsored either by medical schools or professional societies.[15,16] Even though the American Medical Association (AMA) has been trying to mitigate industry-sponsored funding for CME, cooperation between industry and health care practitioners continues to be strong and probably—in the best interest of patients—should be even stronger! The trend to rely more and more on industry resources is partly secondary to stagnant National Institutes of Health funding of biomedical research and development efforts by academic institutions.[17]

Nevertheless, even though industry plays a pivotal role in educating practitioners on the use of the latest medical devices and products, it does not fully satisfy conditions of competent use despite instituting conditions of sale contingencies. Industry-driven CME courses on the use of medical devices often provide complete didactic curricula on the indications for and proper use of their devices. What is often lacking nonetheless is appropriate-level proctoring for the use of the device by a medically trained industry champion. Simply stated, a device expert with a nonmedical background, while possessing an understanding of the technical intricacies of a device, does not necessarily qualify as an expert on its application and effect on patients. Such a scenario applies mainly to smaller companies that may not necessarily have the funds to provide a medically trained product expert and instead have to rely on sales representatives as the sole educational resource for a nonexperienced user.

Exceptions to this paradigm may be found within the setting of companies that have the financial means to support properly structured CMEs. Mentor's Paragon symposium (Mentor Worldwide LLC, Santa Barbara, California) employs plastic surgeons to teach other plastic surgeons ways to optimize their use of silicone implant technology in breast augmentation and reconstruction. Allergan Academy (Allergan, Incorporated, Irvine, California) offers similar insights to plastic surgeons by way of specialty-trained industry champions. LifeCell's Abdominal Wall Reconstruction Summit (LifeCell, Company, Branchburg, New Jersey) offers cadaver laboratory courses that are run primarily by surgeons. Future educational endeavors should follow the latter models, and professional associations such as American Society of Plastic Surgeons (ASPS) and American Society of Aesthetic Plastic Surgeons (ASAPS) should encourage the designation of medically trained and qualified plastic surgeons as champions of industry. Realizing this objective goal of physician and surgeon as champion of industry and dominant CME vessel will only happen when strong partnerships between professional medical associations and industry are forged (**Fig. 1**).

Similar to ACGME-set competency guidelines for plastic surgery residents, the ABPS-administered MOC stresses procedural-based competency with virtually no emphasis on techno-centric and device-related CME activities. The importance of technology credentialing efforts by the ASPS and/or the ABPS is underscored by the fact that many plastic surgery treatments (ie, stem cell-enhanced fat grafting, liposuction, and off-label use of injectables for cosmetic purposes) are used outside the regulatory sphere of the FDA. A viable model is exemplified by Mentor's Paragon symposium held at the ASPS meetings and reflects a three-tiered approach where industry approaches the ASPS or ASAPS and works with them to sponsor educational and procedural forums to educate practitioners. Professional society involvement is further justified by the growing in-flux of nonplastic surgery-trained physicians and middle-level practitioners seeking

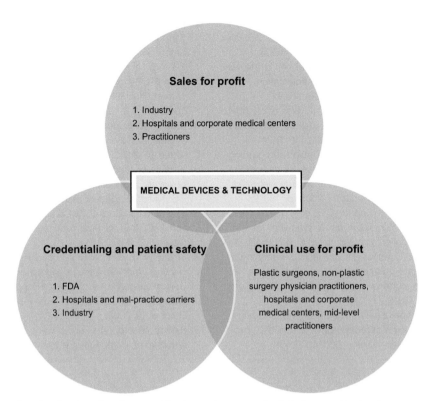

Fig. 1. Inter-related attitudes of various entities toward new medical devices and technology.

to generate greater profits, partly due to government-backed health care reimbursement cuts. Industry, while innovative, must take ownership of the direction of the end user to ensure the product or medical device is used by a credentialed and appropriate practitioner. A laudable example is the newest entry into the breast-implant arena, Sientra (Sientra Inc, Santa Barbara, California). The company's mission states that it will only sell its breast implants to board-certified or board-eligible plastic surgeons, marking a unique milestone of industry selecting the consumer based on safety and qualifications.[18] As a technology-based service industry becomes even more prevalent, core values will be ever-increasingly scrutinized.

SUMMARY

New technology and medical devices are constantly emerging and changing the way in which plastic surgery is practiced by plastic surgery-trained and nontrained practitioners alike. With a reduction in physician reimbursement in many areas of medicine and great potential for profit in aesthetic procedures and surgery, many lesser-qualified or unqualified practitioners are entering a domain of practice that was traditionally occupied by plastic surgeons. Plastic surgery

professional societies have to step up to establish guidelines for the credentialing and monitoring of competence in many of these emerging technologies, just as they do for time-tested surgical procedures as part of the MOC program. Only then can plastic surgeons reliably receive comprehensive product training while safely obtaining consistent results. Not only will this enhance patient safety, but it will provide obligate legitimization of board-certified plastic surgeons as leaders in education of these technologies.

REFERENCES

1. Flanders M, Tischler A, Wise J, et al. Injection of type A botulinum toxin into extraocular muscles for correction of strabismus. Can J Ophthalmol 1987;22(4):212–7.
2. Silberstein S, Mathew N, Saper J, et al. Botulinum toxin type A as a migraine preventative treatment. For the Botox Migraine Clinical Research Group. Headache 2000;40(6):445–50.
3. Binder WJ, Brin MF, Blitzer A, et al. Botulinum toxin type A (Botox) for treatment of migraine headaches: an open label study. Otolaryngol Head Neck Surg 2000;123(6):669–76.
4. Guyuron B, Tucker T, Davis J. Surgical treatment of migraine headaches. Plast Reconstr Surg 2002; 109(7):2183–9.

5. Unal S, Agaoglu G, Zins J, et al. New surgical approach in facial transplantation extends survival of allograft recipients. Ann Plast Surg 2005;55(3):297–303.

6. Pomahac B, Pribaz JJ, Bueno EM, et al. Novel surgical technique for full face transplantation. Plast Reconstr Surg 2012. [Epub ahead of print].

7. Rohrich RJ, Janis JE, Reisman NR. Use of off-label and non-approved drugs and devices in plastic surgery. Plast Reconstr Surg 2003;112(1):241–3.

8. McGaghie WC, Pangaro LN. Evaluation and grading of students. In: Fincher RE, editor. Guidebook for clerkship directors. 3rd edition. Omaha, Nebraska: Alliance for Clinical Education; 2005. p. 180–2.

9. Solyar A, Cuellar H, Sadoughi B, et al. Endoscopic Sinus Surgery Simulator as a teaching tool for anatomy education. Am J Surg 2008;196(1):120–4.

10. Burd A, Chiu T, McNaught C. Plastic surgery in the undergraduate curriculum: the importance of considering students' perceptions. Br J Plast Surg 2004;57(8):773–9.

11. ACGME competencies. In: ACGME website http://www.acgme.org/acWebsite/downloads/RRC_progReq/360_plastic_surgery_07012009.pdf.

12. Rosen JM, Long SA, McGrath DM, et al. Simulation in plastic surgery training and education: the path forward. Plast Reconstr Surg 2009;123(2):729–38.

13. Luce EA. Beyond working hours: part I. genesis and current difficulties. Plast Reconstr Surg 2012;129(4):1015–21.

14. Nasca TJ, Philibert I, Brigham T, et al. The Next GME accreditation system —rationale and benefits. N Engl J Med 2012;366(11):1051–6.

15. Institute of Medicine. Conflict of interest in medical research, education, and practice. Washington, DC: National Academies Press; 2009.

16. Accreditation Council for Continuing Medical Education. ACCME 2010 annual report data. Chicago, Illinois: ACGME; 2010.

17. Smith PW. The National Institutes of Health (NIH): organization, funding, and congressional issues. In: Congressional Research Service Report for Congress. Washington, DC: Congressional Research Service; October 19, 2006.

18. Sientra, Incorporated home webpage. Available at: www.sientra.com. Accessed June 6, 2012.

Erratum

In the July 2012 issue of Clinics in Plastic Surgery, Wound Healing for Plastic Surgeons, Dr Benson Pulikkottil's name is misspelled in the chapter, Negative Pressure Wound Therapy: An Algorithm and in that issue's table of contents and contributor list. We apologize for this error.

DOI of original article: 10.1016/j.cps.2012.05.002.

Clin Plastic Surg 39 (2012) 521
http://dx.doi.org/10.1016/j.cps.2012.08.004
0094-1298/12/$ – see front matter Published by Elsevier Inc.

Index

Note: Page numbers of article titles are in **boldface** type.

A

Abdominal wall procedures, acellular dermal matrix for, 360–363

Acellular dermal matrix, for abdominal wall procedures, 360–363

for reconstructive and cosmetic breast procedures, 363–369

Acellular dermal matrix products, 370

Adipocyte-derived regenerative cells, applications of, 454–455

as mesotherapy agent for alopecia treatment, 460, 461

clinical trials of, 454, 456

description of, 456

for collagen synthesis stimulation, 460

laboratory techniques to obtain, 457–458

safety concerns in use of, 454

to enrich/supplement fat grafts, 456

Adipocyte-derived stem and regenerative cells, in facial rejuvenation, **453–464**

AICAP/SEAP flaps, 487–488

Allotransplants, vascularized composite, 426, 431

complications of, 431–432

Alopecia, treatment of, adipocyte-derived regenerative cells for, 460, 461

Aponeurotic system, superficial muscular, fat grafting and, 455–456, 459

Autologous lymph node transplantation, 387

clinical outcomes of, 394–396

complications of, 396–397

for leg lymphedema, 390–391

in arm lymphedema, operative technique for, 388–390, 391

in iatrogenic lymphedema, indications for, 388

Axilla, management of, in breast cancer, 468–469

B

Biomaterials, description of, 359

in plastic surgery, applications of, **359–376**

Bladder acontractility, catheterization in, 508

functional, treatment of, latissimus dorsi detrusor myoplasty for, **507–512**

functional muscle transfer in, 508

sacral neuromodulation in, 508

Blood vessels, anastomosis of, and total distal ischemia caused by Raynaud phenomenon, 448

couplers for, 447

sutureless, 448

multiple microvascular anastomoses of, 447

Bone, septic conditions of, bone reconstruction for, 445–446

Bone reconstruction, 499, 500–501

in mutilated digits or septic conditions, 445–446

innovative solution for, 445–446

Masquelet technique for, 446

secondary, delayed free flap closure with, 493–494, 496, 497

Botulinum toxin A injections, in distal ischemia caused of Raynaud phenomenon, 448

Breast/abdominal wall healing, synthetic materials for, limitations for, 360

Breast augmentation, autologous, flap design for, 487

pedicled perforator flaps for, 485

indications and contraindications to, 478–485

Breast cancer, advances in treatment of, 468–473

illustrated cases of, concerns and, 473

management of axilla in, 468–469

plastic surgery for, technical advances and, 473

reconstructive and aesthetic advances in breast surgery and, **465–475**

site markers, 468, 469

Breast conservation surgery, 466–467, 468, 469

Breast conservation therapy, 477–478

Breast procedures, reconstructive and cosmetic, acellular dermal matrix for, 363–369

Breast reconstruction, autologous, with pedicled perforator flaps, **477–490**

in delayed partial reconstruction, 481–484

in immediate partial reconstruction, 480–481

in partial mastectomy reconstruction, 478

indications for, 480

delayed partial, thoracic artery perforator flap in, 481–484

experimental techniques for, 470

immediate partial, pedicled perforator flaps for, 480–481

oncological follow-up and imaging following, 470–473

partial necrosis of flap in, salvage procedure after, 484–485, 486–487

postmastectomy, with or without implant, 485

radiation and chemotherapy and, 469–470

United States Postal Service

Statement of Ownership, Management, and Circulation
(All Periodicals Publications Except Requester Publications)

1. Publication Title	2. Publication Number	3. Filing Date
Clinics in Plastic Surgery	0 0 6 - 5 3 0	9/14/12

4. Issue Frequency	5. Number of Issues Published Annually	6. Annual Subscription Price
Jan, Apr, Jul, Oct	4	$448.00

7. Complete Mailing Address of Known Office of Publication (Not printer) (Street, city, county, state, and ZIP+4®)

Elsevier Inc.
360 Park Avenue South
New York, NY 10010-1710

Contact Person
Stephen R. Bushing
Telephone (Include area code)
215-239-3688

8. Complete Mailing Address of Headquarters or General Business Office of Publisher (Not printer)

Elsevier Inc., 360 Park Avenue South, New York, NY 10010-1710

9. Full Names and Complete Mailing Addresses of Publisher, Editor, and Managing Editor (Do not leave blank)

Publisher (Name and complete mailing address)

Kim Murphy, Elsevier, Inc., 1600 John F. Kennedy Blvd. Suite 1800, Philadelphia, PA 19103-2899

Editor (Name and complete mailing address)

Joanne Husovski, Elsevier, Inc., 1600 John F. Kennedy Blvd. Suite 1800, Philadelphia, PA 19103-2899

Managing Editor (Name and complete mailing address)

Barbara Cohen - Kligerman, Elsevier, Inc., 1600 John F. Kennedy Blvd. Suite 1800, Philadelphia, PA 19103-2899

10. Owner (Do not leave blank. If the publication is owned by a corporation, give the name and address of the corporation immediately followed by the names and addresses of all stockholders owning or holding 1 percent or more of the total amount of stock. If not owned by a corporation, give the names and addresses of the individual owners. If owned by a partnership or other unincorporated firm, give its name and address as well as those of each individual owner. If the publication is published by a nonprofit organization, give its name and address.)

Full Name	Complete Mailing Address
Wholly owned subsidiary of	1600 John F. Kennedy Blvd., Ste. 1800
Reed/Elsevier, US holdings	Philadelphia, PA 19103-2899

11. Known Bondholders, Mortgagees, and Other Security Holders Owning or Holding 1 Percent or More of Total Amount of Bonds, Mortgages, or Other Securities. If none, check box ☐ None

Full Name	Complete Mailing Address
N/A	

12. Tax Status (For completion by nonprofit organizations authorized to mail at nonprofit rates) (Check one)
The purpose, function, and nonprofit status of this organization and the exempt status for federal income tax purposes:
☐ Has Not Changed During Preceding 12 Months
☐ Has Changed During Preceding 12 Months (Publisher must submit explanation of change with this statement)

PS Form 3526, September 2007 (Page 1 of 3 (Instructions Page 3)) PSN 7530-01-000-9931 PRIVACY NOTICE. See our Privacy policy in www.usps.com

13. Publication Title		14. Issue Date for Circulation Data Below
Clinics in Plastic Surgery		July 2012

15. Extent and Nature of Circulation		Average No. Copies Each Issue During Preceding 12 Months	No. Copies of Single Issue Published Nearest to Filing Date
a. Total Number of Copies (Net press run)		1281	1100
b. Paid Circulation (By Mail and Outside the Mail)	(1) Mailed Outside-County Paid Subscriptions Stated on PS Form 3541. (Include paid distribution above nominal rate, advertiser's proof copies, and exchange copies)	682	633
	(2) Mailed In-County Paid Subscriptions Stated on PS Form 3541 (Include paid distribution above nominal rate, advertiser's proof copies, and exchange copies)		
	(3) Paid Distribution Outside the Mails Including Sales Through Dealers and Carriers, Street Vendors, Counter Sales, and Other Paid Distribution Outside USPS®	315	332
	(4) Paid Distribution by Other Classes Mailed Through the USPS (e.g. First-Class Mail®)		
c. Total Paid Distribution (Sum of 15b (1), (2), (3), and (4))	▶	997	965
d. Free or Nominal Rate Distribution (By Mail and Outside the Mail)	(1) Free or Nominal Rate Outside-County Copies Included on PS Form 3541	57	44
	(2) Free or Nominal Rate In-County Copies Included on PS Form 3541		
	(3) Free or Nominal Rate Copies Mailed at Other Classes Through the USPS (e.g. First-Class Mail)		
	(4) Free or Nominal Rate Distribution Outside the Mail (Carriers or other means)		
e. Total Free or Nominal Rate Distribution (Sum of 15d (1), (2), (3) and (4))	▶	57	44
f. Total Distribution (Sum of 15c and 15e)	▶	1054	1009
g. Copies not Distributed (See instructions to publishers #4 (page 83))	▶	227	91
h. Total (Sum of 15f and g)	▶	1281	1100
i. Percent Paid (15c divided by 15f times 100)		94.59%	95.64%

16. Publication of Statement of Ownership

If the publication is a general publication, publication of this statement is required. Will be printed ☐ Publication not required
in the October 2012 issue of this publication.

17. Signature and Title of Editor, Publisher, Business Manager, or Owner

Stephen R. Bushing — Inventory Distribution Coordinator

Date September 14, 2012

I certify that all information furnished on this form is true and complete. I understand that anyone who furnishes false or misleading information on this form or who omits material or information requested on the form may be subject to criminal sanctions (including fines and imprisonment) and/or civil sanctions (including civil penalties).

PS Form 3526, September 2007 (Page 2 of 3)

Moving?

Make sure your subscription moves with you!

To notify us of your new address, find your **Clinics Account Number** (located on your mailing label above your name), and contact customer service at:

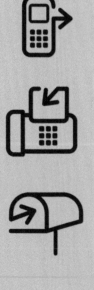

Email: journalscustomerservice-usa@elsevier.com

800-654-2452 (subscribers in the U.S. & Canada)
314-447-8871 (subscribers outside of the U.S. & Canada)

Fax number: 314-447-8029

Elsevier Health Sciences Division
Subscription Customer Service
3251 Riverport Lane
Maryland Heights, MO 63043

*To ensure uninterrupted delivery of your subscription, please notify us at least 4 weeks in advance of move.

ELSEVIER

Printed and bound by CPI Group (UK) Ltd, Croydon, CR0 4YY

03/10/2024

01040358-0010